Therapy Groups Using the Creative Arts

Second Edition

Therapy Groups Using the Creative Arts

2nd Edition

Ann Argé Nathan, Suzanne Mirviss
Deborah Ann Stuart, Carol J. McDowell

Idyll Arbor, Inc.

39129 264th Ave SE, Enumclaw, WA 98022 (360) 825-7797

Cover: Curt Pliler
Idyll Arbor, Inc. editor, Thomas M. Blaschko
Thanks to Roger and Barbara Stuart for support and proofreading assistance.

ISBN 978-1-61158-064-8

Published in the USA

Contents

List of Activities

1

Introduction

Interdisciplinary learning is "learning to know something by its relation to something else."

— Leonard Bernstein

The arts have always been an important part of our culture. Our ancestors produced art by painting on cave walls and carving flutes from animal bone. Perhaps this served as a means of pondering life's mysteries and exploring life's possible meanings (Cornett, 2007). The visual and performing arts continue to provide experiences for people to express themselves, communicate with others, and interact with the world.

The creative arts therapies (art, music, drama, dance/movement, clowning, writing and poetry, puppetry, and integrated techniques) also offer a safe means for people to explore, experiment, and learn about the most important thing: themselves. When a person participates in creative arts therapy, s/he often feels a sense of accomplishment, self-confidence, personal satisfaction, and positive self-image (Edwards, 1997). Children provide the best example. When they draw pictures, explore sounds by tapping on objects, and make objects out of clay, they are learning how to take risks, experiment, and problem-solve. And children almost always have a story to tell about their finished art works.

This book is an introduction to the process of using creative arts groups to help people solve problems and grow. The first part of the book focuses on defining and establishing a basic knowledge of concepts, such as:

- creativity and its expression
- roles a therapist assumes that enable clients to engage in creative arts
- theories of individual growth and development
- group development and dynamics
- logistics of planning and running creative arts groups
- how creative arts relate to the International Classification of Functioning, Disability, and Health

These topics give therapists fundamental information that will help them lead a creative arts group. It is intended to be practical and immediately applicable because it is based on years of experience working with the creative arts in therapeutic and educational settings.

The second part of the book offers guidelines for creative arts groups that have been used with all ages of clients. Many clients have said that participating in these activities impacted the way they viewed themselves both professionally and personally. Research has demonstrated that the activity modalities improve functioning and health.

Students who are learning how to become therapists can use these activities for their personal and professional growth. For students who have been hesitant to lead an arts group, the classroom becomes a laboratory for trying out and processing the activities. Many realize that they could be successful in using arts activities with groups and want to further explore certain creative arts modalities. On a personal level, students experience what it feels like to participate in the activities and can more realistically project what the activities might evoke for clients. Students become more aware of the value of the creative arts and what it takes to facilitate the activities.

Each creative arts modality chapter consists of (at least) four sections:

- a description and history of the modality
- research demonstrating the efficacy of the modality in treatment
- considerations for the therapist on managing a group with that modality

- activities within the modality

The arts offer a unique contribution to society both through their content and through the process by which they are created. Cornett (2007) lists fourteen gifts that the arts provide to the public, whether they are found by students attending school or clients in a therapy session. These benefits may be categorized as follows:

Communication

- **Communication:** providing the ability to understand, respond to, and express thoughts and feelings that cannot be captured through words
- **Content:** providing a source from which to derive new perspectives about how the art was made and how to work backwards from a finished product to understand the kind of thinking and value it represents

Intellectual

- **Creative problem solving:** making mistakes, embracing surprises, experimenting, and brainstorming
- **Critical thinking:** describing patterns, noticing details
- **Comprehension:** trying to make sense of and create meaning by connecting ideas and feelings
- **Composition:** expressing meaning

Social

- **Culture:** recording ways that people lived, what they worried about, and what they valued throughout history
- **Cooperation and collaboration:** working as a team
- **Community:** developing a sense of belonging and building relationships
- **Compassion:** developing concern and sensitivity for others

Personal/Emotional Capacities

- **Commitment and interest:** curiosity and choice, motivation
- **Concentration and attention:** capturing attention and developing concentration

- **Confidence and courage:** developing the courage to take risks and take pride in a finished job
- **Competence and control:** developing skills to control mind, voice, and body

The impact creative arts have on our lives, especially the lives of individuals with disabilities, can be looked at from many perspectives. Individuals who struggle with ongoing challenges often find great benefits in the experiences that the creative arts offer. These benefits, which can be of value to all individuals, can also be described using this taxonomy:

- **Expansiveness and freedom:** The creative arts stimulate our senses, bodies, thoughts, and feelings. In the creative arts experience we can move beyond the bounds of time, space, and physical limitations. Outside our normal realm of existence, we are free to think, feel, and express what seems natural to us.
- **Internal communication:** During creative activity we are linked with our inner selves. We interact with an object or situation and find ways to communicate our thoughts and feelings about what we are seeing or experiencing. While we are involved in creative activity, we are engaged in a sustained union with self that is different from normal consciousness and profound because we are closer to touching our unique self.
- **External communication:** When we express our ideas and feelings through the expressive arts, we have the opportunity to say, "This is me. I exist. This is how I feel and see the world." While the sharing of self is often scary for people, it can also create a bridge to other human beings. Those who thought they knew a client well may react with amazement when they observe a piece of artwork that the client has created.
- **Leisure:** During creative activity, it is possible to escape the hectic, overwhelming external and often internal distractions of life. Creative activity freezes time. Many people experience a sensation of "flow" — of being totally engaged and at peace with self during creative activity. Only the activity of that moment exists. We are given the chance to regroup, rethink, and reenter the world with a fresh perspective (Csikszentmihalyi, 1996).

- **Alternative communication:** Some creative arts involve expression through images, sound, and movement. They bypass left-brain thinking and engage right-brain processing, which is more holistic, less detail-oriented, less logical, but more integrative. This often enables clients to explore and express a troublesome thought, feeling, or conflict in a new way, through an image, a sound, or a movement that communicates it more clearly than ever before. Even when using words, as in a creative writing session, the words have more power and take on an expanded meaning.
- **Self-worth:** The process of expressing creativity involves an exploration of self in order to be able to respond and communicate ideas from a personal perspective. It also involves working materials, words, or movements with one's own hands or body and dealing with one's own evaluation of the work and the evaluation of others. This process can be both frightening and joyful. It takes courage to embark on a creative journey in which there are many "what ifs." What if the work doesn't turn out the way I expect it to? What if it's more difficult than I expect it to be? When one still perseveres, witnessing the product that comes from this energy and inspiration is highly validating. No matter how one might feel about the product, an individual can be proud of the journey, of taking a different, unknown path and not turning back.
- **Healing:** The creative arts can be healing in two ways. First, when an individual is deeply involved in the act of creating, s/he may experience a kind of "mental vacation." Individuals who are normally disturbed by thoughts or anxieties will have noticeably more relaxed faces and bodies during creative activity. Relaxation can occur when the chattering, active mind is occupied, and thoughts and feelings are channeled into positive activity. Second, individuals may experience a surge of energy during creative activity and a feeling of well-being. According to Maslow's (1987) hierarchy of needs, the act of creation fulfills the need to explore and express one's potential and validates one's own ability to do more than just survive.
- **Interpersonal relations:** Interpersonal relations are developed through working out problems together. Perhaps the best way to illustrate that creative arts have an impact on how people relate to each other is through the following example: During an art grant project

involving veterans with psychiatric disabilities at the VA Medical Center in San Francisco, the group was creating a mosaic panel of an orca with ceramic tile. It required the involvement of many clients to lay out pieces and to glue and grout. It took over two months to complete. During the project, there were some very positive interactions between clients. Individuals were seen helping each other problem solve sections of the artwork, assisting in completing sections, taking over responsibility when someone had to leave, and giving each other encouragement and praise for completed work. When the group was having a problem getting the mosaic (which weighed over 60 pounds) into the frame, one client who had done carpentry work offered to help and took over leadership to solve the problem. Now the mosaic hangs in the lobby of one of the VA buildings as a testimonial to the beauty that can be created when people work together.

The Art Part and the Therapy Part (Activity Analysis)

Using the creative arts with clients is really a dual process — one part is carrying out an artistic endeavor and the other part is understanding how to create an environment which will be therapeutic.

The Art Part

- process
- products
- materials

The Therapy Part

- human development
- group dynamics
- conditions and process of therapeutic change
- personal and professional self-knowledge

In any activity, there is a relationship of parts which can change the nature of the activity. This relationship is illustrated in Figure 1-1, where areas that may change and have mutual influence appear.

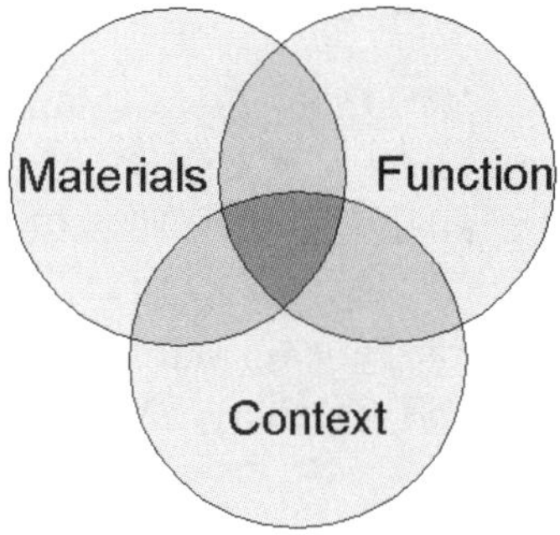

Figure 1-1: Relationship of materials, function, and context.

When any of the variables in the diagram change, it may affect one or both (though sometimes neither) of the others. For example, a game may be played by a group of children as "just a game." It may be played by friends in their leisure time. The function of the game appears to be fun — something to pass the time. If we change the context by playing this game in a therapy session, what else do we change? Perhaps nothing, as we play this game for its own sake. But we could decide to use this game with a group that needs to develop cooperation skills. Now we could add to our list the function of teaching people to work together. The same material is being used but with a new context and function. Context, function, and materials are variables for the therapist and the group to alter as they wish. This is part of the activity analysis process.

The Arts Are Effective

Because they…

- Help us define who we are, expressing our own visions and values
- Allow us to see beyond ourselves as part of a larger culture
- Broaden our perspective, so we see and think differently
- Expand our ability to communicate
- Allow us to escape the mundane and provide a temporary release from ordinary reality
- Develop our imagination

- Allow us to evaluate and make judgments during the creative process (Fowler, 1996)

Art, according to Aristotle (1996), "releases unconscious tensions and purges the soul." It is *cathartic*, that is, the expression of a problem or concern in itself provides relief. This cathartic effect is common to all expressive therapies.

Elements found in the arts, either in individual form or in combination, encourage self-expression and creativity, and bring about enjoyment, insight, and knowledge.

Art therapist Elinor Ulman (1996) defines it as "the meeting ground of the world inside and the world outside."

Creative arts therapies can be a means of both reconciling emotional conflicts and fostering self-awareness and personal growth. The therapy can provide a careful blend of elements adjusted to the specific needs, personalities, and abilities of the individual and the therapist.

References

Aristotle. (1996). *Poetics*. New York: Penguin.

Cornett, C. E. (2007). *Creating meaning through literature and the arts: An integration resource for classroom teachers* (3rd ed.). New York: Pearson.

Csikszentmihalyi, M. (1996). *Creativity*. New York: Harper Collins Publishers, Inc.

Edwards, L. C. (1997). *The creative arts: A process approach for teachers and children* (2nd ed.). Upper Saddle River, New Jersey: Prentice-Hall.

Fowler, C. (1996). *Strong arts, strong schools*. New York: Oxford University Press.

Maslow, A. H. (1987). *Motivation and personality*. New York: Harpercollins College Division.

Ulman, E. (1996). *Art therapy: In theory and practice*. Chicago, IL: Magnolia Street Publishers.

2

Elements of Creativity

Every creative act involves...a new innocence of perception, liberated from the cataract of accepted belief.
— Arthur Koestler, *The Sleepwalkers*

As infants we use our senses to learn where we are and who or what is important in our world. Colors and shapes, sounds, taste, and touch are the indispensable tools of infancy and childhood. Children have the time to wonder and to gaze with curiosity at everything that crosses their paths, from bugs to stars. The young child creates and imagines, spinning dreams and fantasies and then unraveling them in a second.

Adults marvel at these abilities and yet our society often inadvertently squelches them. As the years progress, natural creativity is often squeezed out by pressures to conform to society's expectations — a society that often values an ever-changing set of ephemeral distractions more highly than complex creative expression coming from imagination and sustained concentration. Our technologically advanced, and our post-industrial society has come to believe that artistic creation is in the hands of a few gifted individuals, excluding many people from indulging in artistic processes. Because of this mindset, it is not surprising that the arts could be interpreted as therapy (Warren, 1993).

Many adults have the feeling that something is missing in their lives, when the problem is that their abilities to imagine and to create have become dormant.

This chapter looks at the elements of creativity, from the process itself to the personal qualities that foster it, the nature of the "flow experience," and blocks to creativity. It concludes with a list of the conditions that enhance or hinder expression in groups.

What is Creativity?

Creativity is one of those elusive concepts, like love and justice, that defies definition, though philosophers and artists have been attempting to describe it for centuries. Perhaps one of the most concise definitions comes from Mihaly Csikszentmihalyi (1996), a psychology professor who has extensively researched the topics of flow and creativity. In his book entitled *Creativity*, he writes, "Creativity is any act, idea, or product that changes an existing domain, or that transforms an existing domain into a new one.... What counts is whether the novelty he or she produces is accepted for inclusion in the domain" (p. 28). The "ingredients" (ideas, techniques, materials) may be new, or they may be a new combination of existing ingredients, but the product will be unique to every individual.

The Qualities of the Creative Person

The human qualities that are instrumental to creativity are present in every one of us to some degree. Some individuals are born with physical, cognitive, or emotional challenges that make expressing creativity more difficult. Sometimes circumstances inhibit or damage a person's capacity to experience and express these qualities. Many people in our therapy groups will express the feeling that their creativity has somehow been stifled. For most people this happened sometime in childhood. However, a traumatic event, even in adulthood, can also make it more difficult for a person to risk being creative.

It is one of the tasks of the therapist who uses arts in therapeutic groups to help individuals rediscover their creative selves and validate qualities that spark every aspect of life.

Creative adults were once children, and creative characteristics often emerge during childhood (Csikszentmihalyi, 1996). While it is difficult to discover any reliable pattern within these childhoods, Cornett (2007) established some attributes associated with creativity.

- Curious and questioning
- Likes to explore, seeks adventure
- Spontaneous, impulsive, uninhibited
- Emotionally secure
- Risk taker, but not reckless; courageous
- Nonconforming, opinions of others not a priority
- Confident in own worth and work
- Loses track of time, dislikes deadlines
- Strong sense of destiny
- Independent, unlikely to follow the crowd
- Likes original ideas
- Skeptical of authority, resists "right" answers
- Easily bored with routine
- Heightened sense of humor
- Critical of self
- Not often satisfied, but not easily discouraged
- Likes to work alone, may appear aloof, may not fit in or seek out groups
- Motivated, hardworking, and persistent; not easily frustrated; willing to struggle and sustain effort
- Playful, almost childlike, in their wonder and delight
- Tolerant of ambiguity, doesn't need a right answer
- Broad interests and hobbies
- Empathetic, feels others' pain

These attributes may be helpful when the therapist observes clients, sets goals, and plans therapy sessions.

When we look through the traits, we see that some traits are very straightforward, but there is a curious aspect that is associated with heightened creativity, and that is the phenomenon of paradoxical traits. These traits involve the ability to move from one extreme to the other as the occasion requires — their development expands the boundaries of the personality. The straightforward traits are

- **Curiosity, wonder, and interest** … in what things are like and how they work. Without a good dose of these, it is difficult to recognize an interesting, creative problem.
- **Openness to experience:** A fluid attention that constantly processes events in the environment is a great advantage for recognizing potential novelty.
- **Enjoyment of learning:** Learning brings new information: ideas, thoughts, and feelings that can inspire creative endeavors.
- **Tolerance of ambiguity:** Ambiguity tends to make people uncomfortable. But a tolerance for it lets us perceive a greater complexity in the world than our categories sometimes acknowledge and, with that, to enrich the way we see it. For example, it is possible to mix hundreds or maybe thousands of shades of gray. If the place between black and white is so versatile, why do we keep seeking out the same old colors? Experimenting may produce a gray unlike any other.
- **Risk taking:** Taking risks means accepting challenges that require going beyond a personal comfort zone. It means having the courage to stand alone and make a statement. Why take risks? Success has its own rewards. But even if a risk fails, the individual has sought out an opportunity to learn new things, to increase his/her comfort zone and tolerance for new experiences. Risk taking enhances self-esteem.

The paradoxical sets of traits are arranged as pairs:

- **Playfulness and discipline:** Playfulness is a way of exploring ideas, but after the exploration, it takes perseverance to bring a new idea or vision to completion.
- **Fantasy and realism:** Being creative means alternating between imagination and fantasy at one end and a deeply rooted sense of reality at the other. The individual goes beyond what is considered "real" to create a new reality. To do this means to be able to clearly perceive the present environment and work with it to produce a new vision.
- **Passion and objectivity:** Creative work demands a passion for the subject that motivates an individual to stay with a difficult task, but it

also demands an ability to be objective about the flaws and merits of the work, to recognize the real quality of one's work.

Creative Thinking

Technical advances in neuroscience, along with trends in the arts, cognitive psychology, and the science of learning, have shown great potential to explain how creativity works in the brain (National Endowment for the Arts, 2015). Different areas of the brain are specialized for different tasks. The left hemisphere of our brains is usually better at language functions and time-sequenced events. The right hemisphere synthesizes over space to process information in more holistic, intuitive, and non-linear ways. But both hemispheres are involved in all activities (Bruer, 1999), thus contradicting the left-right brain dichotomy. Depending on the nature of the task, the hemispheres will work together with each taking on the part of the task that is appropriate to its mode of processing. Cornett (2007) cites brain development, environmental influences, experiences, emotion, and common neural networks as elements that can affect arts integration.

In the Western world, there is a tendency to rely too much on verbal processing and not enough on looking at the connections between the elements. If this is an issue for working in the creative arts, there are techniques to quiet the chattering of the left hemisphere. One example is found in Betty Edwards (1989) *Drawing on the Right Side of the Brain.* In that book, she suggests producing a cognitive shift in processing by presenting the left hemisphere with a task that it either can't or won't do. She offers many drawing tasks that cause the right hemisphere to take over, causing an enhancement in the drawing skills of people who thought that they had no artistic talent.

Those who can effectively utilize the abilities of their whole brain will operate on a more creative level. The process of creation involves analysis and intuition, words and mental pictures, and thought and feeling.

The Creative Process

Creativity can really be thought of as more of a process than a talent or an innate gift. As such it becomes accessible to everyone. It is not just the province of geniuses but is practiced in many forms and by many people in a wide variety of disciplines. In a way, it is a form of problem solving, though the problems may be as diverse as expressing a feeling or hypothesizing the structure of DNA.

This process has been explored and written about by countless psychologists and creative people. Csikszentmihalyi (1996) describes the creative process in five phases:

1. **Preparation:** Information gathering. Becoming fully immersed in the puzzle. Learning about the topic by observation, researching, talking with other people.
2. **Incubation:** This is what Csikszentmihalyi (1996) calls "the mysterious time." Internal retreat and synthesis. Ideas are churning below the threshold of consciousness, producing unusual and unexpected connections.
3. **Insight:** Sometimes called the "Aha!" experience — this is when the pieces of the puzzle fall together.
4. **Evaluation:** The phase when a person must decide if an insight is valuable and worth pursuing. This can be an emotionally trying period of self-criticism and insecurity. Is it a novel idea? Will it work? What will others think of it?
5. **Elaboration:** The actual work of creation. This is the hardest work and the most time consuming. Thomas Edison was referring to this phase when he said that creativity was 1% inspiration and 99% perspiration.

Csikszentmihalyi makes the point that in real life there may be several periods of insight, evaluation, and elaboration as the person refines his/her work. It is a *recursive* process, one that is repeated over and over again until the person feels that his creation is "just right."

In a creative arts group, there may be a period of sharing. Sharing work in which one has invested time and effort can be a delicate business. There is no guarantee that the individual's ideas will be communicated or received exactly as they were intended. This is a vulnerable situation for any creator and especially for our clients. If there is time for sharing, the therapist needs to establish ground rules for how feedback is given. There should also be an option *not* to share if a client so chooses. Remind clients to always take what rings true to them and discard what seems like personal taste. If something of value is learned, the individual can note it for future use or return to Phases 4 and 5 of the process.

Creativity and the Flow Experience

Ideally, therapists want their clients to enjoy their creative experience. But what is enjoyment? Csikszentmihalyi (1996) studied those who were engaged as professionals in activities that they seemed to enjoy regardless of money or fame. These optimal experiences were often difficult but stretched people's capacities and involved an element of novelty or discovery. He called these flow experiences. They occur "whenever people deeply enjoyed what they were doing, like being carried away by a current, like being in a flow" (Mark, 2002, p. 202). The description of these flow experiences did not vary much by culture, gender, race, or age. According to Csikszentmihalyi's (1996) research, nine elements describe when an experience is enjoyable:

- **Clear goals:** The person knows exactly what needs to be done next.
- **Immediate feedback to one's actions:** In contrast to everyday life, in a flow experience we know exactly how well we are doing. Each note or brush stroke or move is immediately perceived as right or wrong.
- **A balance between challenges and skills:** If the challenges are too high, people are anxious and frustrated. Too low, and they are bored. In flow, there is the right balance between abilities and challenge.
- **Action and awareness are merged:** In flow, a person's concentration is focused on what s/he is doing, in contrast to ordinary activities, where one may be thinking about one thing and doing another.
- **Distractions are excluded from consciousness:** In flow, we are aware of only what is relevant in the here and now. Flow is the result of intense concentration, one that temporarily relieves us of our fears and the cares of everyday life.
- **No worry of failure:** While in flow, the person is too involved to care about failure. Process becomes more important than product.
- **Self-consciousness disappears:** During the flow experience, we are too involved to worry about protecting the ego. Yet after an episode of

flow is over, we generally emerge with a stronger self-concept. We have successfully met some challenge. Paradoxically, the self expands through acts of self-forgetfulness.

- **The sense of time becomes distorted:** Generally, in flow we forget time. Hours may pass in what seems like moments. Or time may stretch out — a motion may be fast in clock time but feel much slower in experience time. The sense of time becomes dependent on what we are doing.
- **The activity becomes *autotelic*:** Whenever most of the conditions of flow are present, and as skills increase, an activity begins to become *autotelic*, which is Greek for something that is an end to itself. Many things in life are *exotelic,* not done for themselves but in order to get to some later goal. Some are both. The violinist, for instance, gets paid to do what he loves. In many ways the secret to a happy life is to learn to get flow from as many of the activities that we do as possible.

It should be apparent that flow experiences are exactly what we are after when we describe the benefits of engaging in creative arts experiences. Yet people are not always ready or willing to engage in creative experiences; they may be blocked or fearful. In order to help people to break out of these self-imposed limits, it is necessary to understand exactly what blocks their creativity. The next section addresses this issue.

Blocks to Creativity

Why aren't people more creative? In *A Whack on the Side of the Head* Roger Von Oech (1993), a successful business consultant in creative thinking, suggests two reasons. First, people develop routines — thought paths that get them efficiently through the day. Without such routines it would be impossible to get very much accomplished. Secondly, it is our own attitudes (thoughts or feelings that spring from our belief systems) that prevent us from being creative. Von Oech calls these "mental locks," defining them as "certain attitudes which lock our thinking into the status quo and keep us thinking 'more of the same' " (p. 14). It is hard to be creative if our thinking is under the influence of any of these. He identifies the following 10 "mental locks" and then refutes them:

1. **The right answer:** Our educational system often stresses this, and it becomes deeply ingrained in our thinking. Real life, though, is more complex and there may be many right answers.
2. **That's not logical:** So called "lateral thinking" makes connections across diverse categories and not just within one, generating many novel concepts and ideas.
3. **Follow the rules:** Rules are often arbitrary — they can be changed, broken, or bettered. Rules help us become socialized but can keep us playing games that are very limiting.
4. **Be practical:** Probing the possible, the impossible, and the impractical for ideas is often fruitful. Why spend hours on a model airplane or a drawing? Why fly to the moon? This kind of thinking gets us nowhere. Don't limit the imagination when first approaching a problem — brainstorm.
5. **Avoid ambiguity:** In real life, this is difficult. There is usually more than one meaning or interpretation to an object, an event, or a person's actions. Multiple ways of looking at things stretch a person's thinking and lead to a deeper understanding of what's going on.
6. **To err is wrong:** Learning from mistakes can be as valuable, if not more so, than avoiding them.
7. **Play is frivolous:** Play is necessary — it activates different parts of the brain and expands thinking.
8. **That's not my area:** Limiting the scope of one's knowledge and experience can limit creativity. Crossing boundaries and transferring knowledge from one area to another can bring fresh insights to a field.
9. **Don't be foolish:** Giving oneself license to play the fool shakes up thinking and generates ideas and fresh perspectives.
10. **I'm not creative:** Too often this is a self-fulfilling prophecy.

Creative Expression and Our Clients

"Creativity is an expression from the inside which has not been inhibited by societal wants and needs. Once inhibited it is difficult to regain" (Madsen & Kuhn, 1994, p. 40). This concern leads to the question: How then does a therapist encourage creativity?

Many books on becoming more creative are filled with ideas for exercises and experiences that are fun and helpful. These are worth examining as a means of sparking creativity. Some of them may also be useful to our clients in the difficult task of breaking down barriers to creativity. Attitudes, such as the ones discussed above, plus feelings (e.g., fears of failure or of looking foolish) that support these attitudes can be very resistant to change.

Helping clients express creativity involves recognizing and slowly chiseling away at these attitudes when they arise. When clients say they aren't creative, rather than contradicting this creative block, point out ways in which they have already successfully demonstrated their creativity. This may be in the formal sense (a poem, a painting) or informally (putting together an outfit, cooking, doodling).

Provide a balance between structured activities where the outcome is more directed and manageable and open-ended activities in which the outcome rests more heavily on the individual.

Be respectful and compassionate but persistent in dealing with clients' fears regarding creative expression. Fears are real for those who experience them. Many clients have recently experienced a loss, creating fears of the unknown or unexpected. Explain to the client that the trick with fears is often to wait them out rather than running away from them. Stand firm and, with time, they will take on a more manageable form or perhaps even shrink away to nothing. Patience is important.

Everyone experiences creative impasses. A normally enthusiastic participant will suddenly become a stuck and bored individual. Sometimes people can't explain their feelings or don't understand how to move through this state. Try doing something different to change perspective. For example, if you are running a visual arts program, go on an outing and take sketchpads — the zoo is a great place to draw. For a music therapy program, bring in an assortment of junk and suggest that clients recycle it into musical instruments. As a last resort, walk or crawl backwards just to see things in a new way.

Be playful and have fun. Playfulness and creativity are intertwined. Believe that clients are creative, and they will live up to this expectation.

Enhancing or Hindering Expression in Groups

In a group situation, there are three elements that influence creative expression: the therapist, the environment, and members of the group.

Although it is ideal when each of these elements helps enhance expression, it is often enough if strengths in one area compensate for weaknesses in another. A skilled therapist may bring out the best in a group despite limited materials or inadequate space and can still teach clients how to be effective group members.

Enhancing Expression

The following are elements that can enhance expression.

Therapist

The therapist enhances expression by exhibiting the following qualities:

- **Authenticity:** Stay real — be able to react honestly to a situation without masking feelings.
- **Understanding:** A potent quality; a client who feels that s/he has been heard and accepted is likely to feel that s/he can express his/her own individuality and creativity.
- **Respect for privacy:** Be receptive to what clients are willing to disclose and not disclose.
- **Being comfortable with him/herself and the group:** Increases chances that everyone else will relax and be comfortable as well.
- **A non-judgmental attitude and objectivity:** Both qualities encourage people to express their individual viewpoints.
- **Supportive guidance:** Foster self-reliance and risk-taking behaviors in the group.
- **Ability to create a feeling of partnership:** A feeling that "we are all in this together" creates a group bond which facilitates sharing, cooperation, and a sense of participation in each other's growth and discovery.
- **Enthusiasm:** Bring this infectious quality which often energizes group members.

- **Sincerity:** "Say what you mean, mean what you say." This creates trust in the group.
- **Warmth and caring:** Nurturing clients may enable them to open up in ways that they would be reluctant to do in a less supportive environment.
- **Understanding psychological safety:** Know what creates a perception of safety and how to provide ground rules that support this perception.
- **Respect for each person's own pace:** Be aware that group members learn, share, and become comfortable with others and new situations at different rates. Don't force a pace.
- **Participation:** Be an active group member and/or model participation when necessary.
- **Playfulness:** When the therapist is playful, it permits a spirit of playfulness in the group.
- **A neutral position:** The therapist does not become enmeshed in group dynamics but stays on the outside.

Environment

Environmental qualities that enhance expression:

- **A variety of good materials:** Provide the best materials possible given the circumstances of budget and availability. Make sure all tools and supplies (scissors, glue, etc.) are in good working order.
- **Provide choices:** Individual choice lies at the core of leisure. The more options offered, the more empowered the group will be.
- **Availability of inside/outside environment:** Most facilities have a recreation or art room — but using a patio, courtyard, or even a park setting for a program can be exhilarating for clients. Suzanne Mirviss: "One of my memorable experiences with clients was combining a beach picnic with art and music. We made sand candles, then a huge sandcastle, sang, and let our senses absorb the ocean world. There was room to expand because there were no walls to close us in."
- **Colorful space:** If the group meets in an institutional setting, there probably are restrictions on what can be changed in the environment

(e.g., painting walls). At least have a board to display artwork and/or a locked glass display case.

- **Adequate lighting:** Make sure there is enough lighting, particularly for those with visual disabilities.
- **Appropriate music:** Tastes will differ, but select music that is appropriate to the setting, group, and activity.
- **Few distractions:** Elicit staff help in eliminating as many outside distractions as possible. Radios, television, and people going in and out of a room can all hinder creative expression.
- **Workspace:** Keep spaces clean and uncluttered. Allow room to spread out and work. Make sure everyone can establish an adequate personal space.
- **Space:** One that allows for closeness and distance, openness and privacy. Space in which to move and expand when it is called for, yet also space for retreat if someone needs it.

Group

Members of the group help enhance expression through their:

- **Support:** Group members should be encouraged to be supportive, not negative. Negative feelings damage group cohesiveness.
- **Acceptance:** All members, including the therapist, need to feel accepted into the group for the group to function effectively.
- **Willingness to share ideas and feedback:** Members need to be active participants (most of the time) for the group to progress and be fruitful. There may be times when this is not psychologically possible, in which case a person's mental state should be respected.
- **Commitment to being there:** This should be established in the early stages of the group. When members do not show up, their absence affects the rest of the group.
- **Ability to work with the therapist and each other:** A member cannot function if there isn't the ability or desire to work within the established structure.
- **Willingness to engage in the creative process:** If a member doesn't really want to be in the group and/or isn't interested in the activities, it wastes everyone's time and energy.

Hindering Expression

Needless to say, it is important to try to minimize the number of these factors that operate in the group.

Therapist

A therapist may hinder expression in the following ways:

- **Criticism:** Find ways to make positive suggestions rather than criticize.
- **Too much or too little structure:** Too much structure and people feel trapped; too little and they flounder. Create enough structure to allow people room to explore with a purpose.
- **Too much or too little direction:** The therapist must strike a balance so that clients don't feel babied or, at the opposite extreme, feel lost. Continually evaluate the clients' needs for direction.
- **Inappropriate sharing of self:** Know professional boundaries and share only what is needed.
- **Distance:** Being psychologically disengaged or inaccessible to the group or standing apart from group activities leaves clients feeling unsupported.
- **Disrespect for clients' needs:** Not being client-focused in goals and interactions, but imposing goals and expectations limits client's choices.
- **Lack of encouragement:** Without encouragement, confidence may remain low in clients tackling new creative activities.
- **Lack of preparation:** The group's perception will be that they or the activity are not very important to the therapist, though this may be far from true. A one-time problem will not be harmful but being chronically underprepared will.
- **Absence of feedback:** Without feedback on their individual projects and contributions to the group, members may feel their efforts are worthless and underappreciated.
- **Forcing exposure or interpretation:** This is associated with disrespect for clients' needs. Forcing is not only psychologically painful but also counterproductive to creative work.

- **Pushing the process:** Any new process must have enough time to evolve. Efforts to push it in a particular direction or speed it up will usually fail. The therapist who shows patience in letting the process develop will be rewarded with greater — and perhaps unexpected — results.
- **Insincerity:** Clients can usually identify staff who are not sincere. Often this is interpreted as a lack of respect for the client — a definite block to create expression.

Environment

Negative factors in the environment may be

- **Formality:** An overly formal setting discourages clients from feeling that they can be playful, messy, and/or relaxed.
- **Sterility:** A cold and empty space will be barren and unstimulating for clients trying to engage in creative work.
- **Lack of necessary time:** Planning is *critical.* Clients' stress levels rise when they feel rushed. Stress can reduce the ability to be creative. (In some cases, clients are habitually slow as this gets them attention from others. In this situation, it is best to deal with structuring time right from the beginning.)
- **Uncomfortable space:** A cramped, cluttered, or dirty space can be physically and/or psychologically unpleasant for clients. Being too cold or too hot, feeling unsafe or uncomfortable all stop the "creative juices." Maslow (1968) clearly outlined the need for us to deal with human comforts before we can experience creativity.
- **Noise and/or distractions:** These make it difficult to concentrate. Creativity is best experienced in a state of flow. Numerous distractions make it difficult to sustain this state.

Group

Members of the group may hinder creative expression through:

- **Pre-conceived ideas:** Did the member come into the group with an inaccurate picture of the group's purpose and plan?

- **Negative feelings:** Negativity becomes a wall unless the therapist deals with the feelings.
- **Depression or fatigue:** Members in either of these states may cast a heavy shadow over the group. Know group members and check in regularly to see how they are doing. They may need time away from the group to sort out feelings.
- **Disrespect:** This creates anxiety and damages collective and individual self-esteem.
- **Lack of confidence:** Based on fears like "I'm not creative," this can hold back both individuals and groups.
- **Fear of exposure and interpretation:** These fears can make self-expression a nearly impossible task and must be dealt with by the therapist and the individual.

References

Bruer, J. T. (1999). In search of brain-based education. *Phi Delta Kappan, 80*(9), 648-654.

Cornett, C. E. (2007). *Creating meaning through literature and the arts: An integration resource for classroom teachers* (3rd ed.). New Jersey: Pearson.

Csikszentmihalyi, M. (1996). *Creativity*. New York: Harper Collins.

Edwards, B. (1989). *Drawing on the right side of the brain.* New York: St. Martin's Press.

Madsen, C. K. & Kuhn, T. L. (1994). *Contemporary music education* (2nd ed.). Raleigh, NC: Contemporary Publishing Company.

Mark, M. L. (ed.) (2002). *Music education: Source readings from ancient Greece to today* (2nd ed.). New York: Routledge Publications.

Maslow, A. H. (1987). *Motivation and personality.* New York: Harpercollins College Division.

National Endowment for the Arts. (2015). *How creativity works in the brain.* Washington, DC. Available from: www.arts.gov.

Von Oech, R. (1993). *A whack on the side of the head.* New York: Warner Books.

Warren, B. (1993). *Using the creative arts in therapy* (2nd ed.). New York: Routledge Publications.

3

Roles of the Therapist

The therapist who uses the arts as a therapeutic tool for groups embarks on a journey of discovery and wonder. Even with the most meticulous planning, an element of mystery emerges from the minds and spirits of the individuals in the group. The magic of the arts touches the spirit and promotes a level of communication that is different from everyday life.

The therapist who provides the opportunity for creative expression and uses the information that emerges in a therapeutic process takes on many roles. Perhaps the most important is being a willing traveler in a realm that is provocative and mysterious. In order to gird him/herself for this journey, the therapist must examine the variety of roles required for this therapeutic process. The primary roles are facilitator, teacher, artist, and therapist.

Facilitator

To facilitate, or ease the way, the therapist must give up the traditional position as the only knowledgeable authority in the group.

It is important to create a group climate where members derive support from one another as well as from the therapist. Since creative experience is often an enigma, it puts all group members on equal ground. By the very nature of the process, each group member must work to grasp its meaning. An effective facilitator enables clients to be authorities on what is true for them, give and receive information, and support each other's growth and discovery. Being an effective facilitator means being able to:

- **Create safety:** For individuals to become functioning members of a group, they need to feel safe with each other. Specific ground rules established at the start of the group describe how members participate, show respect to other group members, respond to each other in sharing their insights and feelings, and behave as vital members of the group. If the group environment is safe, then individuals are comfortable. They can explore and express what they discover in the art experience.
- **Role model:** People often learn more from what is done than what is said. It is important for the therapist to go beyond telling clients how to be effective members of the group. S/he needs to show them by example what that entails. Group members look to the therapist to show them, for example, how to give or receive feedback.
- **Participate:** As an effective role model, the therapist must be an active participant in the group. Standing back and observing while members are engaged in an activity may be necessary in some circumstances but not helpful on a regular basis. As in the case of role modeling, participation is best facilitated by participating — doing the activities as a part of the group — rather than just talking about it.
- **Take risks:** Taking risks invites change. In a group, a risk may be anything — from encouraging a client to say more about his/her work to admitting to not knowing how to do something. Taking a risk and succeeding can encourage others to take more risks of their own. Clients who see failure as non-fatal feel encouraged to take risks. Even if the therapist's risk-taking is a failure, it may allow clients to see the therapist as human and accessible. By risking vulnerability, the therapist opens him/herself to the possibility that s/he will be allowing other people to shine. This communicates a willingness to strengthen others' self-esteem — a powerful mechanism for accomplishing that task. Suzanne Mirviss: "One of the most poignant moments I have ever had was taking the risk of admitting that I didn't know how to solve a problem with a group art project. That admission allowed a group member with some related experience to come forward and lead us through the dilemma."

- **Be genuine:** If the therapist is not genuine, s/he is perceived as not trustworthy, which affects the climate of safety in the group. What the therapist says within the group should feel real to others. For example, if the therapist says to a client, "You're doing great!" when it is obvious that the individual isn't actually doing all that well, the individual may question the genuineness of the therapist and mistrust any subsequent feedback. Accurate and caring suggestions for improvement are more therapeutic than dishonest praise.
- **Be friendly and open:** Part of effective facilitating is to be a welcoming presence, friendly and genuinely happy to be there for clients. If a therapist is burned out or fears self-disclosure, for example, s/he will find it difficult to create a warm and supportive group environment. Being open to others, feeling honest compassion, and caring what happens to people is the medicine of true healing.
- **Encourage freedom within structure:** One of the challenges of group work is to create a comfortable amount of structure for the group members (e.g., a plan of activities for each session) and still maintain a climate of freedom. Being flexible, paying attention to clients, and being open to changing activities or direction allows clients to experience feelings of freedom. Many therapists have come to a group armed with what they felt were wonderful activities, but received blank stares that said, "I don't want to do this." The reasons may have little to do with the therapist and everything to do with the clients (e.g., pain, adjustment of medications, lack of sleep). Effective facilitating means being willing to abandon a plan in favor of trying to discover what group members need.
- **Maintain proper boundaries:** A therapist needs to participate, take risks, and have compassion. But s/he must also maintain proper personal boundaries. This means not disclosing personal struggles or sharing life histories with clients. The clients, not the therapist, are there for help. Becoming socially involved with clients in a group can also jeopardize boundaries and confuse roles. Clients can't decipher where *friend* ends and *therapist* begins.
- **Be a catalyst:** A catalyst makes things happen. Many clients are overwhelmed by life changes or have a disability which impairs their ability to initiate action. Facilitating may at times mean being the spark,

providing the energy or ideas that will help clients initiate changes in their lives.

Teacher

Being a teacher is an integral part of a being a therapist. The therapist who makes use of the creative arts will be actively involved in instructing, demonstrating, evaluating, and looking for new ideas to motivate clients. The teacher needs to know:

- **Learning styles:** The growth of our clients is the measure of our success. In order to be client-focused, we need to understand that people learn in different ways. Some are visual learners who need to see information to learn it. Others are auditory (hearing) learners who learn and remember best through what they hear. Kinesthetic learners learn by doing. Most people have one or more areas of strength. A skilled teacher recognizes that everyone has their own learning style and addresses more than one learning style when teaching an activity.
- **Presentation:** Presentation refers both to the style of the teacher and the timing and methods of introducing activities. A quiet activity may need to follow a high-energy one. Activities which impact clients emotionally may need to be introduced slowly and be preceded by warmup activities. There are many effective styles of presentation. Some teachers are exuberant and create that kind of energy in a group. Some quietly command attention. Regardless of style, the following techniques apply:
    - Say what needs to be said in several different ways and at different intervals in order to make sure clients understand what they need to know.
    - Summarize what has been said.
    - Practice using techniques and materials in advance of using them in the group — familiarity will save time and prevent mistakes.
- **Resources and techniques:** Having a grab bag of ideas and techniques allows the therapist to be flexible and responsive to group needs. Keeping up to date on new developments in the field and

creating an expanding repertoire of ideas and activities will increase the therapist's effectiveness as a teacher.

- **How to continue learning:** The best teachers are those who love to learn. Inspiring a love of learning and a desire to explore new ideas is a great gift to those in our care. The teacher who is a learner is also sensitive to what it feels like *not* to know, which is a vulnerability that every learner experiences. This knowledge can motivate the therapist to find effective ways of helping clients grasp what you are teaching them.

Artist

Is it necessary to be a painter, musician, or other accomplished artist to use the arts as therapeutic tools? Therapists are often concerned that they are not creative. They may be interested in the arts, but they aren't comfortable or don't feel capable of successfully leading arts-based therapeutic activities. While it certainly helps to have expertise in some aspect of the arts, it isn't mandatory for group work. What *is* needed is a clear idea of what the arts can accomplish for clients and the ability to see oneself as a facilitator of creative expression. The artist needs to:

- **Believe in creativity:** We all have the need, right, and ability to express creativity in our lives. People are naturally creative. As children we are encouraged to use art materials, explore our ideas, and feel free to create. At some point, many people receive the message that other activities are more important than creative activities. Their energy is diverted away from the arts. Some people receive damaging messages like, "You'll never be an artist." or "You have to be really talented to succeed in the arts. Work on practical skills instead." What results is a culture of people cut off from an important aspect of themselves — and missing that passionate engagement they felt in childhood. Expressing creativity is necessary for all human beings. The therapist's job is to assist clients in using their creativity to heal and attain fulfillment.
- **Understand everyday creativity:** Creativity, self-expression, and playfulness go hand in hand. Daily activities can be seen as creative

choices, from putting together clothes to developing ways of making clients comfortable in a new activity. Broadening the definition of creative expression can lead to an increased awareness of creative choices for the client.

- **Know his/her barriers to creativity:** A therapist needs to be aware of his/her blocks and negative messages about creativity. These messages affect our attitudes, infiltrate our being, and cause doubt and fear. Finding ways to break down these barriers will enable the artist aspect of the therapist to express its own creativity and help clients to do the same.
- **Explore the arts:** There are huge numbers of ideas, materials, and processes. If one technique doesn't inspire the therapist and/or the group, there are many others to try. Explore books, craft magazines, newspapers, courses, and the Internet.

Therapist

As therapists, we try to show our clients how to live fuller, more balanced, and joyful lives. One method is promoting the experience of leisure. The leisure experience touches every aspect of life and is potently present during creative activity. Using the tools of creativity is a natural avenue for therapeutic healing. Regardless of their therapeutic orientation, therapists may incorporate processes that come from a variety of allied health therapies such as art, psychology, drama, dance, music, recreational, and occupational therapy.

In using processes from allied professions, we must be clear about our professional goals and boundaries. An art therapist, for example, has specialized training primarily focused on psychology, art development, and art modalities. S/he is qualified to interpret art, diagnose, and recommend treatment. Therapists who are not trained as art therapists must not perform these functions. Drama therapy, dance therapy, and music therapy also require specialized training and experience.

Other therapists can, however, use creative arts techniques for exploration in groups. How these therapists use these processes and how they deal with the information that emerges is different and must lie within the boundary of their profession. For example, rather than interpreting a client's artwork, a recreational therapist would have the client *tell us* what it means. We may discover something important about a client during a group and may take it to a treatment team meeting for information and discussion even if we ourselves cannot establish an art therapy or drama therapy treatment plan. It is our responsibility to remember our professional boundaries and also to appreciate our roles as therapists. A therapist needs to know about:

- **Group purpose:** Has the group formed to learn an art skill, to celebrate their lives, for personal exploration, or for a more therapeutic goal? The purpose sets the tone of the group, the manner and style of the therapist, the interactions among all members of the group, and the way information is gathered and processed within the group.
- **Group goals:** What should be accomplished during the group and ultimately by each client? Once the goals of the group have been clearly defined, it is possible to choose and incorporate creative arts activities that will be intellectually and emotionally appropriate. Success in the group is directly related to clear and realistic goals.
- **Observation skills:** Just as clients learn from observing our actions, we learn from observing their behavior in the group. Good observation skills enable the therapist to catch an important body posture, a facial expression, an emotional reaction, or a subtle behavior. These unconscious reactions are often more revealing than what people say with words.
- **Psychosocial development:** To recognize and understand issues that clients are dealing with, a therapist must be familiar with the psychosocial tasks associated with different stages of life. Then the therapist can assess a client's current level of development and provide therapy to deal with unresolved issues.
- **Group dynamics:** A therapist who works with groups needs to understand how they function. Significant aspects of group dynamics include:
    - how individuals become a group
    - the stages of group development
    - styles of leadership and their effect on the group

  - conflict resolution
  - how to be effective with the varying chemistry of groups

- **Intuitive understanding:** What am I feeling? What is the client really asking for? What would bring closure to this group? Being intuitive is often referred to as a sixth sense, as an ability to read between the lines. It is not so much taught as developed.
- **Least restrictive interventions:** These allow the client to process personal change with as much freedom and personal expression as s/he and the group are comfortable with.
- ***Not* analyzing:** Participants will find their own answers in the images and work they produce and sometimes in verbalizing their private explanations. It may be enough to allow the client his/her own private insights and revelations without further explanation.
- **Setting priorities:** Just as facilitating means creating freedom within structure, being an effective therapist means finding a balance between prescriptive activities and choice. Some activities have more therapeutic value and carry more therapeutic weight than others. Schedules may need to be rearranged to fit the psychological needs of members, but if the purpose of the group is to work through problems, there may be activities that are not optional.
- **Activity analysis:** Activities should be carefully chosen to meet the goals of the group. Activity analysis allows a therapist to judge the physical, cognitive, emotional, and social demands of activities. It can help answer questions such as: Is this activity age-appropriate? What knowledge, skills, and abilities are required to complete the task? What leadership style will I assume? As therapists we should always plan and choose our interventions responsibly. Everything we do has an impact on the people with whom we work.
- **Leisure theory:** Understanding the importance of leisure as part of a person's experience enables the therapist to empower clients. It lets clients find and express their own answers about shaping their time in a way that improves their integrity and self-esteem.

Legal Requirements

Several places in this chapter, and elsewhere in this book, we describe how therapists must be open and non-judgmental regarding a client's contributions. We also say that the therapist must maintain a client's trust by keeping information disclosed in the group confidential. These are important aspects of practice. However, there are two situations where a therapist is required to follow a different set of standards.

The first is when the therapist learns about abuse of children or vulnerable adults. This could be abuse towards the client or by the client. A client may also report abuse that is happening between two other people.

Different states and provinces have different laws, but most of them require therapists to report what they have found to designated authorities within a very short time after finding out about possible abuse. Even if there is no proof of the abuse, most jurisdictions require reporting suspicions or when the possibility is based on reasonable cause. When a client tells the therapist about abuse between other people, some jurisdictions require the therapist to make a report based on this second-hand knowledge. Other jurisdictions require a report from the client. If the requirements are unclear, both should make a report.

The location to file the report and the form of the report, e.g. verbal or written, also depend on the state or province. The authorities who receive the report will investigate the situation. RAINN (2020) has a database that describes the laws in each state. This is available at https://apps.rainn.org/policy/.

Your agency may have policies that require more than the governmental reporting. Be sure you know what is required at that level, too. You may be required to report to more than one place.

The second situation is when therapists learn about a potential for self-harm or harm to others. Therapists usually are allowed more discretion in these situations because threats that clients make may not always be serious. Recreational and arts therapists are not the team members who are responsible for deciding if suicidal or homicidal ideation is or is not serious. It is best to discuss a concern with the rest of the healthcare team. This should not affect the level of trust in the therapist-client relationship.

Agencies usually have guidelines for when you need to report a threat and who will receive the report.

The bottom line is that the safety of the client and those the client may be harming, neglecting, or threatening is more important than possibility that the client's trust in the therapeutic relationship may be disrupted, shakes, or broken. It is always possible that a client will experience relief and increased trust when the therapist makes a report and thereby sets a limit.

References

RAINN (2020). State law database. https://apps.rainn.org/policy/.

4

Individual Development

Every individual who joins a therapy group is a unique composite of personal experience, psychological development, personality, biology, culture, age, gender, mental abilities, and physical abilities. One of the challenges of creating a group is to understand how these components impact the expectations and roles of a person in a group setting. Each person in a group affects the chemistry of the group and how it functions.

Another challenge is to understand the relationship of the individual to the therapist (the helping relationship). As therapists, our task is to manage all the emotion and interactions of the group. But this is a complex puzzle — one that takes time to put together.

This chapter provides a framework for understanding behavior in groups by looking at the developmental stages of the people who are part of them. It will look at the kinds of information we need to know about clients, the stages of psychological development, and the development of artistic skills. The next chapter continues the discussion by studying the structure of therapy groups.

Assessment of Individuals

The process of understanding clients and their needs is complex and ongoing. Understanding what someone needs involves gathering information, conferring with other staff, listening to the client, and observing his/her behavior. Our understanding of the client is dynamic and evolves as we interact with the individual.

Assessment is done to gather information about clients in order to design a program that addresses their needs and interests. The keys to assessment are using appropriate tools, listening, observing, and analyzing.

General information that can be gathered about an individual client includes:

- **Age:** Calendar and functional
- **Gender:** Birth, physical, self-identification, and sexual orientation
- **Current stay:** How long has this person been at the facility? Is this a first stay or a return?
- **Length of treatment:** How much time is available to work with this individual? Consider hours per day, days left in the current stay, and likelihood of a return to the therapeutic environment for another stay.
- **Level of social functioning:** How well does this individual function in a group setting? If relevant, what provokes negative responses or behaviors in the client? Has the treatment team established a consistent approach in response to the client's negative responses or behaviors?
- **Disabilities and abilities**
- **Health status:** Is the individual often in pain, on medication, or affected by a physical or mental condition? Is the person's general condition stable and predictable or erratic and somewhat unregulated?
- **Interests:** Current and past
- **Support systems:** What types of support does the client have outside of the facility? What types does s/he have inside the facility? Where will this client be discharged to?

In addition, the therapist will often interview prospective members of a group before the first meeting, to assess each person's behavior, interests, and motivation for being in the group. The meeting is kept brief and friendly. This is where the skills of listening for verbal clues and observing non-verbal behavior come into play.

By the end of the information-gathering process, the therapist should have a good sense of appropriate groups for the client and an understanding of how the client can be expected to behave in each group.

Psychosocial Development

Understanding a client's current stage of development is an important first step in determining how the client will function in a group setting. Individuals change dramatically as they grow older. The descriptions on the following pages provide an overview of typical growth and development milestones.

These milestones are only general guidelines. It is important to remember that a person's chronological age (how many years s/he has been alive) is only one measure — and probably not the most important one. The biological age, how much the body has developed and aged, is a better measure of a client's physical abilities. The functional age is the best measure of the skills that can be expected in a group.

Cultural norms and environment also impact an individual's development. Young girls in first-world nations who have plenty (or too much) to eat tend to start puberty earlier than girls from third world countries who lack good nutrition. The life span of individuals in certain cultural and socioeconomic groups may be as much as thirty years longer because of lifestyle and healthcare options.

Probably the most important way to use developmental charts is to anticipate the individual's next step toward maturity and help him/her prepare for that step.

The following pages contain information that is grouped by developmental age. Theorists like Piaget, Freud, Erikson, Kohlberg, and Sullivan have all added to our understanding of the developmental process and their works have helped structure our developmental levels. The following information includes a short description of each of these theorist's ideas along with information about typical play behaviors, physiological events, common fears, and medical preparation concerns for each developmental level. The information is from *Idyll Arbor's Therapy Dictionary, 2nd Edition* (2001).

Developmental levels do not end at adulthood. However, clear-cut levels after the age of 20 years have not been studied by many researchers. Eric Erikson has done the most complete work in looking at older ages, so his levels are provided.

Developmental Age: Birth to 12 Months

Psychosocial Stage of Development (Erikson)
Stage One: Infancy
Trust: Ability to trust others and a sense of one's own trustworthiness. A sense of hope.

vs.

Mistrust: Withdrawal and estrangement. Emotional dissatisfaction if needs have not been consistently met.

Moral Judgment (Kohlberg)
Kohlberg does not recognize moral judgment awareness at this age.

Radius of Significant Relationships (Sullivan)
Maternal person — may be either unipolar or bipolar. Given the amount of childcare used today, this distinction is slipping.

Cognitive Stage (Piaget)
Piaget calls this stage the *sensorimotor stage* and extends the chronological age of this stage to two years.

Psychosexual Stage (Freud)
Oral-Sensory — One of the major sources of pleasure at this age comes from exploring the world through oral activities such as vocalizing, sucking, and chewing.

Play Behaviors
Engages in playful activity alone and independently. Will engage in play with someone who is older but play behavior is centered around what interests him/her. Explores world visually by random movement. As ability to grasp and ability to put things in his/her mouth develops, explores the world this way also.

Basic Physiological Events

Develops basic control of body through space (hand to mouth, sitting up, pulling self to standing, crawling, rolling from back to abdomen when lying down). Develops basic fine motor control (palmer grasp, radial-digital grasp, scissor grasp, 3-jaw chuck grasp, and pincer grasp).

Common Fears

Loss of trusted adults' care or support, strangers, animals, loud noises, sudden movements, and bright lights.

Medical Preparation Concerns

Patients who are functionally under one year of age rely heavily on the support of a parent or familiar staff to survive unknown and scary situations. Explain the procedure to a parent or staff person who has a trusting relationship with the patient and is willing to stay with the patient through the procedure. Patients, lacking the general ability to control their environment, are soothed by the physical presence of a parent or staff person that they can trust. These patients are also extremely limited in their ability to adjust quickly to new environments. Provide the patient with familiar objects from his/her room along with the company of the parent or familiar staff person while a procedure is being performed.

Developmental Age: 1 Year to 3 Years

Psychosocial Stage of Development (Erikson)

Stage Two: Late infancy and early childhood

Autonomy: Self-control without loss of self-esteem. Ability to cooperate and to express oneself.

vs.

Shame and Doubt: Compulsive self-restraint or compliance. Defiance, willfulness, shame. Doubt: feelings that nothing one does is any good.

Moral Judgment (Kohlberg)

Pre-conventional (pre-moral). External morality directed and imposed by authoritarian figures. There are two levels associated with the pre-conventional stage. The first one, punishment-and-obedience orientation (where actions are labeled as "good or bad" based on the consequences received), covers this age group.

Radius of Significant Relationships (Sullivan)

Parental Persons (tri-polar)

Play Behavior
Plays alone and independently. Others may be playing nearby but their actions have little influence on the child's play.

Psychosexual Stage (Freud)
Anal Stage. Individuals learn to withhold or expel fecal material at will. Future personality traits such as stinginess, stubbornness, expansiveness, over-generosity, and orderliness or messiness are developed and fine-tuned.

Basic Physiological Events
Turns pages in books, can build a tower of blocks up to nine blocks tall, walks up and down stairs, stands on one foot for a few seconds, in artwork is able to copy circles and crosses.

Common Fears
Separation from parent/primary caretakers, injury, certain persons or locations (e.g., doctor, dentist office), loud or sudden noises, dark places, large machines.

Medical Preparation Concerns
Patients rely heavily on the gross and fine motor ability that they have. Restricted movement may increase the patient's level of stress. Simple procedures like a blood pressure check may produce anxiety. For painless procedures, showing the equipment, performing the procedure on an anatomically correct doll, or teaching the patient how to imitate the procedure on the doll may reduce fear. Play may need to be done a few times prior to the actual appointment. This group does not understand what is inside the body. Avoid lengthy discussions about what is going to be "fixed" or "examined." Concentrate on how the treatment or procedure will feel. Intense emotional upset and physical resistance is developmentally normal. A procedure should be done as quickly and gently as possible with a trusted staff person or parent physically close. After a painful procedure, there should be numerous opportunities to work out fear and misunderstanding. Frequently this group equates pain directly with punishment. If the patient is verbal and talks about the doll being "bad" or needing a time out prior to having the procedure, the staff can direct the patient's play to reflect a truer picture of what happened.

Developmental Age: 3 to 6 Years

Psychosocial Stage of Development (Erikson)
Stage Three: Early Childhood
Initiative: The courage to try to achieve desired goals tempered by a sense of conscience.

vs.

Guilt: Self-denial and self-restriction.

Moral Judgment (Kohlberg)
Pre-conventional (pre-moral). Morality is external, being directed and imposed by authoritarian figures. There are two levels associated with pre-conventional stage. The second one, the instrumental-relativist orientation (where behaviors are considered to be "right" if they bring pleasure), covers this age group.

Radius of Significant Relationships (Sullivan)
Basic Family

Play Behavior
Child plays with toys; engages in activities similar to others nearby, but plays next to, instead of with, others. Engages in make-believe and dramatic play.

Psychosexual Stage (Freud)
Phallic Stage. Freud noted that it is during this developmental period that children begin to recognize that there are differences between the sexes. They also discover that their genitals are interesting and sensitive. He speculated that penis envy and castration anxiety were important concerns for children in this age group. Freud states that personality traits such as shyness vs. brashness, blind courage vs. timidity, and stylishness vs. plainness develop during this stage.

Basic Physiological Events
Skips and hops on one foot, throws and catches balls well, walks backward, ties shoelaces, uses seven to nine parts when drawing a stickman, constantly active.

Common Fears
Monsters, ghosts, or other supernatural beings; injury; death; "bad" people; the dark.

Medical Preparation Concerns

Material in this section is based on the developmental needs of patients between the ages of three years and seven years of age. Around the age of seven years children are more able to understand medical and health issues. Patients tend to think egocentrically and explain unknowns through magical thinking. Without adequate preparation, their minds can become quite active with imagination, making the procedure more exaggerated, bizarre, and frightening than it actually is. Explain the procedure to them using dolls, puppets, and other visual aids. Allow them to take the part of the practitioner prior to the procedure until they feel more relaxed. This reduces the need for both physical and chemical restraints. Children of this age tend to have concerns about mutilation, especially fears of castration. While some adults who function at this developmental age don't exhibit this behavior, many patients will still experience this fear. Be very explicit about the part of the body that the procedure will be done on. Frequently patients want to act like "grown men and women." To them this means that they are not allowed to express their fears, cry, or scream. With the use of the puppets or dolls, staff can help the patient learn appropriate ways to express feelings.

Developmental Age: 6 to 12 Years

Psychosocial Stage of Development (Erikson)

Stage Four: Middle Childhood

Industry: Realization of competence, perseverance.

vs.

Inferiority: Feeling that one will never be "any good," withdrawal from school and peers.

Moral Judgment (Kohlberg)

Conventional Stage where conformity, loyalty, and maintenance of social order is paramount. This stage closely corresponds to the child's operational level of cognitive function. The two levels of this stage (stages 3 and 4, building upon earlier stages) are 3. the interpersonal concordance (one earns approval by following norms and being a good girl or good boy) and 4. the law-and-order orientation where following the rules set out by authority equals correct behavior.

Radius of Significant Relationships (Sullivan)

Neighborhood and School.

Play Behaviors
Plays with others in an organized manner for a purpose (e.g., sports teams, to make something). Feelings of belonging to the group. The youth plays a role (leader/follower) and the others support that role to some degree.

Psychosexual Stage (Freud)
Latency Period. Freud identified this time of maturation to be one of polishing previously acquired personality traits and using energy to acquire knowledge.

Physiological Events
Can follow three-step commands, repeats performances to improve skill, prefers to play with members of own sex, dresses self completely, generally likes competition, pubescent changes may begin to develop.

Common Fears
Storms, the dark, staying alone, failure in school and tests, supernatural beings (esp. seen on TV or in movies), death.

Medical Preparation Concerns
Material in this section is based on the developmental needs of patients between the ages of seven years and thirteen years of age. Around the age of thirteen years adolescents are confused with the physiological changes and also want to have a say in what happens. Patients who function in this developmental category are at least somewhat aware of different illnesses and how people cannot live without certain body organs. When preparing this group for invasive procedures, explain the procedure in a non-hurried manner first. Some of the patients will ask many, many questions to gain a sense of control. Please be patient. Understanding what is going to happen will reduce the need for restraints. Use scientific terminology for body parts and medical procedures. Unlike patients functioning below seven years or above 13 years, this group of patients may be embarrassed by having other people know that dolls were used to explain the procedure. If they don't want to use dolls or similar training props, explain the procedure with pictures.

Developmental Age: 12 to 19 Years

Psychosocial Stage of Development (Erikson)
Stage Five: Adolescence & Post Adolescence. "Identity Crisis."

Identity: Sexual maturation/individuation. Coherent sense of self; plans to actualize one's abilities.

vs.

Role Diffusion: Feelings of confusion, indecisiveness, antisocial behavior.

Moral Judgment (Kohlberg)
Postconventional. Social-Contract, legalistic orientation. Moral judgment tends to reflect generally accepted social standards and follow community laws. Individuals tend to believe that they can influence changes in standards if changes need to be made to increase fairness to and rights of the community in general.

Radius of Significant Relationships (Sullivan)
Outgroups. Relationships during this time tend to be an outgrowth of previously developed close friendships, first with individuals of the same sex, then branching out to members of the opposite sex.

Play Behaviors
Generally, both sexes engage in activities which involve their peers; females tend to spend more time talking than males. Sports, hobbies, social media, and entertainment (computer games, videos, and music) tend to make up much of the adolescent's play behavior.

Psychosexual Stage (Freud)
Genital Stage. This stage begins at the onset of puberty and the production of sexual hormones. While interactions tend to move toward developing a significant relationship, a major source of pleasure comes from sexual pleasures and tensions.

Basic Physiological Events
Top age group for participation in sports, a need for independence and freedom from authority, likely to take risks, very strong need for approval from peers, girls generally two years ahead of boys developmentally.

Common Fears
Social isolation, physical changes in body and own sexuality, divorce of parents, gossip, speaking in public, making mistakes in public.

Medical Preparation Concerns
Use visual aids to provide visualization of the procedures. Include a description of the expected external appearance after the procedure if the patient's normal appearance will change (e.g., cast, stitches). Patients functioning at this developmental level prefer not to have any familiar staff or

a parent with them as the procedures are being explained. Respect their wish for privacy. Additional feelings of control, which should reduce the need for restraints, can be gained by having patients make their own appointments.

Developmental Age: 18 to 25 Years

Psychosocial Stage of Development (Erikson)
Stage Six: Early Adulthood
Intimacy: Capacity for love as mutual devotion; commitment to work and relationships without loss of self.

vs.

Isolation: Impersonal relationships, prejudice.

Developmental Age: 25 to 65 Years

Psychosocial Stage of Development (Erikson)
Stage Seven: Adulthood. around 40, mid-life crisis; 42-65, middle age.
Generativity: Creativity, productivity, concern for others and the next generation.

vs.

Stagnation: Self-indulgence, impoverishment of self.

Developmental Age: 65 Years Plus

Psychosocial Stage of Development (Erikson)
Stage Eight: Old Age.
Possible loss of social and economic status, diminishing physical stamina, institutionalization, disengagement from commercial and professional activities; relatives, family, and friends may become more important.
Ego Integrity: Acceptance of the worth and uniqueness of one's life. Emotional integration. Able to honor the past while preparing to relinquish leadership to younger people.

vs.

Despair: Sense of loss, contempt for others. Life has been too short to achieve one's desires and it is too late to begin again.

Artistic Development

Knowledge of developmental levels in art is useful for many reasons. If the target group includes children, the therapist can choose activities and materials more appropriately and will have more realistic expectations about what the children in a particular age group can successfully accomplish.

Even with an age-appropriate activity, there will be variations in children's abilities. Some first graders will struggle with tracing and cutting through an entire art session while others glide easily through these tasks and move on to the next phase of an activity.

Understanding stages of art development also aids the therapist in guiding the child or adult with emotional or developmental challenges. Art therapists are often able to pinpoint delays or interruptions in development by examining artwork.

Listed below is an overview of artistic tasks which are generally accomplished from ages one to seven. By age seven, most individuals have acquired basic art skills: experience in the use of a variety of media; drawing with lines, shapes, and textures; cutting, tracing, and pasting. During the realistic stage, or beginning at ages seven to ten, children become more interested in representational art. By late childhood or early adolescence, children in our culture begin to master linear perspective or creating the illusion of three-dimensional depth on a two-dimensional surface (Winner, 1986). But it is the drawing of childhood which is the heart and soul of many people's experience with art.

There is, of course, much more to art than drawing. There are color, light, emotion, and media — a myriad of techniques and combinations to explore in order to communicate an idea or feeling. This section on the development of artistic skills covers only a small set of developmental milestones associated with art.

Age 1: Whole Arm Drawing

At this age a child is engrossed in learning to walk and acquiring gross motor skills. Drawing, a fine motor skill, is performed by the one year old with little motor control, by making large motions with the whole arm.

Ages 2-3: Scribbles and Scribbling

This is a stage of pure exploration of the materials, colors, and the movements of hand and wrist. Scribbles are the building blocks of children's art and lead to formation of more recognizable shapes. In the art of drawing there is a form of preliminary sketching called "gesture drawing" that might be thought of as controlled scribbling. The child has about 20 basic scribbles in his/her repertoire and, by adding color variations, a lot of exploring can be undertaken through scribbling. Scribbling is spontaneous, since a child at this age doesn't start out with a plan in mind. The child takes pleasure and interest in the pattern his/her markings make against a background.

Ages 2-4: Secrets of Shape

Discovering the hidden shapes within the scribbles: circles, ovals, squares, rectangles, triangles, odd shapes, and crosses.

Ages 3-4: Art in Outline

The child grasps the crayon and, with a single line, draws a form that s/he likes in scribbles. S/he now can outline a shape. For the child a shape is pleasing, so a child's response may include that fact that the drawing has, for example, nice lines or pretty circles. A child may scribble and proudly say, "This is a tractor, here are the wheels, here is the man." The adult's job is to listen, be enthusiastic, and not impose direction on the child. It is a time when a child is his/her own art teacher and explorer.

Ages 3-5: The Child and Design

Almost from the moment they can draw shapes in outline form, children begin to combine the forms into designs. For example, a circle may be placed inside a square or vice versa. When a child uses more than two shapes, the combinations become almost unlimited. At this stage children are developing a real style of their own — with favorite colors and shapes, ways to begin artwork, or fill the page. Three is a very confident age.

Ages 3-5: Mandalas, Suns, and Radials

Radials can be common asterisks, plants with waving fronds, Fourth of July explosions, a sun, a mandala wheel, or a smiling face. This stage is an important departure from which the child may proceed to draw human figures.

Ages 4-5: People, People, People

Often the human face comes from drawings of the sun. Children also begin to create their first image of a human — the universal "tadpole" — consisting of a circle and two lines for legs (Winner, 1986). At first the head is huge in relationship to the stick legs. At this stage the child is not trying to draw a human likeness but only to place things in a way that looks right and is personally pleasing to him/her.

Ages 4-6: Almost Pictures

Once children begin to draw people, their designs start taking shapes that adults recognize, for example a boat or flower. Drawings of the human figure are followed, after a while, by pictures of animals which stand up on two legs instead of crouching down on all fours.

There is great charm and fluidity in childhood drawings. Encouragement to create clouds with faces or animals standing on two legs is reserved for the pre-school child. Often artists wishing to bring back the imagery of childhood have to "...work hard to do consciously and deliberately what they once did effortlessly and because they had no choice." (Winner, 1986, p. 35) "I used to draw like Raphael," Picasso is quoted as saying, "but it has taken me a whole lifetime to learn to draw like children."

Around age five, as children develop intellectually, they become more interested in drawing representationally. There is a desire to picture something from their own lives, from stories read to them, or from their fantasy world. This focus of drawing will naturally begin to evolve, without adult interpretation.

Ages 5-7: Pictures

Usually until the age of five or six a child's pictures do not begin to tell their own story. Now we can begin to see the house with flowers, a rainbow, and a smiling sun — a picture of life as they see it.

While ability to complete fine-motor tasks varies within an age group, generally children between five and seven have increased dexterity. They can draw within an outline and vary the pressure of their marks from lighter to heavier for different effects. They can use almost any art medium now.

This five-to-seven-year-old stage is one of the critical periods in a child's art development. The child who feels free to use the colors and basic shapes which please him/her will continue to grow artistically when s/he moves into more pictorial work. This is when adults begin to give children more "formulas" for making their art more representational. Often children lose interest in art at the age of seven because they feel the disapproval or lack of encouragement from adults who may try to press them into creating neat and acceptable art. Sometimes people abandon art in childhood only to rediscover it later in life in a new form.

References

Idyll Arbor's Therapy Dictionary, 2nd ed. (2001). Ravensdale, WA: Idyll Arbor.
Winner, E. (1986). Where pelicans kiss seals. *Psychology Today, 20*(7) 25-35.

5

Therapy Group Dynamics

In this chapter we will look at the dynamics of a therapy group — how individuals interact and how group processes evolve through time. To run groups effectively a therapist must understand the awareness of members of a group, patterns of interaction, stages of psychological development within therapy groups, the helping relationship, and aspects of separation after engagement. This chapter provides the therapist with information on each of these topics, focusing on the way they improve running a group.

Johari Windows: A Self-Awareness Model

One vital aspect of working in a group involves the clients' awareness of themselves. Johari windows are a way of representing how aware a person is of him/herself and how aware other people are of him/her. To use the model, you ask yourself two questions:

- How well does this person know him/herself?
- How well do other people in the group know this person?

From those answers you can create a Johari window. Draw a box to represent the person. Draw a line from the top to the bottom of the box to represent the relative amounts the person knows about him/herself versus the amount that s/he does not know. Then draw a horizontal line from the left to the right to represent how much other members of the group know about the person versus how much they do not know. Obviously, the lines will move during treatment as the group learns more about the person and the person learns more about him/herself.

There are four quadrants in the box as shown in the diagram below. Q1 (open) is information that is known to both the person and the group. It is called open because it is information that everybody knows. Q2 (blind) is information that the group has discovered that the person is still not aware of. An addiction that a person is in denial about is one possible kind of knowledge that goes in this quadrant. Q3 (hidden) is information that the person knows about but has not shared. Q4 (unknown) is information that no one is aware of yet. Repressed memory would be in this quadrant.

	Known to Self	**Not Known to Self**
Known to others	Q1 Open	Q2 Blind
Not Known to others	Q3 Hidden	Q4 Unknown

Johari windows are useful for thinking about the dynamics of a group because they provide a graphic representation of the amount of sharing that a person has done and the amount of understanding a person has into his/her problems. In most therapeutic groups it is necessary to understand who is willing to share and who is not. It is also important to consider

Group Awareness Configuration

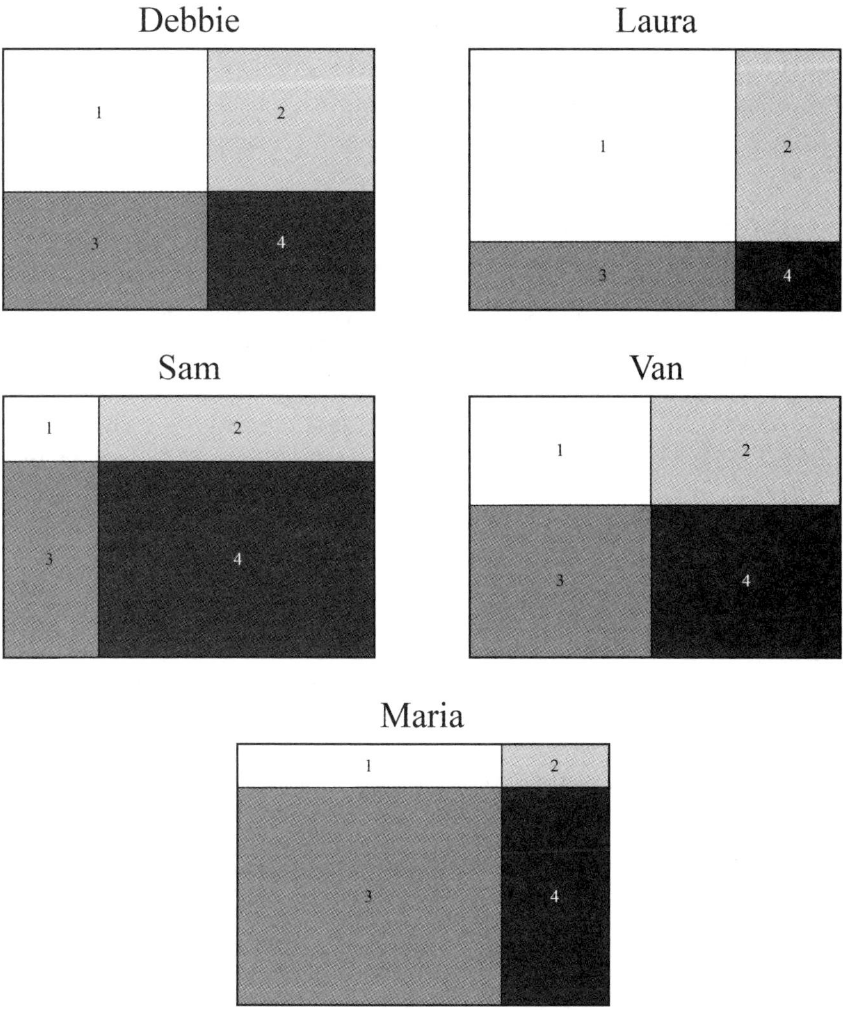

whether the person has the self-awareness to be able to share. The course of treatment is very different depending on the situation.

In the group shown above you can see several patterns. Laura is the most open because she knows a lot about herself and has shared it with the group. Maria and Sam both have very little open information, but the reasons are quite different. Maria knows a great deal about herself but is not willing to share it. Sam doesn't understand himself well, so even if he were willing to share information, he would not have very much to share. In the course of treatment, the therapist would probably want to work with Sam on self-awareness and with Maria on being willing to share — two very different directions in therapy even though the problem of not sharing with the group is the same. The graphic representation makes it easier to visualize the interactions of the group and the best course of treatment.

Interaction Patterns

Any activity can be classified as belonging to an interaction pattern. What follows is a progression of interaction levels. A psychologically healthy adult can interact on all these levels. When forming a group, plan to work at the interaction level where the group members are comfortable. Then develop activities that generate success at the next higher level. This process allows for sequencing of activities to build social and interaction skills.

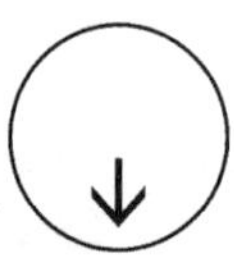

Internal

Action taking place within the mind or action involving the mind and a part of the body.

- Requires no interactions or contact with another person or external object
- Normal behavior unless taken to extreme

Examples: Twiddling thumbs, scratching your nose, fantasies, daydreaming, meditation, and yoga

Problematic Behavior: Characterized by internal activities taken to the extreme. Potential group members who have these problems may include children who are autistic; adults with psychiatric diagnoses such as severe depression, psychosis, or schizophrenia; or individuals with moderate to severe mental retardation exhibiting self-injurious behaviors.

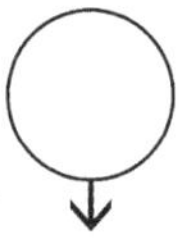

Object-Oriented

Action directed by a person towards an object.

- Requires interaction or contact with an object but not another person
- Requires awareness of and interest in inanimate objects

Examples: Jigsaw puzzles, solitaire, pogo-stick jumping, knitting, weightlifting, punching bag, watching TV, reading, arts, crafts, guided imagery, recorded visualizations, walking, computer games, gardening, and individual creative arts activities.

Problematic Behavior: Characterized by an interaction based on compulsive behavior instead of interest or an extreme amount of time spent in object-oriented activities to the detriment of other levels. Potential group members who have these problems may include individuals with compulsive disorders, mental retardation (especially moderate to severe levels), dementias, autism, or individuals with pathological patterns of using social media, computers, or videos.

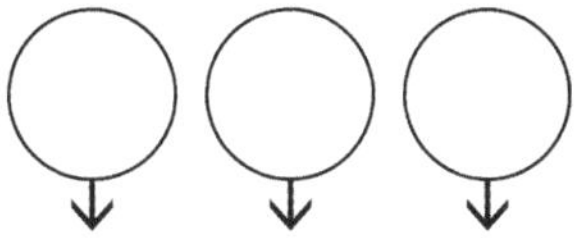

Aggregate

Action directed by a person toward an object while in the company of other persons who are also directing actions towards objects; physical proximity may allow for interaction, spontaneity, and parallel play.

- Action not directed toward each other; no interaction between participants is required or necessary; may respond to leader

- Typical of large group leisure activities including spectator sports, aerobics classes, pedagogical learning activities, and performance activities

Examples: Bingo, roulette, watching a movie, watching a play, crafts, mind-assisted therapy, gardening, walking, watching a baseball game, many classroom situations, and step-aerobics.

Problematic Behavior: Characterized by an individual who, for the most part, ignores other participants and only pays attention to the leader to the detriment of other participants. May be seen with some sensory input disorders including hearing impairment and some types of attention deficit disorders. May also be seen in individuals who feel acutely uncomfortable in social situations.

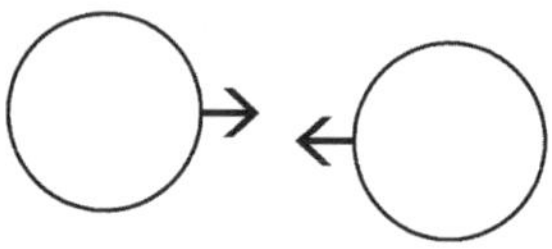

Inter-Individual

Action directed by one person toward another. It may or may not be competitive. The first dyadic relationship. Ability to interact continuously with another; may be cooperative. If the focus is competition, may simulate interpersonal encounters in which individuals need to stand up for themselves against others.

- When the pattern is competitive, has the quality of assisting people to deal with stress, pressure, and concepts of winning and losing. Therapist must focus on this part and plan accordingly.
- Continuous losing is not beneficial.
- Characteristic of these activities is playing by the rules and regulating one's behavior according to the rules. To participate successfully, players agree to behave in certain ways.

Examples: Chess, checkers, tennis, ping-pong, wrestling, mirroring, cooperative drawing, leader/follower, and one-to-one conversations.

Problematic Behavior: At times there is a fine line between individuals who are pathologically inadequate in this skill and individuals who are making normal errors in interaction. While inter-individual interactions occur for most of us daily, this is an extremely complex process of sending messages and receiving feedback both verbally and with body language. An individual's expectations as s/he enters an interaction, his/her level of commitment to pay attention to what is said, and his/her ability and desire to adhere to social norms all play a part. If the expectations do not match between participants, the sender of the message may have his/her train of thought momentarily interrupted by a response. The sender can tell that the receiver is on about the same page but can't figure out how the receiver came up with the response. More extreme mismatches happen with individuals who have thought process disorders such as aphasia or hallucinations, or who have vocal tics.

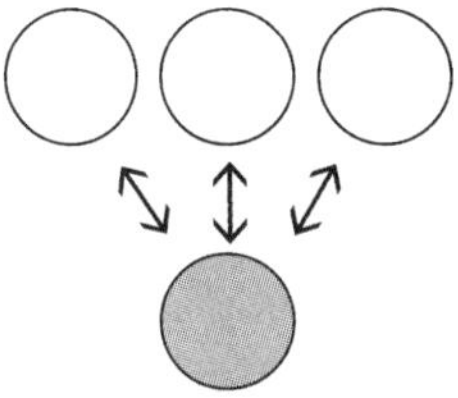

Unilateral

Action among three or more persons, one of whom is the center of attention. Beginning of role differentiation.

- Simultaneous dyadic relationships vying for the attention of the person who is the focus of the interaction

Examples: Tag, dodge ball, blackjack, Simon says, red light/green light, group mirroring with a leader, psychodrama, appreciation line-up, and children vying for a parent's attention.

Problematic Behavior: Characterized by exceptional attempts to obtain the attention of the person who is the focus of the activity — frequently seen in sociopathic disorders; potentially in individuals with head injury or perseveration disorders.

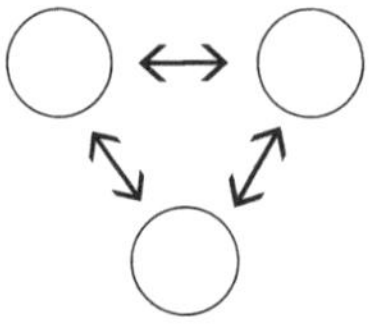

Multi-Lateral

Action among three or more persons, with no one person as the center of attention. Give and take from a lot of people at the same time. Having to react and/or initiate. Requires each person to initiate with the others.

- Activities of this kind allow for a diffusion of effort.
- Must deal with interaction from several people simultaneously as in life situations.
- Responsibility for control is on each individual: decision making, strategy, action not shared by team members. Requires a feeling of self-sufficiency.

Examples: Scrabble, Monopoly, poker game, encounter groups, theater games, and casual socializing (e.g., going out for coffee).

Problematic Behavior: Characterized by the individual who cannot tolerate sustained competitive or cooperative action with just one person.

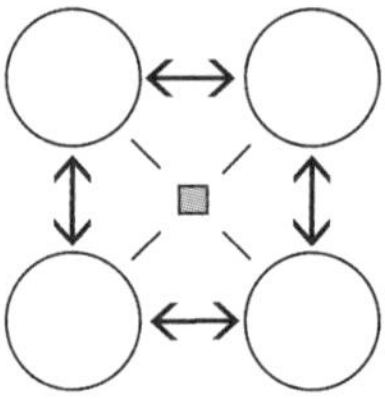

Intra-Group

Action of a cooperative nature by two or more persons intent upon reaching a mutual goal.

- Action requires positive verbal and/or non-verbal interaction.
- Helps to build social skills; may require compromise and cooperation.

Examples: Choir singing, playing music in a band, group dancing (e.g., the Hora), service projects, building a human pyramid, group puzzle, and mural creation.

Problematic Behavior: Characterized by individuals who *must* have group cooperation or input when individualized responses are more appropriate or by individuals who have difficulty interacting with more than one person at a time. Individuals with sociopathic personalities have a hard time working in an intra-group setting.

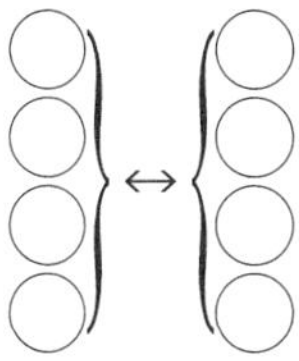

Inter-Group

Actions of a competitive or noncompetitive nature between two or more intra-groups.

- Most difficult to perform since participants must cooperate with other team members and may compete with other team(s).
- Action requires cooperation with some — competition with others.
- Most complicated, many not ready for this level of interaction.
- May produce peer pressure which can be beneficial.

Examples: Scrounge, "laugh it up," basketball, football, other team sports, charades, and many vocational settings.

Problematic Behavior: As with the inter-individual level, there is a fine line between individuals who are making normal errors in the cooperation and competition required at this level. Group norms or expectations, rather than exact universal measurements, determine acceptable levels of performance at this level. Problematic behaviors include significant undesired actions that impede the performance of the others.

Group Structure

Groups provide a space for all the interpersonal interaction patterns described above. Therapists need to recognize that each group has its own dynamic where any and all types of interactions may occur. One of the tasks of the therapist is to shape the group dynamic so that it fosters the types of interactions each client needs to reach the his/her next therapy goal. If it is done well, the group becomes a powerful agent of support for individual change.

For the most part, human beings choose to work with one another, and have always bonded together for safety, security, and empowerment.

Andrew Weil summarized it as follows, "Human beings are social animals and have evolved to thrive in bonded social groups" (Weil, 2011, p. 5).

Groups and Circles

In a therapy context, therapists often need to formalize the interactions of the group. This is important, on one hand, to control the processes of therapy. On the other hand, appropriate formalization will help clients learn more about interpersonal connections that they may not fully understand. One structure that works well for creative arts groups is the circle.

A circle is symbolic of the human need to connect with other people. Gathering in circles of trust, safety, sharing, adventure, learning, dancing, and fun has been important for people throughout time. Therapists can use this human tendency to enhance their practice.

The circle has many modalities including talking stick, drum, sharing, healing, and dance. The circling process can include conflict resolution; improved interpersonal understanding and tolerance; personal, social, and spiritual growth; and appreciation of a shared experience or skill. At its best it can empower individuals and communities to create more healthy connections in the world.

As the group develops, participants begin to relax. As participants become comfortable, they can play and laugh together. "Laughter is more than a pleasurable activity. When people laugh together, they tend to talk and touch more, and to make eye contact more frequently" (Rubin, 2001, p. 6). These are markers of improved social interactions.

The small group circle can provide the opportunity to experience self. Personal growth and personal values can be explored. Through discussions and experiences participants also have an opportunity to change focus from being me to being we. Participants can learn how to cooperate, empathize, and safely depend on others.

Circle groups provide the possibility for participants to experience community. "When a number of individuals form a harmonious group, and thus become psychologically close to one another, there is much energy to be released, which can then be turned outward to useful and creative purposes" (Vargu, 1978, p. 7).

Raccoon Circles

In the early 1990s the psychologist Tom Smith started to facilitate small groups through a sequence of activities with a tubular nylon web loop. The activities involved trust, cooperation, problem solving, risk taking, and fun. Because Tom had studied with Native American elders and had been given the name Raccoon, a friend suggested the web loops could be named Raccoon Circles.

Smith's exploration of Raccoon Circles found that connecting to the web circle was an effective method for small group debriefing and processing. A professional friend of Native American heritage told Tom that he used the knot of the web circle as a talking knot after the tradition of the talking stick.

Although the traditions of the talking stick vary from tribe to tribe, all the rules are basically the same. When one holds the sacred talking object (stick, feather, or knot) that person is allowed to speak and everyone else is to listen in a unilateral relationship.

"[In the traditions] there were three guidelines: a) speak from the heart, meaning speak honestly and sincerely, b) listen with your heart, meaning to listen intently and with interest, c) be lean of expression, meaning to say what you want to say simply and briefly" (Cain & Smith 2006, p. 7). These guidelines are appropriate for most small group processing sessions.

When a group is in a circle sitting or standing and everyone is connected to the web circle, the knot can be passed. If someone has a comment, the person grasps the knot and has the right to speak. If someone has no comment, the person passes the knot to the next person. Using the talking knot format and following the three guidelines brings symbol and ritual into the task of processing.

"Every time we encourage people to 'circle up' and move through a series of activities and then gather in debriefing to share thoughts and feelings, we are giving them an opportunity to know the need, the value, and the joy of being fully human in connection with other people" (Cain & Smith, 2006, p. 8).

Whatever the name or intentions of a small group, gathering in a circle offers wisdom and healing power for the people involved. "The challenge before us is to find our own circles. Each of us has to find our own life companions, right here, right now. All of us need friends with whom we can build community" (Cahill & Halpern, 1998, p. 9).

Cahill and Halpern (1998) go on to say, "People need the ballast of the earth, and this is provided by the circular form. To survive the coming changes to which our earth is heir we have to join together. We may, if we keep to the circling process, be able to provide the living fuel for what will be known as one of the most profound revolutions of all time… to build a renewable, sustainable, culture" (p. 9).

The therapist may not have changing culture as a primary goal. However, improving the abilities of clients to work and play together with others, which often is a therapy goal, will have that effect anyway. In addition to the therapy provided by a specific intervention, doing the intervention as part of a group adds to the benefits for the client.

Therapy Group Phases

In addition to group structure, there are predictable phases for working with individuals or families in groups. Each group will have an initial, middle, and ending phase. It is important to understand the sequence groups normally go through to make sure all phases are covered appropriately.

As the length of time allowed for treatment shortens due to managed care, it is harder for the therapist to move clients successfully through each phase. For this reason, it is vital for the therapist to understand this sequence and know how to facilitate smooth, continuous progress for each client. There is no longer enough time in treatment for the therapist to work without purpose. Several of the issues that are listed here are dealt with in more depth in the next section, The Helping Relationship.

Initial Phase: Development of Trust in the Structure and the Therapist

- Establishment of a therapeutic alliance
- Clarification of roles
- Clarification of the nature of work to be done together
- Conditions and structure for the group to work together

- Group agreements: agreements made by the group and/or requests made by the group and/or by the therapist
- Setting firm, clear, consistent behavioral limits
- Therapist's increased understanding of client(s)
- Enhanced comfort level: the supportive phase
- What to call the group (optional)

Middle Phase: Evoking Expression and "Working Through"

- Development of trust in other group members. The progression of trust may be rapid for some, slow for others — respect each person's pace.
- Periods of resistance. An inability or unwillingness to reflect or to engage, limited self-disclosure, superficial disclosure, and/or regression. Resistance may be seen as a natural defense mechanism, a way to protect the self.
- Transference/counter-transference issues.
- Process of risking, exploring, and confronting ideas and affects (attitudes). Looking many times at the same issues. This is the period of facing, understanding, and, perhaps, accepting a problem.
- Cyclic patterns. An "open" session will often be followed by a "closed" session. The therapist should provide a sustained, empathic reminder that people experience a great amount of anxiety regarding change. It is as if the psyche needs to balance disclosure with privacy. The therapist wants to help sustain the tension of this working-through phase.
- Change takes time. It is best if the therapeutic contact can continue long enough for genuine working through to occur. Defenses may reemerge. Clients may experience inertia.

Ending Phase: Termination Process

There is a consolidation phase followed by a termination phase.

- Consolidation

- Development and integration of a new image or definition of the self. Practicing new ways of behaving, mourning of the old ways and old fantasies.
- A separation of therapist and group is in process. It may be emotionally charged. There may be re-experiencing of past separations.

- Termination
  - Why is it happening — is this a natural process or does it have other causes (insurance cuts, a discontinued program, parents withdrawing a child)?
  - The therapist may review or summarize the therapy process and/or make referrals for continuation with another group or therapist.
  - Recognizing completion of the process or that this is as far as the client(s) can go, or may choose to go, for now.
  - Client re-defining his/her role separate from support offered by the therapist.

The Helping Relationship

A professional helping relationship is a unique association of two people, with its own set of rules and expectations. Unlike a friendship, it concentrates on meeting the needs of only one person — the client. The therapist is expected to have the knowledge and skills to assist the client in meeting a problem or a need so the client can accomplish what s/he could not do alone. The focus is on assisting. The therapist doesn't problem solve for the client but rather helps the client to grow psychologically and cognitively and become more self-sufficient.

How does a helping relationship develop and how is it maintained? Both the therapist and the client need to be willing to engage in certain behaviors that will make a helping relationship productive.

There are three basic phases to the helping relationship: The first phase is building of relationship. The second is facilitating a positive change in the client. The third phase is the ending of the relationship. Each phase progresses through different stages. The eight stages of a helping relationship are described below. Though much of the advice in this section is addressed to the therapist, there are areas (particularly the termination phase) that address concerns of the client as well. These might be shared with the client(s), if appropriate, at the start of the group.

Initial Phase: Building Relationships

Stages one through four involve the therapist's growing understanding of how the clients see the world, through listening, clarifying, and structuring information coming from the clients.

1. Entry: Opening the Relationship (Cornerstones of the Therapeutic Alliance)

- Open the meeting.
- Help to create an environment where individuals may, as clearly as they are able, feel free to state needs, requests for help, and invitations to work together.
- Assess: How do the individuals regard being helped? Is asking for help seen as a weakness?
- Remember that people have a natural reluctance to confront their feelings.
- Note the distance between chairs.
- Remember that psychological discomfort must be great for some before they seek assistance.
- Make use of open-ended questions and statements:
    - "Please tell me what is on your mind."
    - "What do you wish to discuss with me?"
    - "I'm interested in knowing how you are, please fill me in."
- Remember, some situations seem too overwhelming or too unbelievable for clients to share easily.
- Be aware of cultural implications regarding sharing of vulnerabilities.
- Some clients will be better able to disclose information if there is some object (e.g., a Nerf ball or Rubik's cube) nearby which is acceptable for them to pick up and play with. This seems to help release some nervous energy. A knot or talking stick, as described earlier, can also serve this purpose in a way that makes holding the object less socially awkward.

2. Clarification: Reasons for Seeking Help (Statement of Problem or Concern)

- Be mindful of all questions; the individual may feel interrogated. Asking for elaboration on a situation and "how" questions may be helpful.
- Evaluate the degree of desire and motivation for change in each client.
- Is there an awareness of the potentials and limitations of a helping relationship?
- Many clients will not reveal the true problem or need until they present some superficial problems to see how the therapist reacts. Trust is established through this process before the client is willing to reveal his/her primary concern.

3. Structure: Formulating the Contract and the Structure

- What are the conditions under which we will work?
- The goal for this (initial) stage is to decide whether to proceed.
- The following questions need to be answered by both parties:

  Therapist Questions:
  - Do I want to work with this person/group (comfort, compatibility)?
  - Can I meet the expectations (given my skills, knowledge)?
  - What am I expecting (time, place, effort, commitment, responsibility)?
  - What kind of structure do we need (informal understanding, counseling contract, or leave the issue open)?
  - Am I able to work with this person/group (skills, knowledge, experience)? Do my mind, heart, and gut feelings agree?

  Client Questions:
  - Am I willing to commit myself to a relationship agreement, and if so, will we work it out together?
  - Will this relationship get me more involved than I want to be?
  - Will this person be helpful on my terms?
  - What are his/her terms?

- o Is this person able to understand who I am, my culture, and my closely held beliefs? Will we be able to work on my agenda — not the therapist's agenda?
- o If I agree to a contract to do specific things, can I get out of it if I want to?
- o Is this a person I can trust?

4. Relationship: Building the Helping Relationship

- A gradual but steady increase in the depth of the relationship.
- A commitment has been made by the client and the therapist to work for change together. A level of trust has been reached.

Middle Phase: Facilitating Positive Action

Stages five through seven bring about desired changes in the client(s).

5. Exploration: Exploring Problems, Formulating Goals, Planning Strategies, Gathering Facts, Expressing Deeper Feelings, Learning New Skills

- Therapist may become more active and assertive.
- There is a strong tendency on the part of the client to turn inward when describing feeling and delineating problems.
- Sometimes clients feel so good that they experience a flight into health.
- Issues of transference (attitudes towards the therapist that have been transferred from earlier attitudes towards important figures in the client's life) and countertransference (therapist towards client) emerge. Freud said that transference can be a therapist's most effective tool. It can help the client recapture the past by re-experiencing and enacting feelings.
- The specific process goals for the therapist at this stage are as follows:
    - o Maintain and enhance the relationship (trust, ease, safety).
    - o Deal with feelings that interfere with progress towards goals.
    - o Encourage exploration of feelings to expand the client's self-awareness.

- o Gather necessary facts that will contribute to the solution of the problem.
- o Decide to continue or terminate the relationship.
- o Teach skills required to reach goals (demonstrating, modeling, coaching).
- o Initiate homework activities that move towards goals.

6. Consolidation: Exploring Alternatives, Working through Feelings, Practicing New Skills, Breaking Old Patterns

- The client broadens his/her perspective and worldview.
- The client realizes that past ways of thinking and acting did not work. Some trepidation mixed with excitement about trying new things causes the client to struggle anew.
- This is the point at which the client must decide to act or not, to operationalize the insights gained into his/her behavior.
- This can be a Catch 22: if clients change, they won't need the therapist. They may feel that the therapist will reject them because they don't need him/her anymore.

7. Planning for the Future: Planning Strategies to Resolve Conflicts, Reducing Painful Feelings, Generalizing New Skills or Behaviors to Continue Self-Directed Activities

- Plans are formulated for termination/discharge and continuing alone.
- Goals for this stage are to crystallize discussions of earlier stages into a plan of action and to decide that growth has proceeded to the point where termination of the relationship is indicated.
- Best results and decreased readmission or relapse tend to occur if the client has practiced the alternative modes of thought or behavior at least once in the community with the therapist's support (in cases where the helping relationship was established when the client was an inpatient).
- Bringing up new topics is discouraged.

Ending Phase: Termination Process

8. Termination

- Summarizing the process.
- Evaluating the outcomes.
- There are many methods of termination. The therapist:
    - may decrease the frequency of sessions to de-escalate the involvement.
    - may want to leave the door open for follow-up.
    - may refer the client(s) to another therapist, agency, and/or networking situation.

Separation Activities and Rituals

A variety of activities can be used to mark the ending of the therapy group. In addition to the following, many of the closure activities in other sections of the book (*Drama* or *Poetry and Writing*) would also be appropriate to use at this point in the group.

Gift

Each participant receives gifts from the group. Participants are sitting in circle. The one who speaks uses the format "I give you the gift of ________." The gift may be a wish for something material or something abstract, a fantasy, a quality, or an experience.

Collage Messages

Each participant puts his/her name on an approximately 11" x 14" or larger piece of paper. On separate small pieces of paper, members write messages to one another. The messages are then glued to the appropriate person's paper.

Secret Friend

As in the traditional game, each participant chooses a name anonymously and leaves surprises for his/her secret friend.

Group Appreciation

The group forms a circle with the person in the center receiving appreciation.

Sufi Heart Dance

Participants form a circle. The Sufi Heart Dance done with soft music (such as Pachelbel's Canon) is a ritual movement to be done over and over. First, right arm down as an offering; then left arm down as an offering, lastly, lift your two hands together as receiving and place over your heart.

Pennies Activity

Each participant receives two pennies for making wishes. The group forms a circle with a penny pot in the center. Each participant makes one wish for him/herself, one wish for the group.

One Word Sharing Cards

Each participant is given index cards equal to the number of other participants in the group. On each card, one for every other participant, the person writes a word which s/he feels best describes that person. If there are twelve participants, each person will write eleven cards. Once this is completed, the participants exchange with each other the word that they have chosen for one another and a brief explanation of why they chose that word.

Circle Form

X

X X

X O X

X X

X

Person in the center receives appreciation from others and then without responding verbally, moves to the outer circle for the next person's turn.

Line Form

O X X X X X

Each **X** gives feedback to **O**. Then **O** goes to the end of the line and becomes an **X.**

Medal of Honor

Names will be drawn, and no one will know who has what name (until the end, if they choose). Each person will design a medal of honor for the person whose name s/he drew, making it as flashy as possible. The medal will have the person's name and a brief description of the quality of the person that it is honoring (e.g., "always considers the feelings of others," "makes people feel welcome in any group"). The medals will then be given out in a ceremony, presenting each person and his/her honor with great importance and putting the medal on him/her (pinning it or hanging it on a string around the neck), followed by applause from the group. Afterwards, solicit comments regarding how it felt to be honored or to have the spotlight on you.

Appreciation Gift

Put all participants' names in a hat. Each participant picks a name other than his/her own, and then creates an ornament or card for the person s/he picked. Have participants, as they give their gifts, share what they made for their chosen person, why, and perhaps what they wish for that person, or what they see as a positive quality — something that stands out about the person.

Wish

Divide the group in two and pick a volunteer facilitator for each group. The group facilitator writes down names of people in each group on pieces of paper then puts them in a container. Each person picks a name (not his/her own) and doesn't reveal the name that was picked. Each person draws a picture of what s/he wants the other person to have as a farewell present (about 5-10 minutes). Give the picture to the person.

Ceremonies for Change

All cultures have special ceremonies or rituals that celebrate changes in seasons, in government, or in individual status such as marriage or coming of age. Don't wait for a major event. Make a large or small change a reason to celebrate!

Change Celebration

Here are some questions you can ask to plan your change celebration:

- How do you want to celebrate?
- Will you celebrate privately — or do you want to involve others? A small or large group?
- Where and when will your celebration take place?
- How will you name or express the change? What personal symbols and symbolic actions will you use or create to illustrate the change and its positive effect on your life and therefore the lives of people you know?
- How will you begin your celebration? How will this set the tone for what will follow?
- Who do you want to be there? Will they take an active part in your celebration or be observers? Will you surprise them, or will they help you plan the event?
- Will you speak spontaneously about your change or prepare remarks?
- Will you include any of the following? Songs, dance, music, poetry, stories, anecdotes, quotes, prayers, gifts, food, decorations, souvenirs, or tributes.

- How will you connect your change to the power and love that exists in the world? How will you inspire your guests to make progress in their own lives?
- How will your ceremony end?
- Who's on the clean-up committee?

References

Cahill, S. & Halpern, J. (1998). *The ceremonial circle*. New York: Harper.

Cain, J. & Smith, T. (2006). *The revised & expanded book of raccoon circles*. Dubuque, IA: Kendall/Hunt Publishing.

Rubin, K. H. (2001). *The play observation scale (POS)*. University of Waterloo.

Vargu, (1978). in Smith, T. (2017). Power of the circle. Presentation for Midwest Therapeutic Recreation Symposium, St. Louis, MO.

Weil, A. (2011). *Spontaneous happiness*. New York: Little, Brown, and Company.

6

Planning a Creative Arts Group

For a program or group to be successful it is important to invest time in planning. Time spent posing thoughtful questions and working out glitches in advance frees time and energy later that can be used for running the program rather than dealing with crises. Additionally, funding for programs is competitive and resources are limited. Administrators are continually faced with demands for funds and support for a myriad of basic services, personnel, and facilities. In order to give supervisors confidence that resources for a creative arts group will be used wisely and successfully, it is important to propose a well-developed plan based on the anticipated or assessed needs of the clients.

Justifying a Creative Arts Program

Why should a facility support a creative arts program? What needs are not currently being met by the facility? What benefits will a creative arts group offer clients over another kind of group? These are questions that the therapist should be able to answer, formally on paper or in his/her own mind, if s/he wants to start a creative arts program in his/her setting. Being clear about why a proposed creative arts program benefits and enhances therapy services helps communicate the program's value to supervisors, staff, clients, and the public.

Benefits are the basis for explaining why a creative arts program is valuable to clients and the foundation for developing its goals. It may be helpful to gather information from journal articles and from books such as *Recreational Therapy Basics, Techniques, and Interventions* (Porter, 2016). These provide information that can be given to supervisors about outcomes of creative arts programs. Benefits which may be mentioned include:

- Creativity is important to the developmental aspects of life. Creative arts improve the development of physical, cognitive, emotional, social, and vocational abilities.
- Creative arts encourage expressions of thoughts and feelings in a tangible form that can be viewed by self and others. The creation of a product that is an extension of self can bring about insight, joy, and feelings of self-esteem.
- Creative arts foster self-awareness and personal growth. Individuals experience a deepening understanding of themselves and their environment.
- By engaging the emotions, individuals are aided in moving to new levels of experience.
- Creative arts provide an opportunity to communicate both verbally and non-verbally, involving different thinking processes and abilities.

Role of Formal Assessment

The most important justification for a program is that it provides measurable improvement in the level of functioning for members of the group. The best way to demonstrate the improvement is through formal assessment tools to measure the change in abilities.

It is important to choose assessment tools that are appropriate for the members of the group and the goals you expect them to achieve. You need to assess clients before the group starts and at the end of the group to demonstrate the efficacy of the group. You can use assessment tools that are based on your observations — such as the Comprehensive Evaluation in Recreational Therapy — Psych/Behavioral (CERT-Psych) or the International Classification of Functioning, Disability, and Health — during group sessions to monitor client changes. Other tools that require client input should be used less frequently because they use time that would be better spent in group activities.

There are many kinds of assessment tools that measure many different aspects of client abilities. For more information about available assessments and choosing the best tool for your group you can look in *Assessment Tools for Recreational Therapy and Related Fields* and journal articles related to specific kinds of functional skills.

Writing Goals and Objectives

When interacting with clients, it is important to keep in mind the purpose of the group and what you intend to accomplish. Putting goals and objectives on paper helps clarify intentions before beginning to work with clients.

Goals are global statements of intent and lend direction to the program. The therapist should make sure that the goals for the program reflect the goals of his/her employer and the facility. Some sample goals that might be legitimately used in a creative arts program are

- To provide opportunities for wellness through creative self-expression
- To enable clients to explore either individual problem areas and/or problems common to the group

The list of goals should consider physical, mental, social, and emotional domains.

Objectives, particularly behavioral objectives, are specific statements which define the outcome or behavioral changes the therapist and client expect as a result of the program. These objectives must be measurable, realistic, and represent small, meaningful chunks of learning or change that the group can comfortably manage. An objective contains the conditions under which the behavior will take place, the criteria for knowing the client has achieved the desired behavior, and the timeline for achievement. The following are sample behavioral objectives for a creative arts program:

- Client will attend to activity 5 (10, 20) minutes for 1 (2, 3) times per day.
- Client will maintain control and wait until staff is able to assist him/her in 50% (75%, 100%) of episodes.
- Client will tolerate activity 5 (10, 15) minutes without demonstrating anxious behavior 50% (75%, 100%) of the time.

Objectives will often be connected to the formal assessments that you are using to measure the efficacy of the group. For example, you may have an objective for a client to have no scores greater than one in the Group Performance section of the CERT-Psych during a 30-minute activity.

Here are some questions you can ask yourself as you plan the goals and objectives for the program:

- What are the expected effects or outcomes of the program?
- What activities will be used to achieve each goal and objective? The activities should be arranged in a sequence that allows for the development of the most basic skills first and progresses to the development of higher-level skills that require the use of previously learned skills.
- What are the major components of the program to be evaluated?
- How will the program be evaluated? There may be several instruments and/or techniques for the ongoing evaluation.
- When or how often will the program be evaluated? There may be different schedules for each goal or objective.
- Who will evaluate the program?
- How will the data be analyzed?
- What is the acceptable evidence of having achieved goals?

Here are some questions you can ask yourself as you plan the goals and objectives for each client:

- What instruments and techniques will be used for the evaluation? Possibilities include formal assessment, leader's or other professional's observations, client self-reporting, reports from family or other group outside of the facility, and monitoring.
- When or how often will evaluations be done?
- Which goals and objectives will be measured?
- What else needs to be measured and evaluated?

- Who will evaluate the program?
- How will the data be analyzed?
- What is acceptable evidence of having achieved goals?

Planning the Logistics

Logistics are the practical aspects of the program that allow it to operate smoothly. Not considering logistics before the program starts may mean that valuable time must be spent fixing a problem that could have been avoided. Some logistical questions important to planning include:

- Where and when will the group meet?
- What is the starting date?
- What is the length of the program?
- What is the most desirable size for the group? What are the minimum and maximum numbers of members?
- How will clients learn about the group? Is there a facility newsletter, bulletin board, monthly calendar, or community meeting to get the word out?
- How will clients get to the group? Is this well coordinated? If clients depend on staff to get them to this program, it is necessary to work with the staff to make sure this happens smoothly.
- What will be required for appropriate infection control for the members of this group?
- How might the need for infection control change during the time span the group meets (contacts outside the group or outside the facility, other risks of change in disease status)?
- What requirements are there for the area the group will use (appropriate social distancing, accessible to wheelchair users, accessible to restrooms and drinking water)?
- What items are available at the facility (e.g., running water, CD player, chairs, pillows, tables)?
- What additional supplies are needed for each meeting and throughout the program?
- Where can additional supplies be gotten and what are the costs (e.g., art materials, props such as hats, journals for writing)?

- How will supplies be used to avoid spread of infection?
- How will objects that need to be reused, such as musical instruments, be cleaned between sessions to prevent spread of disease? Can participants safely keep their own tools, such as paint brushes, and bring them to each session?
- Are adaptive devices needed (e.g., mouth apparatus for painting)?
- What are the emergency and fire safety plans? Are there first aid supplies? Who should be contacted in case of illness or injury?
- Will volunteers or assistants be present? What training needs to be done? Will the leaders, volunteers, and assistants need to meet before or after sessions?

Creative Arts Group Considerations

The following list consists of questions and considerations which can help in planning a creative arts group. Use it as a guideline, adding questions and categories as needed. The therapist should ask him/herself:

Leader Responsibilities and Considerations

- What role will I have in this group? A therapist? A play leader? A therapist specialist in drama, art, music, movement, or dance?
- Have I had the training required to run this group? (Be careful not to take on more responsibility than you are trained to handle.)
- What are my supervisor's expectations? Are they realistic or do they need to be modified before the group begins?

Standards

- What (if any) city, county, state, and/or federal treatment regulations will I need to comply with?
- What (if any) voluntary standards (e.g., Joint Commission, CARF, American Camping Association) will I need to comply with?
- What facility or agency policies and procedures will I need to comply with?
- What kind of documentation will I need to complete before the group starts? Before and after each session? At the end of the group?

- What professional standards will I need to comply with?
- What infection control standards that apply to this group?

Before the group meets…

- What are the likely needs of this group?
- Written plan with goals for the group: For a new program or new facilitator of an existing group, it helps to write out your plan. Some settings have a planning form but, if none exists, the proposal should include the name of the group, what is to be accomplished (the goals), how logistics will be dealt with, and information on how the program will be evaluated.
- What are the strengths and limitations of the place where we will be meeting and of the resources available?
- Do I have good resources for activities or know where to find them or someone who might help brainstorm ideas?

Who is in the group?

- Do I have all the information I need about group members? Do I have some sense of who each person is as well as the composition of the entire group?
- Have I obtained the best information possible from observation, other staff, family, participant, through interviews, questionnaires, and formal assessments?
- Do I know the diagnoses listed for group members — including the definition, impact on functional ability, and precautions to take?
- Do I understand the possibilities for changes in diagnosis from contacts that occur between group sessions?
- Is this a voluntary or mandatory group?
- Is membership in the group fluid? Can members drop in?
- Is this a newly formed group? If not, how can I find out its history?
- Do group members know one another from another setting?
- What might be the cohesive factor in the group? Is it a group for women, teens, veterans?
- Make sure to identify the characteristics of the population to be served. This will assist others in making appropriate recommendations for

clients who might benefit from the group. Consider age, sex, functional level, and skills required.

Planning the Sessions

- What are the objectives for sessions?
- What kind of behavior is anticipated for each session?
- What kind of behavior is desired for each session?
- Groups need a different kind of structure based on the members of the group. How much structure does this group need? Does the group need a more directive style of leadership (leader more authoritative in giving specific directions) or a more facilitative leadership approach (leader trying to include more client ideas to set direction)?
- What activities are most appropriate to the needs and potential of the group? It may be helpful to use some aspect of the activity analysis process to be sure an activity will have the desired outcome. Activity analysis is the systematic application of a set of variables used to break down and examine a given activity to understand its inherent qualities, participation factors, or outcome possibilities.
- How do sessions change as members of the group meet their objectives? If the activities are not challenging enough, members will start to lose interest and not be invested in meeting new objectives.
- How do sessions change if members of the group are unable to meet their objectives? Groups that are too difficult will reduce engagement and will not help your clients meet their therapeutic objectives.
- Can the activities that have been planned be modified to meet individual situations which may arise during the group?
- What will I be looking for as I lead and observe the group?
- Do I have a budget and a detailed list of materials and supplies which need to be purchased?
- For new groups, how will I: Handle introductions of members and the leader? Discuss what the group will be doing? Discuss rules, agreements, and mandatory behavior? Encourage group suggestions and reactions?
- What warmup activity/activities will be used?

- What criteria will I use to assess the group at the start of each session? (e.g., Will I ask a question at the beginning of each group or do the same song or activity each time and observe the group's energy and response?)

Space Considerations for a Creative Arts Program

Ideally, a therapist should be able to walk into a facility and have the perfect setup for doing creative arts, but that is not usually the case. Most therapists must adapt their surroundings to make the available space work for them. The following are two suggestions for setting up a space that supports creative arts:

Size of Room(s)

If the facility has only one room for all creative arts (art, drama, movement, etc.), it should be a multipurpose or flexible space. It should be spacious enough for freedom of movement or relaxation but adaptable to more intimate work, such as writing or art. Some facilities have both an art room and a general-purpose room that can be used for exercise or more active movement. Some have a room with dividing walls that give the therapist the flexibility to change the space to suit his/her needs. Consider if social distancing will be required. Look at the room(s) available and determine what program(s) can be feasibly offered in that space.

Privacy

No matter what kind of space is available at a facility, it needs to be private while the creative arts group meets. Freedom in creative expression comes from continuity of activity without distractions or interruptions.

Planning Summary

The following checklist summarizes the steps described in this chapter for planning a creative arts group (Stuart, 2018).

1. Justify the need for a program with a statement of purpose based on an assessment of the participants' needs.

2. Write specific goals and objectives for the program and each session in the program.
    - o Needs of the facility
    - o Required resources and program costs
3. Document the overall program.
    - o Program name
    - o Target population
    - o Departments involved
    - o Purpose of group (a concise statement of the general purpose)
    - o Formal assessments to demonstrate efficacy
    - o Program description
    - o Specific goals and objectives for the program
    - o Length of group and meeting times
    - o Staff and resources required
4. Document each session. The activities to be used should be arranged in a sequence that allows for the development of the most basic skills first and progresses to develop higher-level skills that require the use of previously learned skills.
    - o Description of session — activities, equipment, grouping, method, etc.
    - o Goals addressed in the session
    - o Value of goals for each participant
    - o Processing — relating session to daily life and clients' behaviors, problems, assets, etc.
5. Describe program evaluation procedures.
    - o Data collection system
    - o Feedback from clients and other staff
6. Obtain approval for the program.
7. Write specific goals and objectives for each participant based on abilities and needs.
    - o Determine which clients will be in the program
    - o Program goals and participant goals must match

8. Create a detailed set of logistics for each implementation.
    - Time, place, and length of the program
    - Facility area to be used
    - Resources for staff and funding
    - Coordination with other staff

Multicultural and Lifestyle Choice Considerations

We live in a social environment that is increasingly complex and culturally diverse. As a therapist you will probably be working with people whose first language is not English and/or whose life experiences, values, norms, and family support systems may be different from your own. What it requires from you is a more honest and astute level of consciousness. Just as people make suppositions about individuals with disabilities, they also make subconscious judgments about people whose lives and histories are different from their own. The following are suggestions to help you be not just politically correct but, more importantly, humanely conscious in your attitudes and interactions:

- Remember that all of us are products of culture. We have values, attitudes, and ways of dealing with situations that we learned through our families and support systems. Respect the differences between people while also looking for commonalties.
- Become aware of unrecognized assumptions that you and others have. Treat everyone as an individual, not as a member of a sub-group. Get to know how each individual thinks, feels, and lives.
- Creative arts have the capacity to overcome differences in language, background, abilities, and experiences. Music, dance, and art speak to all of us without the need for one language. Celebrate multicultural richness by choosing activities from different cultures.

People Resources and Supportive Funding

These days, many facilities have just enough staff to get by. In many situations it is appropriate to have volunteers that can help clients get set up and can assist clients as needed. A successful volunteer program takes organization, thought, time, and good public relations. Do not initiate a volunteer program if staff are too busy to listen to volunteers' concerns or provide needed training. A good volunteer program, once created, can enhance the quality of a therapist's individual contact with clients. Some reminders about successful supervision:

- Think about what kind of help will be needed. Make sure that you are clear about the tasks you want each volunteer to complete. Take the time to write a job description for each volunteer position.
- Create a scrapbook of photos, artwork, and background information about the program or develop a volunteer handbook. Take these recruitment materials to college classes or community organizations so that interested people can get a better feel about the nature of the program.
- Structure a training process for volunteers to introduce them to the agency, clients, and their duties. Make sure you have the right person doing the right kind of job.
- For volunteers completing college fieldwork, be clear about the requirements (e.g., number of hours, nature of client contact) and make sure that the contract is being upheld.
- Listen to and observe volunteers in order to assess how their experiences are proceeding and make adjustments before problems arise.
- Don't think of volunteers as "fill-in help." Treat them with respect, reward them with praise or other benefits, and write thoughtful letters of recommendation if asked.

Whenever volunteer or financial support is needed, it is important to know where to find the appropriate resources. The following are ideas to help start the search:

Fieldwork and Internships for Colleges and Universities

Many students must complete fieldwork hours to graduate in their major. Check with professional schools such as education, recreational therapy, occupational therapy, social work, psychology, art, or other media to find out if they require fieldwork hours. A responsible student brings fresh energy and ideas to the program. Additionally, if directed properly, a college student who has a fieldwork requirement will be available on a regular basis for at least a semester's time.

Volunteer Bureau

A community volunteer bureau sees many people in the course of a day and might be able to locate a retired artist, music teacher, dance instructor, or even an art lover who might be a valuable volunteer. Make sure the volunteer bureau has a clear job description of the position so they can refer the right person to the program.

Personal Resources

If you are comfortable with these activities, public speaking and/or writing can augment other funding.

Community Organizations

Some organizations will donate time or money to help a program in their community. For example, if the facility is having a special hands-on arts program for children with disabilities, it may be possible to approach local organizations and ask them to sponsor some aspect of the program. This involves some time and energy in making presentations and coordinating funding, but it is the kind of involvement that benefits everyone.

Corporate Funding or Arts Support

Many corporations create philanthropic foundations which often focus on supporting programs in their own communities or counties. Some corporations will exhibit art in their buildings — they get some lovely art for their walls and good public relations and the arts group receives a space to exhibit and public awareness for the program.

Government Funding for the Arts

Arts funding trickles down from the federal level to state, county, and city governments. Each state receives funding for arts programming which is distributed through the arts councils (county and city commissions) in that state. Check for the kinds of programs that are being funded by local arts councils. Some county arts councils, for example, will fund artists to teach their craft to clients in community nonprofit organizations.

VSA

VSA is an international organization on arts and disability. It was founded in 1974 by Ambassador Jean Kennedy Smith to provide arts and education opportunities for people with disabilities and increase access to the arts for all. They are part of the John F. Kennedy Center for the Performing Arts. With 52 international affiliates and a network of nationwide affiliates, VSA provides arts and education programming for youth and adults with disabilities around the world, including festivals, school programs, special projects, performances, and exhibitions. You can learn about them on their website: http://education.kennedy-center.org/education/vsa/.

Planning for the Visual Arts Group

Up to this point the planning ideas for arts groups have been very general and could be applied to any type of group. This last section addresses the concerns of a group that requires specific materials and appropriate space.

A Space for Art

Most facilities do not have perfect art spaces. Most therapists will have to make do with what is available. The following are required for a room that is used for creative arts that require materials:

- adequate lighting — for all individuals but especially for those with visual impairments
- ready access to a sink and water
- an area adequate for the group, with enough table space and chairs to accommodate everyone comfortably. Do your best with this requirement given the limits of your facility.
- storage space (locked) — enough space to enable good organization and easy access of materials
- good ventilation — some people (especially those with respiratory problems) are very sensitive to chemicals in paint. Make sure to keep air circulating through the space.

- capability for privacy — if involved in an art therapy technique or an activity that involves guided imagery, it will be necessary to block out exterior distractions.
- display area — at times it is appropriate to display some of the art created by clients. Make sure there is at least a bulletin board for this purpose.

Materials for Art

Art materials can be expensive. The key is to be smart about how to stretch the budget and resourceful in finding materials that can be gathered cheaply. Many people who lead art groups are pack rats by nature. They see rejected stuff as potential material for art. Students in our classes have brainstormed in groups about household items to save for visual art projects and amazingly the list has grown every year.

Materials to Spend Money On

If the program does have a budget, considering spending some of the money on these items:

- **Paint brushes:** It is a waste of money to buy cheap brushes. After limited use the hairs often come out and the brushes lose their shape. There are great brushes now for smaller children that have flexible but durable brush tips and easy-to-hold handles that will take a lot of beating from small children. If you are working with adolescents or adults, it is important to have a variety of sizes in brushes and tip shapes (e.g., flat or round) for satisfying results. Build up a supply slowly, if necessary, and teach clients how to clean and store brushes properly.
- **Scissors:** Nothing is more frustrating than scissors that don't cut properly. Buy good, sturdy scissors that are appropriate for the age of the clients and, if possible, have some scissors for people who are left-handed — they'll be deeply appreciated.
- **Paper:** There are a wide range of papers and uses to be considered:
    - *butcher paper* — Purchase a large roll of butcher paper for general use and casual scribbling.

- recycled computer paper, old stationery, and leftover posters — for scribbling and idea building.
- *newsprint* — good for pencil and charcoal work, some can take a little wet media.
- *construction paper* — try to get a non-fading variety, if possible. Scraps can be recycled for collage and other uses.
- *drawing paper* — Some varieties can also handle ink, markers, or watercolor. Get the most diversity out of the paper.
- *tracing paper* — you can work out a drawing on tracing paper and transfer it to good paper without damaging the surface of the good paper by erasing and reworking it.
- *fancy paper* — for watercolor or acrylic painting. Use a weight of paper that can handle some working, at least 60 pounds.
- *handmade paper* — beautiful paper can be created using a blender, paper scraps of all sorts, and even leaves. These papers can be used for painting and collage and are all the more special because they are handmade.

- **Paints:** Keep a supply of basic tempera paints in plastic jars. If working with children, use containers with color-coded tops and snappable, non-spill lids to keep paint ready for use. If cake watercolor is used, buy the kind that can give you more variety in value (i.e., lightness or darkness of color). Some only give you pale color. Markers are fun (as long as the tops get put back on!) — children love the scented ones. For older children or adults, add things like chalk or oil pastel. Oil pastels are a great alternative to oil paint — they are less messy and can be blended with turpentine for interesting effects. Acrylics, watercolors, or oil paints in tubes are expensive — look for student grade supplies. They are a bit cheaper and fine for group artwork.

Being Resourceful

Packrats will be in heaven when they read this list of things to save from around the house for art projects. The only limitation is storage area, but this can usually be cleverly organized as well.

Materials to Save

- alphabet soup letters
- baby food jars
- bag twisties
- beads (old necklaces from thrift stores and flea markets)
- beans (dried)
- bottle caps
- boxes (little to as big as you can store)
- broken crayons
- broken toys
- buttons
- calendars (for photos or pictures)
- cardboard scraps (corrugated and other interesting surfaces)
- chop sticks (great for scooping paint or mixing materials)
- coffee cans
- computer paper (quick, casual drawings)
- corks
- cotton balls
- dried flowers
- egg cartons (for paints, sorting beads and sequins)
- fabric scraps (for collage, masks)
- game pieces from old games
- gloves (for puppets)
- ice trays (palette)
- jars (all sizes for storage)
- magazines (for collage, ideas for topics)
- margarine containers (for storage)
- newspaper
- noodles and other pasta (for collage)
- oatmeal boxes
- old jewelry (for masks, collage, puppets)
- old socks (for puppets)
- paper bags (for masks, puppets)
- plastic bubble packing material (for collage)
- polished glass or rock from beach (for masks, sculpture)

- rags (for cleaning)
- rocks and twigs (for masks, sculpture, collage)
- rubber bands
- salt (for use in recipes for sculpture materials)
- shoe boxes
- string
- Styrofoam (for collage)
- tiles (for sculpture)
- tissue paper and wrapping paper scraps
- wallpaper scraps
- wood scraps (for sculpture)
- yarn and ribbon ends (for collage, puppets)

Where to Find Resources

Most communities are goldmines for leftover materials that can be recycled as art. Brainstorm a list of places to check for help in stocking art supplies. Some ideas that have been contributed by our students:

- appliance stores (for very large boxes that can be used for sculpture)
- plastics stores that sell plastic tubing and sheeting may allow rummaging through their remnants for sculpture supplies
- garage sales (for beads and other reusable items)
- lumber yards (for wood scraps)
- fabric stores (for throw-away scraps and remnants)
- cardboard or packing companies (will donate unusable remnants)

The community might even have an art recycling center where manufacturers can donate materials for use by non-profit agencies for a minimal fee. Being creative about collecting resources is both fun and wise. Money saved in one area means being able to obtain a greater quantity or better quality of materials (like brushes) that must be bought.

Reference

burlingame, j. & Blaschko, T. M. (2010). *Assessment tools for recreational therapy and related fields* (4th ed.). Enumclaw, WA: Idyll Arbor.

Porter, H. R. (2016). *Recreational therapy basics, techniques, and interventions.* Enumclaw, WA: Idyll Arbor.

7

Running a Creative Arts Group

Having a well-planned group is the beginning step in the process of running a group. As you run the group, you will need to adapt your plans to meet the needs of the clients who are in this group. Each group has its own dynamics. It is important to analyze and document what happens in each session. We'll look at how to do that in the first part of this chapter.

There are two questions you must ask when you are running any therapeutic group: Is each client making progress toward his/her therapeutic goals? Is there a way to change an individual's experience so objectives can be met more effectively? We'll look at these after the discussion about the overall analysis of each session. The way you answer those questions and the adaptations you make to the group process will determine the success of your group.

Group Process

Planning the First Session

The first session is crucial to the success of the group. Some of this was discussed in more detail in the previous chapter about planning a group, but it is so important that we list the important points again.

- Understand your role in the group and how you will help each client to meet his/her treatment objectives.
- Understand the needs of each person in the group. In a therapy group each client must have clear, agreed-upon objectives.
- Have a clear plan for the first session and understand how the structure you create will continue through later sessions.
- Explain the purpose and structure of the group, its rules, agreements, unacceptable behavior, and mandatory behavior.
- Introduce yourself and explain your role in the group.
- Chose how to introduce members of the group to one another and begin the process of creating appropriate interactions among group members.

Running the Creative Arts Group

While you are running a group, you will need to pay attention to how the session is going. If you stay open to small changes, a session that is not going optimally can be improved. Rigidly following your original plan is usually not the best solution. Here are some questions that may help you make changes while the group is going on.

- What is the general mood of the group?
- What are the group's concerns and goals right now?
- Are there blocks to individual engagement or meaningful group interactions?
- Does the process seem interesting? If the answer is no, probably no one else is challenged either. How can I make this material or activity more motivating?

Post-Session Evaluation

When the session is over and you can reflect on what happened without the pressure of making changes on the fly, analyze what happened. Look for what went well and what you might want to change if you run this session again.

- How did it go? What happened that was unexpected? Positive? Negative?

- Was the program implemented as designed? If not, do the design or implementation need to be changed?
- What was the group response to the therapist, helpers, the material, and to each other?
- Did the goals and objectives of the session seem appropriate and productive? Were they achieved?

Documentation

Required documentation depends on the facility and the state and federal laws it operates under. How and what you document depends on many things including the program, the status of the clients, and the methods you have chosen to measure progress toward goals and objectives. Be sure to meet documentation standards of governments, employer, profession, and accrediting agencies.

You need to write something in every client's chart. If an intervention isn't documented, it didn't happen. Some of the time it will be enough to write only a description of the session. Usually, though, you will need to add something about a client's reaction to the session. Any evaluations regarding progress toward objectives, including discussions with clients about their progress, need to be included, too.

Planning for the Next Session

Analyzing group and individual dynamics will help you make the next session more effective. Small — or even large — changes may be needed in upcoming sessions to meet the goals and objectives of the group. This is also a time to consider if the goals and objectives, themselves, need to be changed. Here are some of the questions you can ask:

- Do I want the group to continue in the same basic direction?
- Are there changes I want to make in approach, use of time, use of space, degree of supervision or explanation, degree of intervention?
- Are individual members being well served?

Compare your initial, pre-meeting impressions and perceptions of the group members with those you have now.

- What insights does this give me about myself as the group's leader?

- Do I have a changed understanding of the group itself?

Client Progress toward Objectives

Each client (or the client's guardian) has agreed to a set of goals and objectives related to treatment. Some of these objectives are being worked on in this group. It is important to let the client know about your evaluation of progress toward meeting the objectives.

If the objectives were written well, they will be measurable, realistic, meaningful chunks of learning or change. They will be ordered so that each objective is placed in a developmental sequence. The basics are first, and later objectives are accomplished with the skills learned in earlier objectives.

During the planning process the following decisions were made:

- Instruments and techniques for evaluation
- How often goals and objectives will be measured
- Other things that need to be measured and evaluated
- The person evaluating the program
- Methods of data analysis
- Acceptable evidence for achieving goals

The participants review their progress with the therapist. This may be after each session, but it is more likely to be once a week or once a month. Each client needs to see how the current program is helping (or not helping) him/her meet his/her goals and objectives.

If goals and objectives are being met as planned, then there is no need to do anything differently. If they are not being met, it's time to make changes.

Possibly, the client needs a whole new set of goals. This is a question that the whole treatment team needs to address in a timely manner.

Other times there may be a mismatch between the program and the goals or objectives. This problem may mean that the program is not appropriate, and you should find another program for the client. The client may be able to stay if the program can target another set of his/her goals and objectives. If many clients are failing to meet their goals and objectives, that suggests that the program needs to be modified.

Therapists have a responsibility to make sure their clients are meeting their expectations for treatment. An important part of running a group is evaluating whether each client is meeting expectations. When the client is not, the therapist needs to do what is necessary to make the goals, objectives, and treatment techniques compatible, including involving other members of the treatment team when that is required.

Modification of Experiences

Our job as therapists is to create opportunities for individuals to participate in our programs as fully as possible. We must be flexible in our thinking and willing to modify a program as needed. Sometimes a formerly successful activity will not work with a new group and needs revision. The following guidelines taken from *Closing the Gap* (Department of Recreation and Leisure Studies at San Jose State University, 1989) are basic considerations to keep in mind to help modify your program, if needed:

- Think *abilities*. Base modifications on what participants can do. For example, if some members have limited vision, consider their abilities to hear, smell, and touch. Add auditory and tactile cues to a visual experience to enable everyone to participate. Everyone's experience will be broadened.
- Take your *cues* from participants. For example, never remove crutches from a person when that person is seated, unless a request is made. Wheelchairs, artificial limbs, crutches, canes, and walkers are part of what the person needs to function as fully as possible. There are enough challenges without creating unnecessary ones. If one of your participants falls, do not panic or rush over like a paramedic. The person will let you know if and how much assistance is needed, and how to do it. Common sense and preservation of dignity must combine to create a good solution. With time, everyone will read each other's cues accurately, and routines will be worked out for dealing with various situations.
- Change a *location* if necessary, to minimize the limitations of environmental barriers. Think of the surface you will be using if there are

participants who use wheelchairs. A harder surface is easier to maneuver on than a soft one. Anticipate potential barriers. Always verify wheelchair access. File appropriate complaints if access is not provided where the law requires it.

- *Preserve* the experience and its components as close to the original activity as you possibly can. Modify only those elements that need to be adapted. In this way the skills learned in this environment will be more easily applied to situations at school, work, the park, or in the world at large.
- *Involve* those who know — your clients — in the adaptation process. This not only encourages them to create their own leisure experiences outside the group, but they often have ideas about what would be useful. They often know or have heard of something that works well. They will also reap the good feelings of finding alternatives for others as well as themselves.
- *Learn* everything you can about adaptive and special equipment that helps participants with physical disabilities participate fully in daily living. Try to use adaptive equipment that will include an individual in an experience. Become an advocate for inclusion of these items in the budget of your facility.
- *Create* and introduce new experiences in order to encourage group cohesion, build self-confidence, and widen participants' interests. Occasionally these experiences can require that all participants experience a limitation in common. For example, games can be played in the dark or with blindfolds. Another possibility is to instruct the participants to communicate only through non-verbal use of their face and body from the waist up. They will provide a new perspective on gestures, facial expressions, drawing, and writing, for example. In this as well as other activities, adaptations must be individualized whenever possible.
- The Bottom Line. Ask yourself these questions as you modify the activities for your participants. Your answers are *critical factors* in the decisions you make. If you find that you are not thrilled with some of the answers, take up the challenge to overcome your limitations as you work to make life fuller and more inclusive for others:

- Are you overprotective and too ready to jump in? Do you become so anxious that you don't allow participant enough time to do something without assistance?
- Do you wait until your assistance is requested?
- Do your assumptions limit your participants before you have really had a chance to fully know them and their situations?
- Is your idea of a successful activity realistic and optimistic at the same time?
- Do you focus on a person's eyes and general presence rather than the wheelchair or other indicator of disability?
- Is one of your goals to sometimes forget that the person has a disability?

Compensatory Techniques and Useful Tips

There are a number of compensatory techniques which can help clients with disabilities participate more fully and successfully in creative arts experiences. Specific adaptive devices are also available online and in catalogs to assist clients who would benefit from modified techniques.

General Techniques

- Use masking tape to fasten paper, fabric, cardboard, or other flat items to the worktable.
- Attach suction cups to the bottoms of plates, cups, jars, and bottles to be decorated. Suction cups are also useful for bottoms of paint jars to prevent knocking over and spilling. Especially useful are suction soap holders, modeling clay, or floral putty. The non-slip pads used under throw rugs also work well when they are cut to size.
- Build up the handles of tools and utensils such as paint brushes, screwdrivers, utility knives, or crochet hooks by wrapping sponge or foam rubber around the handle until it is a comfortable diameter. Tape the foam firmly into place. Tape the end of the foam to the tool handle to avoid slipping.

- Build up the arm of a chair to a comfortable working height by taping foam or folded towels onto the top of the chair arm. A hand tremor may be reduced when the elbow is supported on the chair arm.
- To assist someone with limited motor control to cut paper or fabric, insert the paper or stiff fabric into the center of a thick book and cut with bent-handled scissors.
- Avoid skin abrasion by attaching sandpaper to smooth blocks of wood with tacks. You can also use sanding blocks available in hardware and paint stores.
- Use C-clamps to fasten looms, stretcher frames, or weaving frames to the worktable, holding the frame in a convenient, upright position.
- Hold work for sewing by attaching one edge of the work to a table with masking tape and weighing down the work in the lap with a book or other suitable object.

Tips for People with Limited Vision

- Work with bright colors. Neutral, pastel, or subtle colors are frequently difficult to identify or differentiate.
- Use thick yarns, large-eyed needles, and larger beads. Think bigger to reduce frustration in working on projects.
- In painting or drawing with color, think of creating simple patterns with large areas of color and little detail. Rather than detail, work with shape, color, and texture. These alone can create interesting pieces of art. Abstracts are particularly suitable.
- Investigate the market of aids such as magnifiers that clip onto eyeglasses, magnifiers on stands, and magnifiers worn around the neck. Consult a physician about the suitability of any of these aids for a particular individual.
- Develop the client's sense of touch by experimenting with arts or crafts that are particularly suited to people with vision problems: working with clay, weaving, and mosaic tile work are examples.

Tips for People with Arthritis

- Electric scissors are easier to use than hand scissors.

- Macramé, rug hooking, weaving, and working with clay are particularly good exercises for the fingers.
- Knitting and crocheting should be avoided because the fingers are held stiffly for long periods of time.
- Handles of tools can be built up to avoid the necessity of holding the fingers in a tight grasp.

Tips for People with Sensitive Skin

- Use plastic gloves, preferably the thin, disposable surgical type, for any messy work. (Be careful of latex sensitivity.)
- Ask clients if there are any materials which cause reactions and avoid them or use substitutes whenever possible.
- Use acrylic yarns instead of wool.
- Avoid handling abrasives such as sandpaper. Mount sandpaper on a wood block or in a plastic holder to keep it away from the skin.
- Keep hand cream available and use it to keep the skin as supple as possible.

Tips for People with Respiratory Problems

- Work in a well-ventilated room. It is possible to purchase excellent air purifiers that are quiet and very effective in maintaining a high quality of air in the room.
- Use water-based paints and adhesives that have no objectionable odors or harmful fumes. The brushes, sponges, and cloths for these products are cleaned in water, thus eliminating the use of harmful thinners such as turpentine.
- Avoid projects involving sanding unless you can work outdoors or in a room with an exhaust fan. Use a mask as added protection against inhaling dust.
- Avoid all aerosol products.
- Hunched over postures reduce lung capacity. Good air exchange happens in positions that allow the head to be held up and the shoulders back.

Tips for People with Attention Deficits

- Reduce competing stimuli in the workspace.
- Limit the variety of tools and supplies available at any given time.
- Have the clients sit around a table so that their attention is always focused inward (toward the center of the table) and not around the room.
- If possible, put the light source directly over the table leaving the walls of the room darker.
- Soothing music, with little variation in the melody, may help.
- A fan in the background may produce enough white noise to mask other, more distracting background noises.

Program Evaluation

At the end of the program you need to evaluate the effectiveness of the program. The most important measure is whether the clients met their goals and objectives. In the planning process, you made goals and objectives for the program. Now it is time to decide if they were met.

- Did the program meet its expected effects or outcomes?
- Did the sequence of activities achieve each goal and objective with the most basic skills first and higher-level skills later?
- Did each important component of the program succeed based on the chosen instruments and/or techniques for the evaluation?
- Was each goal or objective evaluated in a timely way?
- Did the appropriate person evaluate the program?
- Was the data analyzed appropriately?
- Did the evidence show that the program achieved its goals?

If the answer is no to any of these questions, you will need to go through the planning process before the program is run again. Don't discard a program out of hand when it doesn't meet all its goals. Look at possible changes to the program or the way you ran the sessions. Improving a program that had some success is easier than starting again from scratch.

Also consider whether the goals and objectives assigned to the program were appropriate. It's possible that the program will work when you have different goals for what you want it to do.

It's also possible that you selected an inappropriate set of clients. In that case work for a better match of clients and programs.

The most important thing to remember is that you must evaluate each program you run to determine its efficacy. Because you have measurable client objectives and formal assessments to determine changes, you can answer the questions about whether the program works. In today's healthcare environment, these are powerful tools to demonstrate that the programs you run are a valuable part of the treatment plan.

References

Department of Recreation and Leisure Studies, San Jose State University. (1983). *Closing the gap: An in-service training guide for mainstreaming recreation and leisure services.* A Project of the Department of Recreation and Leisure Studies, San Jose State University, San Jose, CA. Distributed by the Office of Special Education, US Department of Education.

8

Therapy Groups and the International Classification of Functioning, Disability, and Health

The *International Classification of Functioning, Disability, and Health* (called the ICF for short) was released by the World Health Organization in May 2001. It is updated periodically. This book discusses the codes in the 2016 version of the ICF. Descriptions of what codes cover are taken from the ICF (World Health Organization, 2016).

Governments, providers, and consumers can use the ICF to describe the current condition of anyone in a way that others working with the person can understand. The model includes a person's health and other health-related domains. These include body functions, body structures, activities and participation, and the person's interactions with the environment.

The ICF is a classification system with over 1400 codes for recording the current condition of clients. The terms in the model and the classification system provide a common language for describing functioning and health. Having a common language across disciplines and countries allows comparison of data, which can strengthen research, policy, and practice.

Therapists leading creative arts groups can describe their clients using this model and can base their treatment on what others have assessed. This chapter includes all the codes in the ICF down to the three-digit definitions. Some codes have as many as five digits to describe finer details of a category, e.g., b16701 Reception of Written Language.

This chapter is not intended to provide detailed information about the ICF. That is covered in Heather Porter's (2016) book, *Recreational Therapy and the International Classification of Functioning, Disability, and Health*. The information provided here is from Porter's book. The following brief introduction to the structure of the book will help therapists navigate the ICF codes and connect them to treatment.

The ICF is divided into four components: body functions, body structure, activities and participation, and environmental factors.

Body Functions: Body Functions are the physiological and psychological functions of the body. Many of the codes in this component are part of the scope of recreational therapy practice. There are eight chapters that look at all the functions of the mind and body from mental functions to skin functions. Body Functions codes all begin with a lower-case b. If a person has difficulty with a body function, it is called an impairment.

Body Structures: Body Structures provides a list of anatomical parts of the body such as organs, limbs, and their components. There are eight chapters. Typically, a physician or nurse practitioner codes a client's status in Body Structures. Recreational therapists seldom score Body Structures codes, but they are very important when deciding whether a client can participate in a group. Body Structures codes all begin with a lower-case s. If a person has difficulty with a body structure, it is called a deficit.

Activities and Participation: "Activity" is the execution of a task or action by an individual. "Participation" is involvement in a life situation. Activities and Participation lists the activities that people commonly perform in real life, such as taking care of plants, maintaining health, handling stress, preparing meals, swimming, shopping, using transportation, recreation and leisure, and spirituality. There are nine chapters. The scores assigned by the therapist reflect a client's ability to engage or participate in those activities in a standardized environment (capacity) and in his/her current real-life environment (performance). Activities and Participation is different from Body Functions. Body Functions reflects the function in isolation, while Activities and Participation reflects the client's ability to do an activity. For example, a client may have moderate difficulty with short-term memory but no difficulty managing a daily routine. The Activities and Participation component allows us to look at the level of difficulty that a client has with a specific activity, not just the level of body function impairment. Recreational therapists usually work within the context of an activity. As a result, many of the codes used by recreational therapists are in this section. In creative arts groups these codes can be used to decide if a group is appropriate for a client. Improvements in a code can also be used as a measurable objective. Activities and Participation codes all begin with a lower-case d. If a person has difficulty in executing an activity, it is referred to as an "activity limitation." If a person has difficulty with involvement in a life situation, it is referred to as a "participation restriction."

Environmental Factors: Environmental Factors are things in the person's environment that affect his/her health and functioning, such as adaptive equipment, attitudes of other people, or physical structures of buildings. There are five chapters. Problems in the environment are called barriers. In the ICF therapists can score the extent that environmental factors are barriers, and they can also score the extent that environmental factors are facilitators for activities. For creative arts groups, the codes can be used to keep track of required adaptations and how successful they are. Recreational therapists can attach Environmental Factors codes to Activities and Participation codes to show the connections. Environmental Factors codes all begin with a lower-case e.

Therapists can use the codes and suggestions in the rest of the chapter to decide if a client will be able to participate successfully in a group. Appropriate creative arts group modalities are also suggested for many of the codes.

Body Functions

Chapter 1 Mental Functions

These functions can be used to decide if a client has appropriate mental functions for being in a creative arts group. Many, but not all, of the functions described in ICF Chapter 1 can be treated with group activities.

Global Mental Functions (b110 - b139)

Evaluating global mental functions is important for deciding if group work is appropriate for a client. To work in a group a person must be able to interact appropriately with others. Some impairments in mental functions may make group work impossible.

b110 Consciousness Functions

Usually, clients who have disabilities related to consciousness functions are not able to function in groups because they are unable to process ongoing activities. Underlying causes usually need to be addressed before asking the client to join a group.

b114 Orientation Functions

Orientation to time, place, and person is required for some group activities, but not all. Creative arts groups do not usually focus on improving function in these areas. Other groups will probably be more relevant.

b117 Intellectual Functions

Intellectual functions refer to ongoing development and integration of the other mental functions. Impairments in this area will limit a client's ability to learn from creative arts activities, so the client may not be appropriate for groups.

b122 Global Psychosocial Functions

These are mental functions that lead to formation of interpersonal skills. Deficits in this area suggest that a client may not be appropriate for creative arts groups.

b126 Temperament and Personality Functions

This code looks at functions of extraversion, introversion, agreeableness, conscientiousness, psychic and emotional stability, and openness to experience; optimism; novelty seeking; confidence; and trustworthiness. A therapist needs to consider findings in this area when deciding whether a client should be invited into a group. Many of these issues can be addressed in creative arts groups that emphasize interpersonal interactions.

b130 Energy and Drive Functions

This code looks at functions of energy level, motivation, appetite, craving (including craving for substances that can be abused), and impulse control. These areas can be evaluated for a client's suitability for a group. Energy level and motivation may be addressed in creative arts groups that focus on discovering new possibilities for activities.

b134 Sleep Functions

Sleep issues are not addressed by creative arts groups. Poor sleep patterns leading to falling asleep in groups can make participation difficult.

Specific Mental Functions (b140 - b189)

This area looks at specific mental functions such as attention and memory. Deficits in some of these areas suggest that a client is not appropriate for creative arts groups. Creative arts groups can improve functioning in some of these areas.

b140 Attention Functions

The ability to attend to the group process is required for participation. Initial treatments for deficits in attention are better handled one-on-one. Creative arts provide more challenging situations when the client is ready for them.

b144 Memory Functions

Clients with memory problems will have difficulty in many creative arts groups. Simple activities in visual and tactile arts can be used for clients with significant deficits. Other modalities will be more problematic.

b147 Psychomotor Functions

These codes involve psychomotor retardation, excitement and agitation, posturing, catatonia, negativism, echopraxia, and echolalia. Therapists should consider whether clients with deficits in these areas are appropriate for creative arts groups. Creative arts do not address these issues.

b152 Emotional Functions

This code looks at areas such as appropriateness of emotion, regulation and range of emotion; affect; sadness, happiness, love, fear, anger, hate, tension, anxiety, joy, sorrow; lability of emotion; and flattening of affect. Therapists should match clients with groups that address the aspects of emotional functioning that the client needs to work on.

b156 Perceptual Functions

These codes look at auditory, visual, olfactory, gustatory, tactile, and visuospatial perception. Therapists look at these codes to decide if a client can participate in a particular group.

b160 Thought Functions

Thought function impairments are generally seen in mental health disorders such as schizophrenia, bipolar disorder, delusional disorders, phobias, depression, dementia, and obsessive-compulsive disorder, as well as physical disabilities that impair the brain including dementia, traumatic brain injury, and cerebrovascular accident. Therapists look at these codes to decide if a client can participate in a particular group.

b164 Higher-Level Cognitive Functions

These functions include abstraction and organization of ideas; time management, insight, and judgment; concept formation, categorization, and cognitive flexibility. Some skills in these areas are required for participation in creative arts groups. These functions can also be improved with many of groups described in this book. Clients in a group should all be working on the same kind of issue.

b167 Mental Functions of Language

This code looks at all the mental functions required for reception, expression, and integration of language. Therapists need to be sure that clients can process language well enough to work in a group. Theater games, writing groups, and music where singing is involved are the most appropriate for working on deficits.

b172 Calculation Functions

These codes look at addition, subtraction, and other simple mathematical calculations and also functions of complex mathematical operations. For most creative arts groups a therapist will be able to find adaptations for deficits in these areas.

b176 Mental Functions of Sequencing Complex Movements

The ability to sequence complex movements is required for many kinds of creative arts activities. Clients with deficits in these areas will be limited to groups that have only simple sets of movements. Visual and tactile arts and music have the greatest number of possibilities.

b180 Experience of Self and Time Functions

These codes look at mental functions related to the awareness of one's identity, one's body, one's position in the reality of one's environment and of time. A lack of awareness limits clients to activities that do not require this kind of awareness. Visual and tactile arts, music, and simple movement are the most likely to be successful and may lead to improvements. Body image issues are seen, for example, in eating disorders and phantom limbs. Clients with these issues will benefit from groups that are concerned with perception of self and more complex movement. Therapists should choose clients with similar issues for a group.

Chapter 2 Sensory Functions and Pain

This chapter is about the functions of the senses: seeing, hearing, tasting, and so on, as well as the sensation of pain. Creative arts groups do not typically treat these areas. However, therapists must be aware of deficits in these codes when deciding if a client is appropriate for a group. These codes also let therapists know if they need to devise adaptations for clients so they can participate more fully in the group experience.

Balance issues are included in the codes on hearing and vestibular functions. Therapists need to consider the risk of falls whenever they wish to include a client in a group.

Pain is also a concern for clients in groups. Therapists must be aware of the causes of pain and create an experience that is as pain-free as possible.

Three-digit ICF codes are included here to remind you of the kinds of issues to look for related to sensory functions and pain.

Seeing and Related Functions (b210 - b229)

b210 Seeing Functions

b215 Functions of Structures Adjoining the Eye

b220 Sensations Associated with the Eye and Adjoining Structures

Hearing and Vestibular Functions (b230 - b249)

b230 Hearing Functions

b235 Vestibular Functions

b240 Sensations Associated with Hearing and Vestibular Functions

Additional Sensory Functions (b250 - b279)

b250 Taste Function

b255 Smell Function

b260 Proprioceptive Function

b265 Touch Function

b270 Sensory Functions Related to Temperature and Other Stimuli

Pain (b280 - b289)

b280 Sensation of Pain

Chapter 3 Voice and Speech Functions

This chapter is about the functions of producing sounds and speech. The concepts of language and speech are often thought of as being the same. However, they are quite different. Language, as in b167 Mental Functions of Language, is a method of expression or communication, which may or may not be vocal. Speech, as described in this chapter, is using the voice for talking, singing, and other sounds.

Some of the creative arts may seem to not require speech. These include visual and tactile arts, music, and dance and movement. However, all groups are based on participation of the members of the group, and voice and speech are the most common means of sharing. So, therapists need to be aware of any deficits in voice and speech functions as they select members for a therapy group. Adaptations must be available if there are deficits, so that all members of a group have the opportunity to participate fully.

The three-digit codes are included below.

b310 Voice Functions

b320 Articulation Functions

b330 Fluency and Rhythm of Speech Functions

b340 Alternative Vocalization Functions

Including production of notes and making a range of sounds.

Chapter 4 Functions of the Cardiovascular, Hematological, Immunological, and Respiratory Systems

This chapter is about the functions involved in the cardiovascular system (functions of the heart and blood vessels), the hematological and immunological systems (functions of blood production and immunity), and the respiratory system (functions of respiration and exercise tolerance).

General physical endurance, aerobic capacity, and fatigability can significantly limit or enhance a client's ability to participate in therapy groups. Many illnesses and conditions can negatively impact exercise tolerance functions. These include physical disabilities, such as high-level spinal cord injury or multiple sclerosis, psychiatric conditions, such as depression, surgery, general deconditioning from chronic health conditions, inactivity, obesity, respiratory impairments including asthma and chronic obstructive pulmonary disease, and any other condition impacting mobility and movement.

Therapists must consider a client's condition when deciding if the client is a good fit for a group. To the greatest extent possible therapists should provide adaptations so clients can be part of a wide range of groups. When a client's ability to engage in leisure and community tasks or leisure time physical activity is compromised due to such dysfunction, health and quality of life are negatively affected.

Creative arts groups will generally not have objectives related to these ICF codes, except that objectives for increasing exercise tolerance may be part of groups that require active physical participation. The three-digit codes for this chapter are provided below.

Functions of the Cardiovascular System (b410 - b429)

b410 Heart Functions

b415 Blood Vessel Functions

b420 Blood Pressure Functions

Functions of the Hematological and Immunological Systems (b430 - b439)

b430 Hematological System Functions

b435 Immunological System Functions

Functions of the Respiratory System (b440 - b449)

b440 Respiration Functions

b445 Respiratory Muscle Functions

Additional Functions and Sensations of the Cardiovascular and Respiratory Systems (b450 - b469)

b450 Additional Respiratory Functions

b455 Exercise Tolerance Functions

b460 Sensations Associated with Cardiovascular and Respiratory Functions

Chapter 5 Functions of the Digestive, Metabolic, and Endocrine Systems

This chapter is about the functions of ingestion, digestion, and elimination, as well as functions involved in metabolism and endocrine glands. Therapists need to consider issues in these codes when selecting participants for groups.

Digestive, metabolic, and endocrine functions can impact group participation. These negatively affect health, quality of life, and social participation. A team approach, including recreational therapy groups, can address the systemic issues. For example, difficulty with fecal incontinence in adolescents and adults with spinal cord injury is associated with depression, anxiety, and significant impairments in quality of life (Hocevar & Gray, 2008). Difficulties with digestive functions post stroke that result in eating smaller pieces or the need for only soft food can result in avoiding social activities out of concern for eating safely and properly. Theater games and drama therapy, for example, may provide ways for clients to explore techniques they can use to increase social involvement when they have these kinds of issues.

Deficits in other functions discussed in this chapter signal therapists that they need to structure creative arts groups in ways that take the conditions into account. Treatment will usually be the responsibility of other members of the treatment team. The three-digit ICF codes are shown below.

Functions Related to the Digestive System (b510 - b539)

b510 Ingestion Functions

b515 Digestive Functions

b520 Assimilation Functions

b525 Defecation Functions

Fecal continence and flatulence are included in this code. Therapists need to provide appropriate ways to handle problems in these areas.

b530 Weight Maintenance Functions

b535 Sensations Associated with the Digestive System

Nausea, bloating, and cramping may need to be addressed during a group.

Functions Related to Metabolism and the Endocrine System (b540 - b559)

b540 General Metabolic Functions

b545 Water, Mineral, and Electrolyte Balance Functions

Therapists must consider issues with hydration and mineral and electrolyte balance when planning strenuous groups activities and when the weather makes these functions more likely to be an issue.

b550 Thermoregulatory Functions

b555 Endocrine Gland Functions

Chapter 6 Genitourinary and Reproductive Functions

This chapter is about the functions of urination and the reproductive functions, including sexual and procreative functions. Discussion on each part of the chapter is shown below.

Urinary Functions (b610 - b639)

Urinary incontinence deficits are the most likely to affect creative arts groups. In general, these codes are treated by other medical team members.

b610 Urinary Excretory Functions

b620 Urination Functions

b630 Sensations Associated with Urinary Functions

Genital and Reproductive Functions (b640 - b679)

Individuals who have a disability related to reproductive functions may face physical, mental, behavioral, psychological, emotional, social, communication, and spiritual challenges. All of these have the potential to affect sexual functioning and relationships. Creative arts groups are unlikely to have objectives related to these codes. The groups are much more likely to provide treatment related to Activities and Participation codes in d7 Interpersonal Interactions and Relationships.

b640 Sexual Functions

b650 Menstruation Functions

b660 Procreation Functions

b670 Sensations Associated with Genital and Reproductive Functions

Chapter 7 Neuromusculoskeletal and Movement-Related Functions

This chapter is about the functions of movement and mobility, including functions of joints, bones, reflexes, and muscles. Gait patterns, voluntary and involuntary movement, balance, mobility of bones and joints, and the endurance, strength, and tone of muscle are basic functions that support body movement. Individuals may have difficulty with these neuromusculoskeletal and movement functions due to illness, disease, disability, or the normal aging process. When a person has difficulty with these basic functions, participation in creative arts groups can be significantly hindered. Therapists need to consider these areas when selecting group members and be ready to provide adaptations, as required, for participation. The three-digit codes and additional comments are provided below.

Functions of the Joints and Bones (b710 - b729)

Issues of flexibility and stability may limit what the client can do.

b710 Mobility of Joint Functions

b715 Stability of Joint Functions

b720 Mobility of Bone Functions

Muscle Functions (b730 - b749)

Therapists need to take muscle power, tone, and endurance into account when matching clients and activities. Issues related to strokes and spinal cord injuries, and other neuromuscular conditions, are documented using these codes.

b730 Muscle Power Functions

b735 Muscle Tone Functions

b740 Muscle Endurance Functions

Movement Functions (b750 - b789)

Movement functions document some of the underlying causes of mobility issues. Art therapy groups will generally be more concerned with d4 Mobility codes, which are Chapter 4 of Activities and Participation.

b750 Motor Reflex Functions

b755 Involuntary Movement Reaction Functions

b760 Control of Voluntary Movement Functions

b765 Involuntary Movement Functions

b770 Gait Pattern Functions

b780 Sensations Related to Muscles and Movement Functions

Chapter 8 Functions of the Skin and Related Structures

Therapists need to be aware of issues related to the skin and related structures to know when to protect clients from possible harm during activities.

Functions of the Skin (b810 - b849)

b810 Protective Functions of the Skin

b820 Repair Functions of the Skin

b830 Other Functions of the Skin

b840 Sensation Related to the Skin

Functions of the Hair and Nails (b850 - b869)

b850 Functions of the Hair

b860 Functions of the Nails

Body Structures

Leaders of art therapy groups need to be aware of issues related to some body structures when selecting members for a group. Adaptations may be required. It is unlikely that any objectives for a group will use these codes. Instead, the objectives will almost always be related to one of the body-function codes, as described above, or to activities and participation codes described later. Three-digit codes are provided.

Chapter 1 Structures of the Nervous System

s110 Structure of Brain
s120 Spinal Cord and Related Structures
s130 Structure of Meninges
s140 Structure of Sympathetic Nervous System
s150 Structure of Parasympathetic Nervous System

Chapter 2 The Eye, Ear, and Related Structures

s210 Structure of Eye Socket
s220 Structure of Eyeball
s230 Structures Around the Eye
s240 Structure of External Ear
s250 Structure of Middle Ear
s260 Structure of Inner Ear

Chapter 3 Structures Involved in Voice and Speech

s310 Structure of Nose
s320 Structure of Mouth
s330 Structure of Pharynx
s340 Structure of Larynx

Chapter 4 Structures of the Cardiovascular, Immunological, and Respiratory Systems

s410 Structure of Cardiovascular System
s420 Structure of Immune System
s430 Structure of Respiratory System

Chapter 5 Structures Related to the Digestive, Metabolic, and Endocrine Systems

s510 Structure of Salivary Glands
s520 Structure of Esophagus
s530 Structure of Stomach
s540 Structure of Intestine
s550 Structure of Pancreas
s560 Structure of Liver
s570 Structure of Gall Bladder and Ducts

s580 Structure of Endocrine Glands

Chapter 6 Structures Related to the Genitourinary and Reproductive Systems

s610 Structure of Urinary System
s620 Structure of Pelvic Floor
s630 Structure of Reproductive System

Chapter 7 Structures Related to Movement

s710 Structure of Head and Neck Region
s720 Structure of Shoulder Region
s730 Structure of Upper Extremity
s740 Structure of Pelvic Region
s750 Structure of Lower Extremity
s760 Structure of Trunk
s770 Additional Musculoskeletal Structures Related to Movement

Chapter 8 Skin and Related Structures

s810 Structure of Areas of Skin
s820 Structure of Skin Glands
s830 Structure of Nails
s840 Structure of Hair
s898 Skin and Related Structures, Other Specified
s899 Skin and Related Structures, Unspecified

Activities and Participation

Activities and Participation contains some of the most important codes for recreational therapy practice. Included in this section are the activities of learning, performing tasks, communication, mobility, self-care, interpersonal interactions, major life areas, and community and social life. Everything we *do* as humans is included here. These are the most useful codes when writing objectives for creative arts groups. Activities and Participation is divided into nine chapters.

Chapter 1 Learning and Applying Knowledge

This chapter is about learning, applying the knowledge that is learned, thinking, solving problems, and making decisions. This section is related to Body Functions b1 Mental Functions. The Body Functions chapter assesses brain functions and the Activities and Participation chapter assesses brain activities. Recreational therapists use activities to determine the functioning of the brain. For example, a therapist presents the client with a problem-solving activity to assess the brain function of problem solving.

Creative arts groups will usually use these codes for writing client goals instead of using body function codes. The earlier codes in this chapter are more concerned with abilities that are required for participating in groups. The later codes are abilities that are more likely to be improved through groups.

Purposeful Sensory Experiences (d110 - d129)

These abilities are necessary for participating in groups. One-on-one activities are better for improving abilities in these areas. The three-digit codes are shown below.

d110 Watching

d115 Listening

d120 Other Purposeful Sensing

Basic Learning (d130 - d159)

These abilities are necessary for participating in creative arts groups. The abilities can be taught one-on-one or in a group setting. The groups will be focused more on instruction of skills than creative arts. The three-digit codes are shown below.

d130 Copying

d135 Rehearsing

d140 Learning to Read

d145 Learning to Write

d150 Learning to Calculate

d155 Acquiring Skills

Applying Knowledge (d160 - d179)

Minimum levels of these abilities are required for participating in creative arts groups. Creative arts groups can be used to improve the abilities of focusing attention, thinking, solving problems, and making decisions. Reading, writing, and calculating are abilities that will be used in creative arts groups, but instructional groups will probably be better at improving the abilities. Note that instructional groups can successfully use creative arts as one of the modalities of instruction. The three-digit codes are shown below.

d160 Focusing Attention
d163 Thinking
d166 Reading
d170 Writing
d172 Calculating
d175 Solving Problems
d177 Making Decisions

Chapter 2 General Tasks and Demands

This chapter is about general aspects of carrying out single or multiple tasks, organizing routines, and handling stress. These items can be used in conjunction with more specific tasks or actions to identify the underlying features of the execution of tasks under different circumstances.

This chapter is about *tasks*. In creative arts groups, a task is the direct effort to complete a goal. A task generally occurs in a sequential order and has a beginning point and a target outcome. This chapter is also about *demands*. A demand is motivation to act to fulfill a need.

The World Health Organization recognizes the ability to complete many different tasks as the basis for taking care of oneself and fitting into one's community. Because of the importance of being able to undertake and complete all types of tasks, the World Health Organization made tasks its own, major chapter in its system of categorization. When problems are seen in a client's ability to perform a task, it is usually a result of an impaired body function, a body structure deficit, or an inappropriate environment.

Therapists must assess the clients' abilities to do tasks when deciding which activities to use in a group. If client goals include improving the ability to undertake tasks, the therapist should choose activities that appropriately challenge clients to improve their task performance. If there are no task-related goals, then therapists should choose simpler activities that let the client focus on what they are intending to learn rather than focusing on the challenges of performing the task.

d210 Undertaking a Single Task

Carrying out simple or complex and coordinated actions related to the mental and physical components of a single task, such as initiating a task, organizing time, space, and materials for a task, pacing task performance, and carrying out, completing, and sustaining a task.

What is done in a creative arts group is usually a single task. It may be simple or complex. All the modalities in this book have some examples of single tasks, both simple and complex. Therapists teach clients the skills listed as part of participating in the group.

d220 Undertaking Multiple Tasks

Carrying out simple or complex and coordinated actions as components of multiple, integrated, and complex tasks in sequence or simultaneously.

In a clinical setting, therapists usually present single task challenges to clients. This is because it is easier to evaluate a client's actual skill level when the therapist looks at one skill at a time. However, life in the community is seldom that simple and planned. The ability to juggle many different demands at the same time requires a complex set of skills that are hard to define and harder to measure. Often, when a client fails to complete multiple tasks, it is hard for the therapist to determine if the client failed because s/he was not able to perform a specific skill in one of the many tasks being evaluated or if s/he was not able to integrate the "higher level" skill of planning and coordinating multiple tasks.

The creative arts modalities usually present single tasks, but some are multiple tasks. If a client goal includes improving abilities related to multiple tasks, look for activities that require members of the group to switch between different actions as part of the process. For example, in the part of Writing for Wellness Groups where clients are reading what they wrote, they need to switch fluidly between the roles of presenting, listening, and giving appropriate support and feedback. But this isn't nearly as complicated as planning and carrying out a four-store shopping expedition with a grandma in a wheelchair and a baby, a toddler, and a preteen. The power of recreational therapy is that it gets out into the real world and presents clients with real challenges that go far beyond what can be taught in groups.

It is important to distinguish between a lack of ability for the single tasks that are being done and the inability to successfully switch between tasks as required. Switching successfully is what this code covers.

d230 Carrying Out Daily Routine

This may be addressed in drama therapy but not in other creative arts groups.

d240 Handling Stress and Other Psychological Demands

This can be addressed in creative arts groups that create situations for studying interpersonal interactions, such as theater games and drama therapy. Other expressive arts groups give the client ways to express stress and psychological demands. Often group feedback looks at ways to improve the situation.

Chapter 3 Communication

This chapter is about general and specific features of communicating by language, signs, and symbols, including receiving and producing messages, carrying on conversations, and using communication devices and techniques. Some level of communication is required for creative arts groups. Creative arts groups can also improve communication abilities.

Therapists need to consider the communication abilities of the clients they invite to the group. It might be best if everyone has the same abilities. But it might also be therapeutic if some of the clients help other clients with communication challenges, for example by reading instructions for a person with poor vision or signing for someone with hearing deficits. Awareness of deficits and how the clients will interact with one another is the key to deciding who will fit in a group.

Communicating — Receiving (d310 - d329)

Comprehending literal and implied meanings of messages. Some ability to receive messages is required for participation in groups. Creative arts groups can improve a client's ability to receive messages as described below. Note that all groups with sharing have some aspect of receiving messages.

d310 Communicating with — Receiving — Spoken Messages

Groups which are especially appropriate to improve receiving spoken messages will be found in theater games, improvisation, and perhaps drama therapy.

d315 Communicating with — Receiving — Nonverbal Messages

Groups which are especially appropriate to improve receiving nonverbal messages will be found in visual and tactile arts, masks, theater games, improvisation, laughter and clowning, music, dance and movement, and puppetry.

d320 Communicating with — Receiving — Formal Sign Language Messages

In any group, sign language can be substituted for spoken language.

d325 Communicating with — Receiving — Written Messages

Writing and poetry groups might be used to improve receiving written messages, but the focus of many of these groups is on content rather than skill of communication.

Communicating — Producing (d330 - d349)

Producing messages with literal and implied meaning, such as answering a question, sharing an emotion, expressing a fact, or telling a story. Some ability to produce messages is required for participation in groups. Creative arts groups can improve a client's ability to produce messages as described below. Note that all groups with sharing have some aspect of producing messages.

d330 Speaking

Groups which are especially appropriate to improve producing spoken messages will be found in theater games, improvisation, and drama therapy.

d335 Producing Nonverbal Messages

Groups which are especially appropriate to improve producing nonverbal messages will be found in visual and tactile arts, masks, theater games, improvisation, laughter and clowning, music, dance and movement, and puppetry.

d340 Producing Messages in Formal Sign Language

In any group, sign language can be substituted for spoken language.

d345 Writing Messages

Writing and poetry groups might be used to improve producing written messages, but the focus of many of those groups is on content rather than skill of communication.

Conversation and Use of Communication Devices and Techniques (d350 - d369)

All creative arts groups have conversations and discussions during the sharing part of the session.

d350 Conversation

Groups that are intended to improve conversations are found mainly in theater games, improvisation, and drama therapy.

d355 Discussion

Groups that are intended to improve discussions are found mainly in theater games, improvisation, and drama therapy.

d360 Using Communication Devices and Techniques

Communication devices should be used as required by clients to allow communication with other members of the group. Training in the use of these devices is usually not the focus of creative arts groups.

Chapter 4 Mobility

This chapter is about moving by changing body position or location or by transferring from one place to another, by carrying, moving, or manipulating objects, by walking, running, or climbing, and by using various forms of transportation. The scope of the term mobility has been greatly expanded by the World Health Organization. Mobility now encompasses walking and moving, using transportation options, and participating in many different types of activities, such as catching and running.

The scope of practice for the recreational therapist includes many elements of mobility training and enhancement. While it is common for a physical therapist to determine the type of walking and moving appropriate for a client after a disabling condition, it is often the recreational therapist who helps the client problem solve barriers to mobility, especially related to moving around the community and using adaptive mobility equipment for recreational activities.

Creative arts groups can be especially important for some of these codes because they provide a place to practice and an activity that is engaging for the client. The recreational therapist also uses his/her specialized knowledge to help clients integrate equipment and techniques into everyday life, as well as identify additional equipment and training that are needed to enhance community and leisure participation. See the descriptions below.

Changing and Maintaining Body Position (d410 - d429)

d410 Changing Basic Body Position

Getting into and out of a body position and moving from one location to another, such as getting up out of a chair to lie down on a bed and getting into and out of positions of kneeling and squatting. Creative arts groups need to be within the abilities of the clients, as assessed by the therapist. The groups may provide a place to practice these abilities.

d415 Maintaining a Body Position

Staying in the same body position as required, such as remaining seated or remaining standing for work or school. Creative arts groups need to be within the abilities of the clients, as assessed by the therapist. The groups may provide a place to practice these abilities.

d420 Transferring Oneself

Moving from one surface to another, such as sliding along a bench or moving from a bed to a chair, without changing body positions. This is not usually part of creative arts groups although the group leader needs to be sure clients can transfer as required for the group.

Carrying, Moving, and Handling Objects (d430 - d449)

Many creative arts groups involve moving, carrying, and handling objects. The therapist needs to be sure that clients who are invited into the group can work with objects as required. The therapist may need to find adaptations for some clients. See the codes below for ideas about which types of creative arts provide the best practice for improving each of the abilities.

d430 Lifting and Carrying Objects

The subcodes for this code discuss using the upper extremities and the head for lifting and carrying. Creative arts groups that involve lifting and carrying include visual and tactile arts, masks, music (for the instruments), and puppetry.

d435 Moving Objects with Lower Extremities

If the lower extremities are used for moving objects in a creative arts group, it will usually be because the client is using them as an adaptation for a lack of ability to use the upper extremities.

d440 Fine Hand Use

The subcodes look at picking up, grasping, manipulating, and releasing. Fine hand use is found in visual and tactile arts, masks, music, and puppetry.

d445 Hand and Arm Use

The subcodes look at pulling, pushing, reaching, turning or twisting the hands or arms, throwing, and catching. Hand and arm use are found in visual and tactile arts, masks, some theater games, clowning, music, dance and movement, and puppetry.

Walking and Moving (d450 - d469)

Some creative arts groups involve walking and moving, including moving using equipment. Most groups do not do a lot of moving from one place to another during the session. The therapist needs to be sure that clients who are invited into the group can get around as required. The therapist may need to find adaptations for some clients. See the codes below for creative arts groups that work with the abilities described.

d450 Walking

Clients may walk when the activity involves moving from one group member to another or from one place to another. This happens most in theater games and improvisation and in some of the mask activities. See the next code for a discussion of dance.

d455 Moving Around

Moving around includes crawling, climbing, running, jumping, and swimming. Interestingly dancing is not included in the mobility codes, except, perhaps, under the catchall "other specified" or "unspecified." Moving around that is not walking is found in theater games and improvisation, clowning, music, dance and movement, and puppetry.

d460 Moving Around in Different Locations

This code discusses the ability to move around inside and outside. It isn't addressed by most creative arts groups.

d465 Moving Around Using Equipment

The equipment includes things like skates and skis, as well as wheelchairs. The therapist must be sure the client can get around sufficiently for the group. It is seldom the purpose of the group.

Moving Around Using Transportation (d470 - d489)

Transportation is not a focus of creative arts groups.

d470 Using Transportation

d475 Driving

d480 Riding Animals for Transportation

Chapter 5 Self-Care

This chapter is about caring for oneself, washing and drying oneself, caring for one's body and body parts, dressing, eating and drinking, and looking after one's health. The actual caring for oneself is not a focus of creative arts groups. Discussing attitudes about caring for oneself might be part of theater games, improvisation, and drama therapy. The three-digit codes are shown below.

d510 Washing Oneself

d520 Caring for Body Parts

d530 Toileting

d540 Dressing

d550 Eating

d560 Drinking

d570 Looking After One's Health

Chapter 6 Domestic Life

This chapter is about carrying out domestic and everyday actions and tasks. Areas of domestic life include acquiring a place to live, food, clothing, and other necessities, household cleaning and repairing, caring for personal and other household objects, and assisting others.

Except for assisting others, these abilities are not taught as part of creative arts groups. Interpersonal interaction abilities required for domestic life are part of the next chapter. Group process in all the modalities teaches a client how to assist others in communication and interpersonal relations. The three-digit codes are shown below.

Acquisition of Necessities (d610 - d629)

d610 Acquiring a Place to Live
d620 Acquisition of Goods and Services

Household Tasks (d630 - d649)

d630 Preparing Meals
d640 Doing Housework

Caring for Household Objects and Assisting Others (d650 - d669)

d650 Caring for Household Objects
d660 Assisting Others

Chapter 7 Interpersonal Interactions and Relationships

This chapter is about carrying out the actions and tasks required for basic and complex interactions with people (strangers, friends, relatives, family members, and lovers) in a contextually and socially appropriate manner. This chapter in the ICF covers one of the major focuses of Art Therapy Groups — interactions with others.

Any group that has an interaction between two or more people has potential for improving abilities in interpersonal relationships. Many of the groups have that as their stated purpose. One of the criteria therapists need to use when selecting clients to be part of a group is that they are capable of maintaining interactions that don't harm the group.

In this chapter there are general interpersonal interactions that apply to all interactions and interactions with specific types of people.

General Interpersonal Interactions (d710 - d729)

The first part of this chapter talks about general interpersonal interactions that apply to all interactions.

d710 Basic Interpersonal Interactions

Interacting with people in a contextually and socially appropriate manner, such as by showing consideration and esteem when appropriate, or responding to the feelings of others. These skills that are required to develop meaningful relationships with others. While they are normally developed when growing up, some conditions, such as autism and intellectual/developmental disability, can limit a person's ability to develop interpersonal skills. Psychological disorders, such as obsessive-compulsive disorder and schizophrenia, are often accompanied by deficits in the ability to interact with others appropriately. These skills can also be lost as a result of brain injury. The creative arts modalities that enhance abilities in these areas include visual and tactile arts emphasizing interactions, masks, theater games and drama, clowning, multi-person dance and movement, and puppetry. The following four-digit codes show the skills listed in the ICF.

- d7100 Respect and Warmth in Relationships
- d7101 Appreciation in Relationships
- d7102 Tolerance in Relationships
- d7103 Criticism in Relationships
- d7104 Social Cues in Relationships
- d7105 Physical Contact in Relationships

d720 Complex Interpersonal Interactions

Maintaining and managing interactions with other people, in a contextually and socially appropriate manner, such as by regulating emotions and impulses, controlling verbal and physical aggression, acting independently in social interactions, and acting in accordance with social rules and conventions. This code explores the development of social skills related to general interpersonal interactions. Most clients who require this level of training have cognitive impairments that reduce their ability to understand and interpret social rules and interactions.

The structure of creative arts groups is, by itself, a model for these types of interactions. Specific creative arts modalities that enhance abilities in these areas include masks, theater games and drama, multi-person dance and movement, and puppetry. The discussions in the first part of this book — especially interaction patterns, group structure, and therapy group phases — are possible ways art therapy groups can accomplish the skills covered by the four-digit codes listed below.

- d7200 Forming Relationships
- d7201 Terminating Relationships
- d7202 Regulating Behaviors within Interactions

- d7203 Interacting According to Social Rules
- d7204 Maintaining Social Space

Particular Interpersonal Relationships (d730 - d779)

The second part of this chapter talks about interactions with specific types of people. Role playing groups from theater games and drama therapy are often used to teach clients how to handle these relationships more effectively. Some writing exercises also focus on these interactions. The three-digit codes are shown.

d730 Relating with Strangers

Engaging in temporary contacts and links with strangers for specific purposes, such as when asking for directions or making a purchase.

d740 Formal Relationships

Creating and maintaining specific relationships in formal settings, such as with employers, professionals, or service providers. Relationships between clients and therapists are part of this code.

d750 Informal Social Relationships

Entering into relationships with others, such as casual relationships with people living in the same community or residence, or with co-workers, students, playmates, or people with similar backgrounds or professions.

d760 Family Relationships

Creating and maintaining kinship relations, such as with members of the nuclear family, extended family, foster and adopted family and step-relationships, more distant relationships such as second cousins, or legal guardians.

d770 Intimate Relationships

Creating and maintaining close or romantic relationships between individuals, such as husband and wife, lovers, or sexual partners.

Chapter 8 Major Life Areas

This chapter is about carrying out the tasks and actions required to engage in education, work, and employment and to conduct economic transactions. This chapter is divided into three significantly different sections: Education, Work and Employment, and Economic Life.

Many tasks and actions are required to engage in informal or formal education. These include learning, gaining admission, engaging in school-related responsibilities and privileges, attending, working cooperatively with others, organizing, studying, completing tasks and projects, and advancing to other stages of education. The ability to engage in meaningful life work has a direct impact on health and quality of life. Economic skills of basic and complex economic transactions and economic self-sufficiency are skills required for independent living, unless another person, such as a guardian carries the responsibility for the individual.

These will seldom be a criterion for accepting clients into a creative arts group and are not usually a focus for the groups. The three-digit codes are shown.

Education (d810 - d839)

d810 Informal Education
d815 Preschool Education
d820 School Education
d825 Vocational Training
d830 Higher Education

Work and Employment (d840 - d859)

d840 Apprenticeship (Work Preparation)
d845 Acquiring, Keeping, and Terminating a Job
d850 Remunerative Employment
d855 Non-Remunerative Employment

Economic Life (d860 - d879)

d860 Basic Economic Transactions
d865 Complex Economic Transactions
d870 Economic Self-Sufficiency

Chapter 9 Community, Social, and Civic Life

This chapter is about the actions and tasks required to engage in organized social life outside the family, in community, social, and civic areas of life. These codes refer to life situations outside of therapy. They are not used to decide if a client belongs in a group, but they may be the focus of a group, especially when the goals of the group include community integration or reintegration.

d910 Community Life

Engaging in all aspects of community social life, such as engaging in charitable organizations, service clubs, or professional social organizations. Ceremonies are included in this code, so termination ceremonies and other presentations of awards may be taught with creative arts groups.

d920 Recreation and Leisure

Engaging in any form of play, recreational, or leisure activity, such as informal or organized play and sports, programs of physical fitness, relaxation, amusement or diversion, going to art galleries, museums, cinemas, or theaters; engaging in crafts or hobbies, reading for enjoyment, playing musical instruments; sightseeing, tourism, and traveling for pleasure. Four-digit codes are shown below.

- d9200 Play

Engaging in games with rules or unstructured or unorganized games and spontaneous recreation, such as playing chess or cards, or children's play.

Play is a necessary component for healthy development, as well as a human right. Play develops imagination; develops dexterity and physical, cognitive, and emotional strength; contributes to healthy brain development; provides a context to engage, create, explore, and interact with the world; provides a context for conquering fears while practicing roles; helps to develop new competencies that enhance confidence and resilience to face future challenges; helps teach how to work in groups, to share, to negotiate, to resolve conflicts, and learn self-advocacy skills; provides opportunities to practice decision-making skills, move at one's own pace and discover areas of interest leading to full engagement in passionate interests; builds active, healthy bodies; creates feelings of joy; provides a context to express views, experiences, and frustrations; helps with adjustment to school and enhances learning readiness, learning behaviors, and problem solving skills; and fosters development of social-emotional learning (Ginsburg, 2007). All the creative arts groups have one or more aspects of this description of play.

- d9201 Sports

Engaging in competitive and informal or formally organized games or athletic events, performed alone or in a group, such as bowling, gymnastics, or soccer. This is not part of creative arts.

- d9202 Arts and Culture

Engaging in, or appreciating, fine arts or cultural events, such as going to the theater, cinema, museum, or art gallery, or acting in a play, reading for enjoyment, or playing a musical instrument. Visual and tactile arts, theater games and improvisation, music, dance and movement, writing and poetry, puppetry, and integration all have group activities that are related to this code.

- d9203 Crafts

Engaging in handicrafts, such as pottery or knitting. Visual and tactile arts, masks, and puppetry could all be considered crafts.

- d9204 Hobbies

Engaging in pastimes such as collecting stamps, coins, or antiques.

- d9205 Socializing

Engaging in informal or casual gatherings with others, such as visiting friends or relatives or meeting informally in public places. Creative groups are not considered socializing, but some of them teach clients how to socialize more effectively. The ones with the most activities include theater games, laughter and clowning, music, and integration.

d930 Religion and Spirituality

Engaging in religious or spiritual activities, organizations and practices for self-fulfillment, finding meaning, religious or spiritual value, and establishing connection with a divine power, such as is involved in attending a church, temple, mosque, or synagogue, praying or chanting for a religious purpose, and spiritual contemplation. Creative arts groups using masks, music, and meditation may touch on religion and spirituality.

d940 Human Rights

Enjoying all nationally and internationally recognized rights that are accorded to people by virtue of their humanity alone, such as human rights as recognized by the United Nations Universal Declaration of Human Rights (1948) and the United Nations Standard Rules for the Equalization of Opportunities for Persons with Disabilities (1993); the right to self-determination or autonomy; and the right to control over one's destiny.

d950 Political Life and Citizenship

Engaging in the social, political, and governmental life of a citizen, having legal status as a citizen and enjoying the rights, protections, privileges, and duties associated with that role, such as the right to vote and run for political office, to form political associations; enjoying the rights and freedoms associated with citizenship (e.g., the rights of freedom of speech, association, religion, protection against unreasonable search and seizure, the right to counsel, to a trial, and other legal rights and protection against discrimination); having legal standing as a citizen. This code is not a focus of creative arts groups.

Environmental Factors

Environmental Factors are things in the environment that facilitate or present barriers for the client. It is divided into five chapters. Therapists who are leading creative arts groups evaluate the environment of the place where the group is being held to make sure that it is as supportive as possible for the clients in the group. Different sets of clients will have different needs for the best environment, so the therapist needs to evaluate these factors for each group.

Chapter 1 Products and Technology

This chapter is about the natural or human-made products or systems of products, equipment, and technology in an individual's immediate environment that are gathered, created, produced, or manufactured. The ISO 9999 classification of technical aids defines these as "any product, instrument, equipment, or technical system used by a disabled person, especially produced or generally available, preventing, compensating, monitoring, relieving, or neutralizing" disability. It is recognized that any product or technology can be assistive. For the purposes of this classification of environmental factors, however, assistive products and technology are defined more narrowly as any product, instrument, equipment, or technology adapted or specially designed for improving functioning of a disabled person. Therapists should consider all these types of manufactured products when assessing what will help clients succeed in the group. The areas below include general products as well as assistive products. The three-digit codes as shown.

e110 Products or Substances for Personal Consumption
e115 Products and Technology for Personal Use in Daily Living
e120 Products and Technology for Personal Indoor and Outdoor Mobility and Transportation
e125 Products and Technology for Communication
e130 Products and Technology for Education
e135 Products and Technology for Employment
e140 Products and Technology for Culture, Recreation, and Sport
e145 Products and Technology for the Practice of Religion or Spirituality
e150 Design, Construction, and Building Products and Technology of Buildings for Public Use
e155 Design, Construction, and Building Products and Technology of Buildings for Private Use
e160 Products and Technology of Land Development
e165 Assets

Chapter 2 Natural Environment and Human-Made Changes to Environment

This chapter is about animate and inanimate elements of the natural or physical environment, and components of that environment that have been modified by people, as well as characteristics of human populations within that environment. Codes e210 Physical Geography to e235 Human-Caused Events are not something a therapist can control. The codes after that should be carefully considered to provide the best environment for clients. Three-digit codes are shown.

e210 Physical Geography
e215 Population
e220 Flora and Fauna
e225 Climate
e230 Natural Events
e235 Human-Caused Events
e240 Light
e245 Time-Related Changes

e250 Sound
e255 Vibration
e260 Air Quality

Chapter 3 Support and Relationships

This chapter is about people or animals that provide practical physical or emotional support, nurturing, protection, assistance, and relationships to other persons, in their home, place of work, school, or at play or in other aspects of their daily activities. The chapter does not encompass the attitudes of the person or people that are providing the support. The environmental factor being described is not the person or animal, but the amount of physical and emotional support the person or animal provides.

Therapists should work to make sure the people clients interact with in creative arts groups provide appropriate support. The most important part of this code is the therapist's support. Interactions between clients are probably better considered in d7 Interpersonal Interactions and Relationships. Dealing with lack of support can be worked on in masks, theater games, drama therapy, laughter, and puppetry. The three-digit codes are shown.

e310 Immediate Family
e315 Extended Family
e320 Friends
e325 Acquaintances, Peers, Colleagues, Neighbors, and Community Members
e330 People in Positions of Authority
e335 People in Subordinate Positions
e340 Personal Care Providers and Personal Assistants
e345 Strangers
e350 Domesticated Animals
e355 Health Professionals
e360 Other Professionals

Chapter 4 Attitudes

This chapter is about the attitudes that are the observable consequences of customs, practices, ideologies, values, norms, factual beliefs, and religious beliefs. These attitudes influence individual behavior and social life at all levels, from interpersonal relationships and community associations to political, economic, and legal structures. The attitudes classified are those of people external to the person whose situation is being described. They are not those of the person themselves. Values and beliefs are not coded separately from attitudes as they are assumed to be the driving forces behind the attitudes.

Therapists should work to make sure the attitudes of the people clients interact with in creative arts groups are the best possible for the client. The most important part of this code is the therapist's attitude. Dealing with the attitudes of others is something that can be worked on in masks, theater games, drama therapy, laughter, and puppetry. The three-digit codes are shown.

e410 Individual Attitudes of Immediate Family Members
e415 Individual Attitudes of Extended Family Members
e420 Individual Attitudes of Friends
e425 Individual Attitudes of Acquaintances, Peers, Colleagues, Neighbors, and Community Members
e430 Individual Attitudes of People in Positions of Authority
e435 Individual Attitudes of People in Subordinate Positions
e440 Individual Attitudes of Personal Care Providers and Personal Assistants
e445 Individual Attitudes of Strangers
e450 Individual Attitudes of Health Professionals
e455 Individual Attitudes of Health-Related Professionals
e460 Societal Attitudes
e465 Social Norms, Practices, and Ideologies

Chapter 5 Services, Systems, and Policies

This chapter is about:

- Services that provide benefits, structured programs, and operations, in various sectors of society, designed to meet the needs of individuals.
- Systems that are administrative control and organizational mechanisms, and are established by governments at the local, regional, national, and international levels, or by other recognized authorities.

- Policies constituted by rules, regulations, conventions, and standards established by governments at the local, regional, national, and international levels, or by other recognized authorities.

They are not part of creative arts groups, except occasionally when the group is looking at how to deal with lack of services. The three-digit codes are shown.

e510 Services, Systems, and Policies for the Production of Consumer Goods

e515 Architecture and Construction Services, Systems, and Policies

e520 Open Space Planning Services, Systems, and Policies

e525 Housing Services, Systems, and Policies

e530 Utilities Services, Systems, and Policies

e535 Communication Services, Systems, and Policies

e540 Transportation Services, Systems, and Policies

e545 Civil Protection Services, Systems, and Policies

e550 Legal Services, Systems, and Policies

e555 Associations and Organizational Services, Systems, and Policies

e565 Economic Services, Systems, and Policies

e570 Social Security Services, Systems, and Policies

e575 General Social Support Services, Systems, and Policies

e580 Health Services, Systems, and Policies

e585 Education and Training Services, Systems, and Policies

e590 Labor and Employment Services, Systems, and Policies

e595 Political Services, Systems, and Policies

References

Ginsburg, K. (2007). The importance of play in promoting healthy child development and maintaining strong parent-child bonds. *Pediatrics, 119*(1), 182-191.

Hocevar, B. & Gray, M. (2008). Intestinal diversion (colostomy or ileostomy) in patients with severe bowel dysfunction following spinal cord injury. *J Wound Ostomy Continence Nursing, 35*(2), 159-166.

Porter, H. (2016). *Recreational therapy and the international classification of functioning, disability, and health.* Ravensdale, WA: Idyll Arbor.

World Health Organization. (2016). International classification of functioning, disability and health (English version). © Copyright 2015, 2016. Used with permission.

Accessed from the ICF Browser June 2015 through February 2016. http://apps.who.int/classifications/icfbrowser/Default.aspx

9

Visual and Tactile Arts

This chapter provides an overview of concepts relating to art and art therapy and offers activity ideas for using visual arts with clients. The term "visual and tactile arts" refers to a product or process that uses art materials to create a form that can be experienced by seeing or touching.

This area can demand a lot of a therapist's time and budget in procuring and organizing materials, but it has the capacity to engage clients with a wide range of ages and backgrounds. Most people who have gone through the school system have had some exposure to art and have some associations that help them connect to the topic when it is introduced. Some clients may have had more positive experiences in art than others, but at least there is some basis for communication with most clients.

Helping clients learn about themselves from these art activities involves several stages of processing. First there is the pure *doing* of the activity, which uses both the thinking mind and the expressive mind.

Once the activity is completed, it is important to help clients decipher and digest what they have experienced. This is achieved by having clients answer questions or reflect on some part of the art activity using writing. Writing uses symbols to communicate ideas and helps bring the ideas into the client's consciousness.

Finally, clients are invited to share what happened or what they learned with a partner or the group as a whole. Expressing ideas in words clarifies thoughts and allows other group members to give feedback and provide more insight for the individual. It is the therapist's job to do whatever s/he can to make the learning real and to plant a helpful concept in the mind of the client, so it has a chance to incubate and grow.

Research has shown a long list of positive effects from working with visual and tactile arts. Specific studies that support the efficacy will be found in the descriptions of experiences and modalities discussed below. Here is a summary of the findings.

- Improved reminiscing
- Increased interactions
- Increased vitality and quality of life
- Increased psychological well being
- Increased self-esteem
- Increased coping skills and resiliency for homeless youth
- Increased attention
- Increased growth developmental level
- Interest in personal aesthetics
- Increased positive behaviors
- Increased cognitive function and memory
- Better decision making
- Better completion of task
- Decreased depression
- Decreased anxiety
- Decreased impulsive behaviors
- Psychological adjustment to loss, change, and cancer survival

Visual Arts Experiences

In visual arts there are a range of expressions that classify the activities, with each activity having its own purpose.

Fine Arts

Traditionally this refers to art, such as painting, drawing, or sculpture, that focuses on the aesthetic (pure beauty) and is created for its own sake. The individual expresses his/her own views and feelings about a subject and takes pleasure in using the materials to create a form that can be experienced by the artist and others. The process of creating the art may have therapeutic value to the artist but this is not a goal for fine arts.

Crafts

This refers to art, such as weaving, jewelry making, and ceramics, that is produced for utilitarian purposes. The artist is making something that can be used by people in their homes and in their lives.

Therapeutic Art

This refers to art therapy or techniques used in therapeutic interventions. In this realm the focus is on *process* rather than on the product. The therapist is a facilitator of experiences that can lead to increased psychological well-being.

While these categories help to differentiate functions of art, there are many examples where the categories overlap. These help us to view the categories more flexibly. For example, a mask created for a therapeutic purpose may have beauty and capture the essence of human experience, so it can also be thought of as fine art. Or an individual engaged in making a craft may experience feelings of well-being and calm that make the art therapeutic.

Skills Involved in Art Activities

Clients are likely to be receiving a therapist's services because they are having problems and are functioning below their optimum level. While engaging in creative arts activities may enhance clients' functional skills and quality of life, asking them to become involved in activities that are beyond their abilities may actually cause harm. The art activities suggested in this chapter assume that clients have a certain skill set. Consult this checklist if there is any doubt about the ability of a group member to participate in art activities in general or in using a particular medium.

- Some degree of muscle and hand-eye coordination
- Reasonable endurance for starting and engaging in activity
- Tolerance and willingness to touch clay and other supplies which make one "dirty" (not tactilely defensive)
- Basic problem-solving skills

- Ability to follow one-, two-, or three-step instructions
- Ability to function independently in a semi-structured environment
- Basic communication and listening skills
- Willingness to relate to others
- Basic social skills
- Capacity to deal with emotions evoked by activities

Art Materials in Therapeutic Situations

The therapist can use art materials to refine behavior as well as to encourage expression and enhance learning. As the therapist develops his/her treatment goals for a group, s/he will need to make sure that the art medium complements the desired goals. Some art media encourage active, expressive movements, while other media encourage expression within very specific limits.

Some of these materials are included in more than one category, being, for instance, both compulsive and expressive. The psychological issues involved in a particular project define the way each type of material is used. In addition to using these materials, drawing is always a possibility, especially with the idea of drawing *feelings* rather than objects.

Compulsive Art Materials

Restrictive, limiting boundaries. These can be ego supporting and help enhance impulse control.

- sticks, wood
- pencils with rulers
- weavings
- mosaics
- monoprints, stencils, rubbings
- manipulating geometric forms

Regressive Art Materials

Can lead to regression due to inability to find or control boundaries, psychological and/or concrete. Can be very satisfying if the client is able to use them.

- clay (has no form)
- finger paints
- watercolors

Aggressive Art Materials

Allow for expression of anger and aggression. These can be used to elicit repressed feelings or as a way of sublimating the action of aggression.

- Torn-paper collage
- wood and nails
- splatter painting
- clay

Expressive Art Materials

Allow for non-verbal expression of thoughts, feelings, and ideas.

- crayon
- collage
- felt-tip pen
- crayon resist
- body outline
- chalk
- string painting
- paper masks
- mobiles
- cut photo paper
- puppets
- pencil
- wood sculptures
- brush painting

Drawing, Painting, and Collage

The activities offered in this section are done using some method of drawing, painting, or collage. It is helpful to focus on how these therapeutic processes promote self-awareness and expression.

Drawing

A line can be a powerful and evocative tool for individual expression. A dark, heavy line could express sadness or, perhaps, anger. A pale, delicate line could communicate fragility or insecurity. Through drawing, the client uses line, color, shape, and texture to help express existing feelings that are difficult to verbalize and communicate.

Have large sheets of paper (at least 18" x 24") available so that group members can be expansive by using more of their bodies in drawing. Colored pencils, felt tip pens, crayons, charcoal, and pastels are all appropriate media. In using painting or drawing have participant(s) answer open-ended questions such as, "How do you feel at this moment?" or "Where are you right now in your life?"

Painting

Making strokes, shapes, and textures on paper using a brush and paint can give clients a feeling of movement and fluidity. It is especially helpful for a client who has blocked feelings and/or modes of expression. When working on opening blocks to expression, have clients paint standing up using a large piece of paper taped to an easel or the wall. This enables clients to see more clearly what they are doing, to use more of their body in the painting process, to feel freedom of movement, and to tap into emotions that are locked up in parts of the body. Have them warm up by painting for five minutes, then ten minutes, and finally give them a time frame for a longer piece of work. In the beginning, clients will need help structuring the time they spend on each painting. The goal is for the clients to eventually become sensitive to when their paintings are finished.

Collage

From the French *coller* — to glue — collage is a technique of art creation. It is primarily used in the visual arts. The artwork is made by assembling many forms, thus creating a new whole. A collage may include magazine and newspaper clippings, ribbons, paint, bits of colored or handmade papers, texts, feathers, photographs, fabric, leaves, and other found objects. They are glued to a piece of paper or canvas. The origins of collage can be traced back hundreds of years, but this technique became a distinctive part of modern art in the beginning of the 20th century.

Research

Hattori et al. (2011) conducted a quasi-experimental study by randomly assigning 39 patients with Alzheimer's disease to either an art therapy group or a control group. The art therapy group had the primary task of coloring abstract patterns with crayons or water-based paint (N=20). The control group performed simple mathematical calculations (N=19). Groups were conducted for twelve weeks. Family members and caretakers accompanied the participants, and group sizes were a maximum of five people. Cognitive function and memory were evaluated using the Mini-Mental State Examination and the logical memory subscale of the Wechsler Memory Scale. Mood and vitality were evaluated using the Geriatric Depression Scale (GDS) and Apathy Scale (Japanese version). The quality of life (QOL) was evaluated using the short form (SF-8) which included physical and mental viewpoints. Behavior abnormalities were evaluated using the Dementia Behavior Disturbance Scale (DBD). Caregiver burden was addressed. The results showed significant improvement in the Apathy Scale for the art therapy group in comparison to the control group (p=0.014) and in the Mini-Mental State Examination score (p=0.0150). There were no significant differences between the groups in the other items. Patients in all groups showing a 10% improvement were then compared between the two groups and significant improvement in quality of life (QOL) was observed in the art therapy group over the control group. The results show that the art therapy interventions improve vitality and quality of life for patients with mild Alzheimer's disease.

Traditional verbal therapy with its emphasis on verbal communication between therapist and client may not be appropriate for patients with dementia due to impaired cognitive and verbal abilities. Stallings (2010) did a qualitative study on the use of collage in art therapy to aid in the process of reminiscence for individuals with dementia. Data were collected and analyzed using a modified Magazine Photo Collage assessment (Landgarten, 1993) with three participants. Findings support the hypothesis that collage gives older adults with dementia an opportunity to express information that they might not be fully capable of verbalizing. Participants' interactions with collage as a therapeutic modality also were examined, as well as their interactions with the researcher.

A study by Julliard (1995) looked at whether a collage intervention would help addicts accept step one of a twelve-step program — admitting powerlessness over the addiction. Six outpatient adult clients participated in the art therapy intervention. Each client made a collage expressive of addiction and recovery. Gilbert's (1991) Steps Questionnaire was used to measure belief in the step. It was administered just before group members started the collages and again nine days later after the collages had been discussed. A factor analytic method was used for scoring along with a Rasch. A direct measure, the Daily Check-In was administered at 5 pm to assess the previous 24 hours. "Patients estimated the percentage of time they spent thinking about using their drug or about their addictive behavior and indicated whether drugs seemed intensely or mildly appealing, neutral, or intensely or mildly unappealing". (The instrument is provided in the article). Patients began using the Daily Check-In one week before the collage activity and this was continued for at least a week after. The Steps Questionnaire was administered once immediately before the collage activity and again after group discussion. The study found that art therapy and role-playing interventions increased participant belief in Step One among individuals who were chemically dependent.

Drawing, Painting, and Collage Activities

Drawing Objects Game (a version of Pictionary)

Players are divided into two teams at equal distance from the leader. Each has a stack of paper and pencils. The group leader has a list of objects (like a Christmas tree or a house) and people (like a cook or fireman) who have distinguishing characteristics. One player from each team comes to the leader in the center. The leader tells the two players one object or person to draw. Each member runs back to his/her team and draws it. The first member on a team to correctly guess the object or person being drawn wins. Remind groups that no talking is allowed.

Picture Mosaic and Enlargement

Choose a colorful and interesting photograph or a picture from a magazine. Cut it into equally sized squares and on the back make an identification so you will know the how to reassemble the pieces. Show the entire picture to the group briefly. Then, give each group member or pair of participants a piece of the picture and a larger piece of paper to depict and enlarge their part. The goal is to recreate the essence of their part of the picture. It does not need to be a duplication. At the end, reassemble the parts and glue them to a large sheet of cardboard.

Combining Art and Music

Butcher paper with a large circle drawn in the middle is laid out on the floor. Each group member draws a picture of an animal with its tail inside the center circle. To play, the leader steps on tails and, when a particular tail is stepped on, the designated participant makes the animal sound or another note until the leader moves off the tail. This activity can also be developed as a storytelling process.

Symphony of Emotions on Paper

Participants are asked to think about how they feel and express their feelings on paper with crayons, markers, or paint. Then, each person is asked to produce a sound representative of their emotion. When a person's picture is touched by the leader, the person makes his/her sound. The leader conducts a symphony of emotions. Everyone must pay attention and begin and end exactly on cue.

Group Mural

Each person picks one colored crayon or magic marker and decides on one shape to draw during the entire activity. Examples include a line, dot, circle, or squiggle. One long, continuous piece of paper is spread out on a table or the floor. People line up on all sides of the paper and draw their shapes on one section of the paper for approximately one minute. The leader says "switch" and each person moves to a new section and draws his/her shape again. The activity is repeated until the mural is completed.

Mural of a Town

Attach a large sheet of butcher paper to a wall with masking tape. Provide a variety of materials: paints, crayons, and felt-tip pens. Scissors, glue, and tactile objects like yarn and crepe paper can also be used. The group, through discussion and compromise, designs a town. A basic outline is agreed upon. Then each person chooses a different part of the town such as a building or park to work on. Each individual will need to look at his/her own needs for food, clothing, safety, and entertainment, for example, in deciding what form the town will take. Suggest that individuals check with their potential neighbors (i.e., other group members) and make necessary accommodations for each other's needs. When the mural is completed, the group can discuss how they feel about their town.

Initials

Provide sheets of paper, pencils, felt-tip markers, and crayons. Each participant draws his/her own initials in the style, size, and color s/he wishes. The initials may be plain or elaborate, large or small depending on what individuals wish to share about themselves with other members of the group. Clients are invited to share their completed drawings and talk about them, if they want to.

Drawing Pass

Each client gets one piece of paper and is asked to draw a few lines on it and sign it. The paper is then passed to the right and the next person adds to the previous drawing. This sequence is repeated until the paper is returned to its original creator. The results can be shared or not. Thoughts and feelings about the task can be discussed.

Collage for Remembering and Reminiscence

(Amanda Stuart, 2017)

Provide magazine pictures, copies of photographs, and colored paper. Feathers, flowers, leaves (real or artificial), fabric, and other materials may be added for depth and texture. Scissors and glue sticks or liquid glue are used for assembly. Hot glue or superglue may be needed for some of the objects. Have the client select one sheet of colored paper as the base for the collage. If they wish, clients can draw designs for the collage before starting to cut pictures. Clients use scissors to cut pictures into shapes of their own choosing. Once the pictures are cut, the client arranges the pictures and other material onto the paper. Remind the client it is all right for the pictures to overlap each other or the sides of the paper. When the arrangement is complete, the client or the therapist applies glue to the back of the pictures and places them onto the colored paper base in the selected positions. The client may choose to add more pictures, objects, and/or colored paper after the first set of material is glued on.

Clay

Working with earth is one of our earliest artistic experiences. As children, many of us made mud pies and even whole mud villages. If you close your eyes and remember the cool, smooth feel of earth, you will understand why clay is an appealing and therapeutic modality. Earth is one of the traditional four elements. In human experience and thought it is an ancient icon of nature, growth, and mother.

Working with clay has a calming influence on many clients, especially if the initial focus of the work is on process rather than product. As clients become more familiar with the medium, the results of their work can be striking.

Objectives

- To become comfortable with and sensitive to the medium of clay through tactile exploration
- To allow for the release of tension and expression of feelings through clay
- To show how the use of clay can be a bridge to interaction with other people

Research

Doric-Henry (1997) used an eight-session pottery class based on Eastern-method throwing techniques to test if it improved psychological well-being. Quantitative evaluation included a forgiveness scale (Hebl & Enright, 1993) self-esteem (Coopersmith, 1981), depression (Beck Depression Inventory, Beck et al., 1961), and anxiety (State-Trait Anxiety Inventory, Spielberger et al., 1983). Twenty elderly residents in a nursing home were compared with 20 nonparticipating residents. Following the intervention, the participating group showed significantly improved measures of self-esteem, and reduced anxiety and depression ($p < .05$) relative to the comparison group.

Elkis-Abuhoff et al. (2008) looked at art therapy as a support for medical treatment and palliative care. A total of 41 patients were placed in two matched groups. There were 22 patients with Parkinson's disease and 19 patients without Parkinson's disease. Each participant completed the Brief Symptom Inventory (BSI) (Derogatis, 1993) in pre- and post-test sessions and was asked to manipulate a ball of clay and to respond to follow-up questions on the experience. Quantitative BSI results and qualitative results showed a positive outcome with significant decreases in somatic and emotional symptoms in both groups. The research supports the value of a therapeutic clay program for patients diagnosed with Parkinson's disease and recommends future studies addressing art therapy with caregivers.

Clay Activities

As with a blank piece of paper, a lump of clay can be very intimidating to clients. It takes a while for people to learn how to work clay and to create a shape that communicates an idea or feeling. When clients first look at the clay, they will want to make something out of the lump in front of them. Try to de-emphasize this desire to create something representational by focusing on process rather than product. By taking the time to explore the clay, a client can experience the meditative and calming value of working with clay. How willing clients are to enjoy the journey (process) rather than the destination (product) is valuable information about each person.

Clay Exploration (Warmups)

- Provide enough clay for each individual and also water and sponges for clean-up.
- Have each person take a piece of clay. Encourage exploring the properties of the clay: Is it wet, cold, elastic? Suggest that group members knead, stretch, flatten, tear, squeeze, and poke holes through the clay. Optional materials: rolling pins, shaping tools, and fabrics (e.g., lace) that will transfer texture to the clay
- Ask group members to create a shape with their clay that shows how they are feeling. The form may be abstract or representational.
- Allow group members to talk about their shape if they wish. This activity encourages self-expression and gives the therapist a clue to each person's emotional state.

Create a Fantasy Creature

Ask participants to imagine themselves as a creature and make that creature with the clay. Encourage each person to describe his/her creature or have it "speak" to the group. Ask each person to be his/her creature and introduce him/herself as "I am…," and/or to speak about what it's like to be that creature.

Variation: Ask group members to imagine themselves as an object or symbol (e.g., star, tree, mountain) and create that image in clay. Continue as above by having each person in the group introduce him/herself. For example, "I am the star burning inside, too hot to get close to..."

Create in Pairs

Divide the group into pairs. Ask the partners to create something together. It can be a place they would like to be or something fun they would like to do together. Ask them to include themselves in the sculpture.

Self-Portrait in Clay

Instruct group members to make their self-portrait in sculpture. Ask participants to depict themselves as they believe they really are, which includes their feelings and current state of being. For example, if anger is a dominate emotion, the sculpture should reflect that emotion. Group members can also depict how they would like to be or feel. Discussion of the activity should deal with the differences between the images of how they are and how they wish to be. Ask what actions might help them reach a more desirable state of being.

Activities Grouped by Therapeutic Outcome

These techniques come from art therapists who use a variety of techniques, depending on the desired outcomes for their clients. The six categories, developed by art therapist James Denny (1972), are classified according to the kinds of effects they are expected to produce in the participant. The outcomes are exploration, rapport building, expression of inner feelings, self-perception, interpersonal relations, and the individuals place in the world.

Depending on the stage of the group's development, some activities will be challenging to introduce to the members. For example, a therapist wouldn't use an activity like *Self-Portrait* with a new group. One of the exercises to explore media would be more appropriate. Each of the six categories is described with suggestions for identifiable behavioral goals.

Research

A study by Alders and Levine-Madori (2010) investigated the efficacy of art therapy to enhance cognitive performance in a sample of 24 elderly Hispanic/Latina members of a community center who participated once a week in a 12-week structured Thematic Therapeutic Arts Program. Participants who attended the art therapy sessions showed greater improvement on a Clock Drawing Test and the Cognitive Failures Questionnaire than those who did not attend. Further testing needs to be done with randomly assigned test and control groups, but the findings suggest that the art therapy sessions may enhance cognitive abilities.

Making visual art (Reynolds, Vivat, & Prior, 2011) has been found helpful in reducing perceptions of pain among people with osteoarthritis.

Wood, Molassiotis, and Payne (2011) conducted a systematic review of literature related to art therapy and cancer. A total of 14 studies were found. They investigated emotional, physical, social, and global functioning, and existential and spiritual concerns. Art therapy was successfully used to manage treatment-related symptoms and facilitate psychological adjustments to loss, change, and cancer survival.

A study by Olsson, Kucharewski, and Fedorenko, (1999) looked at using therapeutic arts in a recreational therapy academic program. Art is utilized by recreational therapists to facilitate function, psychological and emotional health, and quality of life.

Prescott et al. (2008) utilized both quantitative (N=212) and qualitative (n=3) measures to examine the function of creativity and art making with respect to resiliency in homeless youth who were attending a drop-in art center. Quantitative methods identified a strong correlation between an individual's engagement in creative activity and his or her achievement. Qualitative methods included individual stories derived from interviews. Drawings illustrated how participants valued the role of art in making healthy lifestyle choices. Creativity may be a critical component of resiliency in the lives of homeless youth.

Exploration

Exploration activities are especially useful in the initial sessions of a group when the therapist is trying to introduce clients to the art experience. Many therapists will continue to use exploratory exercises throughout the sessions, sometimes as warmup or closure activities. These activities are similar to free association and encourage spontaneous expression. Since they focus not on product but on process, they help release conscious controls on expression. The techniques are simple, direct, and liberating.

Behavioral Goals

- Spontaneous expression by drawing on paper with various art media.
- Become acquainted (or reacquainted) with art materials by using four different types of media in some way.
- Explore the use of these media in making lines, symbols, and forms, and by making a design using at least two different media.

Scribble Drawings

Have clients do these with eyes open and/or shut. Be sensitive to the group and how long they are comfortable doing this kind of open-ended activity. For a number of these freeform activities, start with one minute and gradually add more time.

Finger Painting

For adults this can be a regressive kind of experience and can evoke memories of childhood. It is a kind of scribbling that uses more of the body. Slick finger-painting paper eases the experience and flow of finger painting.

Free Drawings

The choices of subject and media are left to the client. Free (spontaneous) expression is encouraged. Planning the picture is discouraged. Initially, free drawing should be done for one to two minutes. Then the amount of time can be gradually increased. Encourage clients to maintain an empty mind and not preconceive stories or images.

Ink Blot

Using watercolors or ink, create a blob of color on the paper. The paper may then be folded (by client or therapist) like a Rorschach inkblot. Write a story or make a statement about the image on the paper.

Straw Painting

Place a blob of liquid color on paper and gently blow on the color with a straw. The result might suggest an image or evoke a thought or feeling.

Build a Curiosity Picture

Write two letters (e.g., G and H) on a piece of paper. Use crayons, markers, or oil pastels to create an abstract design out of the letters by connecting lines, filling spaces, putting in squiggles, or any other means. Many clients are intimidated by a blank sheet of paper — having something already on the paper can help motivate the client (Landgarten, 1981).

Watercolor/Crayon Resist

This activity encourages exploration of flow and resistance effects. Crayon is used to make designs on paper. Then watercolor paints are applied. The crayon "resists" the flow of the watercolors, creating interesting patterns.

Clay

Exploration is especially helpful when introducing clay to an inexperienced group. This means experiencing the feel of the clay — its texture and movement possibilities. The clients should be encouraged to roll and pound the clay, to form and crumble shapes. Helps to acquaint clients with how the medium works.

Edible Art

This technique is especially good for children or individuals with visual challenges. Introduce finger-painting by using pudding or icing with food coloring. Incorporate the senses of taste, smell, and touch. Sculpture can be made with oatmeal or bread dough. Printmaking can be done with vegetables and fruits.

Automatic Drawing

Good for bypassing the critical mind that wants everything to look "right." Some ideas:

- Make free lines or scribbles on paper first with eyes open and then with eyes closed.
- Draw using the non-dominant hand.
- Draw by not taking the hand off the paper until the picture is complete.

Media and Color Exploration

- Make blobs and dribbles on wet paper with watercolor.
- Make blobs and dribbles on paper with ink.
- Make a non-representational, freeform design with pastels or crayons.
- Make a design using two different types of media.

Rapport Building

This set of techniques is designed to facilitate a more natural transition between creation and exploration. The techniques help prepare the client to express ideas and feelings by connecting with another person.

Behavioral Goals

- Conceptualize ideas that can be shared.
- Share ideas with another person.
- Create something with the support of another group member.
- Encourage exchanges between participants.

- Support development of a group identity.

Pair Scribble

Members form pairs, each has his/her own drawing tool, but they share a piece of paper. They are not to speak but to somehow work together to fill the page during a period of three to five minutes. What occurs depends on the personalities of the group. The natural leaders lead, the followers tend to follow, and the negotiators work out compromise and cooperation. This activity reveals a client's unconscious style of doing things.

Variation: Scribble and Completion. One person makes a scribble and the other person converts the scribble into an image or builds upon the scribble in some other way.

Pictionary

The game of Pictionary™, which involves guessing a word or phrase from an image drawn on paper, is a good way to introduce playfulness into the art process. The game also helps people address the fear of drawing images on a blank piece of paper.

Non-Verbal "Conversation"

Advanced pair scribbling. Create a design in five minutes. Draw shapes, lines, colors, and symbols without talking. This may help reveal how communication works within a family. Parallels may be discovered between the way clients behave in this situation and the way they behave at home.

Something to Do Together

Promotes sharing of ideas and negotiation. Decide on something you and your art partner would like to do together — like taking a walk — and depict it, including yourselves in the picture.

Painting Completion

Begin a free drawing and pass it to a partner for additions. Continue to pass it back and forth until the process feels complete.

Building Together

Build something together without verbal interaction. Recycled materials like cardboard tubes and shapes, bits of fabric, and yarn can be used for this activity.

Back Drawing

One person's back is the canvas. The creator faces the canvas (the partner's back) and "draws" using his/her finger. The "canvas" then transfers onto paper what s/he perceives as the design. Ask the creator to keep the drawing very simple and work slowly to help the "canvas" comprehend the image. Reverse roles.

Message Sending

Using images, symbols, colors, and shapes send a message about yourself to a partner or a message to everyone in the group. Some other ideas include:

- Send a message to your partner that expresses a positive quality you have noticed and appreciate about him/her.
- Create a wish for your partner.
- Share a concern you have about your partner.

Expression of Inner Feelings

These activities are done to encourage exploration of feelings and fantasies and to create visual representations of them. Anxiety may increase or decrease as a client's awareness of his/her feelings broadens. The therapist may assist a client by clarifying feelings and helping to identify problem-solving strategies.

Behavioral Goals

- Express and face feelings at least once during the session by painting or drawing lines, symbols, or forms that represent at least one aspect of how the client feels.
- Express one feeling or mood using at least one color other than black or white.
- Use art to nonverbally express something related to a personal problem at least once during the group.
- Verbally interpret a drawing to one other person.
- Interact with one other person by expressing one idea that comes to mind when viewing another person's drawing.
- Share interest in the feelings of at least two other people by asking each at least one question about each creation.

Affective Words #1

Divide the paper into six to eight sections. The participants are given about a minute to respond spontaneously with images, color, or symbols to key words spoken by the therapist. The words may come from the therapist or be compiled through group brainstorming. Suggestions include words like love, hate, freedom, responsibility, anger, anxiety, faith, father, mother, trust, rejection, hope, etc. It can be interesting to use polarities such as strength/weakness, independence/inter-dependence. Compare similarities and differences in responses within the group.

Affective Words #2

Write words connoting feelings on small pieces of paper. Fold the papers and place them in a box for the whole group. Shake the box and have each member of the group draw out a piece of paper. Have each client draw or paint what the chosen word means to him/her without verbalizing the word to the others in the group. Through discussion, the group attempts to match the words with the pictures. Match the correct words with the pictures. Share feelings about the experience.

How Do I Feel Now?

Participants are asked to fold a paper into three sections. In the first section, the client is asked to depict through drawing how s/he is feeling at this moment. In the third section the client responds to the question, "How would you like to feel?" In the middle section, the client tries to express what is in between or what steps would lead to feeling better.

Create a Care Package for Yourself

Include both tangible (e.g., cookies, music) and intangible (e.g., love, trust, hope) objects that fit your tastes and needs.

Three Wishes

Depict three wishes expressing what you want most out of life. Discussion may then focus on commonalties and differences in the group and also on issues of attainability.

Road of Life (Picture Autobiography) #1

Each participant is asked to depict the road or path of life that s/he has been traveling the past few years. The client may go back further. The therapist may suggest the inclusion of three accomplishments.

Road of Life (Picture Autobiography) #2

Each participant is asked to paint the road or path that s/he has been traveling in life. Then each participant tries to remember how s/he was feeling at certain points along this road. An extension of this work would be depicting, in drawing or painting, the road a participant hopes to or expects to travel in the future.

Want to Do

Using symbols, images, and color draw a picture of yourself doing something you have never done but have always wanted to do. Include in the picture how you think you would feel doing this activity.

Create a Me Collage or Me Box

This project is a kind of autobiography and helps the individual become aware of him/herself in deeper ways. Paint or cover the outside of a box (a small or large box as space allows). Through words, pictures, drawings, stories, and photographs ask the client to use the box to tell about him/herself: friends, likes, dislikes, values, plans, experiences, mistakes, etc. The leader can brainstorm categories with the group.

Joy/Sadness/Wish

Divide the paper into three sections. In the first section think of what it is about the world that brings you joy. It could be the thought that eagles are no longer endangered, or it could be nature in general. In the second section think about your sadness for the world (e.g., hunger, poverty). In the third section draw what you wish for the world.

Anti-Coloring Book

The anti-coloring book was developed as a creative alternative to the traditional coloring book — which may stifle creativity by giving little room for individual input. There are many books in this series. Each page presents an open-ended question or theme along with the beginning of a drawing to get an individual started. S/he has a lot of leeway to complete the drawing in his/her own way. Some examples of open-ended suggestions that fit the "Expression of Inner Feelings" category are

- Do you see your future in the crystal ball?
- If you went away for a long time, whose portrait would you take with you?
- What was the nicest dream you ever had? Your worst nightmare?

Events and Emotion

Using the media of your choice, symbolize some of the events and significant, related emotions you have experienced this week.

Association Drawing

The leader draws an object, event, or feeling which is related to a topic (e.g., alcoholism). The drawing is passed around the group. Each member adds something that further explains, personalizes, or communicates a specific meaning.

Self-Perception — Portrayal of Self

The goal of these activities is to integrate body image with a wider sense of being (e.g., needs, dreams, fears, strengths, values, beliefs).

Behavioral Goals

- Become more aware of body image or self-concept by drawing oneself and other human figures.
- Interact with others by verbally interpreting their drawings of a person to one or more people in the art group.
- Become aware of ideas and meanings that can be expressed as symbols in art and demonstrate understanding of this by using an animal form to express things about oneself.

Hero/Heroine

This is a good activity for identifying qualities that the individual admires and would like to acquire or strengthen. Draw the best man or woman you could be or your hero/heroine. When the drawing is complete, turn the paper over and write a few sentences explaining what it is about this individual you admire. Can you see these qualities in yourself or the potential for developing these qualities or attributes to some degree?

Immediate States of Being

Select one of the following phrases to paint or draw: "I am _____," "I feel _____," "I have _____," or "I do _____." On completion, exchange and discuss paintings or drawings with a partner. Then select a second phrase and do another painting or drawing. Exchange and discuss with a different partner. Exchange impressions about each other's feelings.

Self Book

If you wrote a book about yourself, what would it be titled? Draw the cover and write the forward.

Self-Portrait on Paper

This can be an evocative activity and most likely would be done with a group that has developed some trust in the leader and other members. On one sheet of paper, using any media, depict yourself as you would really like to be (ideal self). On another piece of paper, depict yourself as you believe you really are (perceived or real self). Discussion could include questions like

- What is different about these two images?
- What steps, behaviors, or changes could reduce the gap between these two images?

Animal Side

Ask the clients to choose one or both exercises:

- Depict yourself as the kind of animal you feel you are most like.
- Depict yourself as the animal you would least like to be.

Have the clients discuss or write about their feelings related to their choice(s).

Inside/Outside Box

This activity is a variation on the "Me Box" concept. Use a box to depict two aspects of self. On the outside depict the parts of yourself that you think others see. On the inside of the box show your inside self and your personal qualities. Write about or discuss your feelings related to any differences between the inside and outside.

Body Tracing

This activity requires a lot of floor space. Using a sheet of butcher paper the length of your body, have someone trace your outline as you lie on the paper. Generally, people stretch out full length on the paper, but you could assume a position (e.g., fetal) that has some meaning for you. Embellish the inside with colors, symbols, and images that tell about you, your feelings, and your state of health.

Self Poster

Using any media, make a poster of yourself that addresses the following questions:

- How does your body feel?
- Think of healing. What images come to mind?

Include what is important to you in your life.

Masks

Masks and mask making fall under the category of "Portrayal of Self" and are dealt with extensively in the *Masks* chapter.

Morning Mirror

Draw or paint: What do you look like or feel like when you first get up in the morning?

Positive/Negative Attributes

- Draw or paint three positive characteristics of self.
- Draw or paint one negative characteristic/aspect of self.

Discuss individuals' depictions in the group. Ask how realistic they are.

Variations:

- Express two positive aspects about yourself. Pass papers around for other participants to add qualities.
- Divide a piece of paper in half. On one half depict feelings you would like to get rid of. On the other half show attributes that you would like to develop.

What I Like About Myself

Have each participant create his/her own territory in the room using a piece of butcher paper, making sure his/her name is visible on the paper. Use words, abstract symbols, pictures from magazines, and images to depict your positive qualities — the things you like about yourself. These may be qualities, interests, or accomplishments.

Participants then move around the room and add to another's butcher paper territory the additional qualities they feel that the person has. Post-it Notes work well for this purpose. At the end of the activity, discuss what the individual initially did and what was added and by whom.

Heroic Deed

Draw, paint, and write: You have just performed a heroic deed. This is the picture and the story in the newspaper the next day.

Award

Draw or paint: Award yourself a medal for what you know you do best.

Johari Window Exercise

Depict the proportions that fit for you in various situations and discuss how you might change those proportions. (See Chapter 5, *Therapy Group Dynamics*, for a discussion of Johari Windows and how to determine the proportions for each block.)

Status Change

Through a photo or drawing collage, depict your daily life ____ years ago (your choice) and your daily life now. Write about or discuss your feelings about each situation.

Positive Lifetime Review

This technique will take several sessions to complete. Create an album which shows positive aspects of your life experience. These may include incidents from your past, childhood memories, school activities, family happenings, work experiences, situations which offered pleasure, vacations, friends, social affiliations, hobbies, and sports activities. Any recall which has a positive association can be shown through a representational or abstract portrayal. Memories put into a concrete form may give an individual the opportunity to see the wealth of experience s/he has accrued. This activity may strengthen self-identification, increase self-esteem, and/or stimulate further recall.

Life-Line Drawing

Draw a picture that traces your life from your birth until a time in the future. Mark the important events in your life along the line in some way. This can be done with pictures, designs, or whatever images and symbols you like. You can use crayons, markers, pencils, or whatever is available. It can be as large or as small as you like.

Personal Shield

This shield represents some important parts of you and shows what your goals are. Complete the four sections of the shield:

- Three photos or pictures that describe me.
- (Draw or write) Three things that I'm good at.
- (Draw or write) A present I would give to myself.
- My favorite animal or an animal that is like me.

Colors, size, and shape of any pictures are up to the individual.

I Am a Tree

Draw yourself as a tree — thinking about the kind of tree that most represents who you are. Taking turns, everyone holds up his/her completed drawing and describes the tree, speaking in the first person about the characteristics of the tree. Example: "I am strong, I have lots of energy"; or "I am frail and delicate. I am standing in a storm. Will my roots hold me?"

Then have each member pass his/her drawing to the person on the right, so that everyone has someone else's drawing. Repeat the descriptive process with this new drawing, again taking on the characteristics that you see in the drawing, speaking in the first person.

Each person will see new adjectives for the drawings and will be expressing a new part of him/herself. For example, a strong individual might be exploring a part of herself by expressing the statement, "I am delicate." Descriptions should be kept to a couple of minutes at the most. Just using one or two adjectives is fine. Repeat the process as often as time allows, hopefully until the drawings return to the original owner. You could divide the group to facilitate the process. Follow with a discussion of feelings that emerged.

Variations:

- Depict yourself as a house and describe your characteristics (e.g., size, color, style, outside, inside). What kinds of furniture or objects are there? What does the house feel like when you walk inside?
- Portray yourself as a symbol. Examples: a thunderbolt, a cloud, a heart. Verbally give some clues about yourself without showing the picture. Example: thunderbolt, "I make a lot of sudden noise that unsettles people." The participants will try to guess the aspect of self you are portraying.

Influences

Depict three things that have influenced your life greatly, including people, places, ideas, beliefs, and experiences.

Interpersonal Relationships

To make participants more aware of others and the way others perceive them.

Behavioral Goals

- Become more aware of interactions between people.
- Increase understanding of family dynamics as they relate to the current situation.
- Learn to see oneself from other people's points of view.

Support

Depict a time in your life when you needed support and in what form(s) that support came to you. Example: loss of a family member. The support came from church members who called and sent cards and from grieving sessions with a therapist.

Portraits

In pairs, group members draw one another adding qualities, characteristics, and aspects to create a complete representation of the person.

Care Packages for Others

Create care packages for one another. Include both tangible (e.g., chocolate, furry slippers) and intangible (e.g., love, trust, hope) gifts that fit that individual's personality and needs.

Your Family

Use drawing, collage, photographs, or clay to depict your family.

Family Sociogram

Create a sociogram model of your family. A sociogram is a visual diagram showing the members of a group and how they relate to and feel about each other. You may use circles of colored paper to represent various individuals.

Kinetic Family

Depict the family doing something together or a typical family scene.

Animal Family

Depict family members as animals that most represent their personalities and/or behavior.

Mural

Mural making can be an enjoyable and revealing activity. You can learn:

- How people cooperate (e.g., deciding who uses what space and how much space).
- How boundaries are created (e.g., invasion of "your" space by another member).
- Different styles in approaching the project (e.g., thoughtful and slow or impulsive and quick).

Taking a piece of butcher paper long enough to enable everyone to contribute to the project, create a mural on topics that include:

- Group mural: Portray your ward, community, class, or group. Note positive and negative aspects of the group.
- Nature collage: Depict nature in a way that says something about you. Example: the ocean environment can be stormy or calm. It has riches hidden under the surface.
- Global issues: Have your mural say something about world issues that concern you.

Group Mobile

Each person adds something that expresses an aspect of him/herself. Example: a pair of sunglasses (I am hiding my expressions), a transparent cloth (you all can see through me).

Unfinished Messages

Use the collage method to depict family, friends, or acquaintances with whom you left something unsaid. Write or tell what you wish you were able to say to each of these people.

I Give You

Complete the statement, "I give you the gift of _____" using any medium to express a characteristic or quality.

Circle of Love

Place yourself in the center of a piece of paper. Depict the circle of love that surrounds you — your family (alive or deceased), friends, animals, or energies from nature or places.

Trophy

To whom would you give a trophy and what would it look like? Draw or design the trophy.

Family Crest

Design a family crest that tells something about you and your family.

Birthday

Draw or use other media to answer the question: Today is your birthday. Can you see the gift you want most in the world?

As Seen by Others

Each person receives an 11" x 14" sheet of paper on which each writes his/her name. Arrange the seating into a circle and ask the clients to pass their sheets of paper to the person on the right. All the clients cut something (a word or picture) out of a magazine that reminds them of something they like about the person whose sheet they have. They then paste it on and pass the sheet to the right. Once all the clients receive their own sheets, they look them over for a minute. Next each person holds up his/her collage while other members describe why they chose to add what they did.

The Individual's Place in the World

To increase awareness of our relationships with the world.

Behavioral Goals

- Learn to share space with other people.
- See one's place as part of the whole world.

Sharing Space with Another

Sit facing a partner and draw together on one piece of paper without speaking. Be aware of territoriality and how it is affected by your relationship with another person.

House, Tree, Person

Include all three in a picture.

Elements

Represent the elements of earth, water, air, fire, and spirit in a drawing or painting.

Your World

Using the concept of the sociogram, design your world. Include the people that you feel close to, places that have meaning, and your interests, values, and dreams.

Time Tree

Depict yourself as a tree in three stages of growth — yesterday, today, and tomorrow. After you have drawn these three images, answer the following questions:

- Where are you growing?
- What are your strengths and weaknesses?
- What nurtures you?
- What is your future?
- What might you change?

Create the World

As a group, create an image of the world. Any of the following themes could be used:

- Identify wishes for the world's healing.
- Share sadness for the world.
- Create your ideal world.
- Depict what brings you joy in the world and what brings you sadness.

This activity, with its various parts, could be effective as a mural process.

Then and Now

Depict the world, or your world, as it was and then as it is.

References

Alders, A. & Levine-Madori, L. (2010). The effect of art therapy on cognitive performance of Hispanic/Latino older adults. *Art Therapy: Journal of the American Art Therapy Association, 27*(3), 127-135.

Beck, A. T., Ward, C. H., Mendelson, M., Mock, T., & Erbaugh, J. (1961). An inventory for measuring depression. *Arch. Gen. Psychiatry, 4*(6), 561-571.

Coopersmith, S. (1981) *Self-esteem inventories*. Palo Alto, CA: Consulting Psychologist Press.

Denny, J. (1972). Techniques for individual and group art therapy. *American Journal of Art Therapy, 2*(3), 117-134.

Derogatis, L. R. (1993). *BSI Brief Symptom Inventory: Administration, scoring and procedural manual* (4th ed.). Minneapolis, MN: National Computer Systems.

Doric-Henry, L. (1997). Pottery as art therapy with elderly nursing home residents. *Art Therapy: Journal of the American Art Therapy Association, 14*(3), 163-171.

Elkis-Abuhoff, D. L., Goldblatt, R. B., Gaydos, M., & Corrato, S. (2008). Effects of clay manipulation on somatic dysfunction and emotional distress in patients with Parkinson's disease. *Art Therapy: Journal of the American Art Therapy Association, 25*(3), 122-128.

Gilbert, F. S. (1991). Development of a "steps questionnaire." *Journal of Studies on Alcohol, 52*, 353-360.

Hattori, H., Hattori, C., Hokao, G., Mizushima, K., & Mase, T. (2011). Controlled study on the cognitive and psychological effect of coloring and drawing in mild Alzheimer's disease patients. *Geriatrics Gerontology International, 11*, 431-437.

Hebl, J. & Enright, R. D. (1993). Forgiveness as a psychotherapeutic goal with elderly females. *Psychotherapy: Theory, Research, Practice, Training, 30*(4), 658-667.

Julliard, K. (1995). Increasing chemically dependent patients' belief in Step One through expressive therapy. *American Journal of Art Therapy, 33*(4), 110-119.

Landgarten, H. (1981). *Clinical art therapy: A comprehensive guide.* New York, NY: Brunner/Mazel Publisher.

Landgarten, H. (1993). *Magazine photo collage (MPC)*. New York: Brunner/Mazel Publishers.

Metzl, E. S. (2008). Systematic analysis of art therapy research published in *Art Therapy: Journal of the American Art Therapy Association* between 1987 and 2004. *The Arts in Psychotherapy, 35*(1), 60-73.

Olsson, R., Kucharewski, R., & Fedorenko, J. (1999). Using therapeutic arts in a recreational therapy academic program. *Expanding Horizons in Therapeutic Recreation. 18*, 103-112.

Prescott, M. V., Sekendur, B., Bailey, B., & Hoshino, J. (2008). Art making as a component and facilitator of resiliency with homeless youth. *Art Therapy: Journal of the American Art Therapy Association, 25*(4), 156-163.

Reynolds, F., Vivat, B., & Prior, S. (2011). Visual art-making as a resource for living positively with arthritis: An interpretative phenomenological analysis of older women's accounts. *Journal of Aging Studies, 25*(3), 328-327.

Spielberger, C. D., Gorsuch, R. L., Lushene, R., Vagg, P. R., & Jacobs, G. A. (1983). *Manual for the State-Trait Anxiety Inventory*. Palo Alto, CA: Consulting Psychologist Press.

Stallings, J. W. (2010). Collage as a therapeutic modality for reminiscence in patients with dementia. *Art Therapy: Journal of the American Art Therapy Association, 27*(3), 136-140.

Stuart, A. (2017). Collage activity. Personal communication.

Wood, M. J. M., Molassiotis, A., & Payne, S. (2011). What research evidence is there for the use of art therapy in the management of symptoms in adults with cancer? A systematic review. *Psycho-Oncology, 20*, 135-145.

10

Masks

Man is least himself when he talks in his own person, give him a mask and he will tell the truth.

— Oscar Wilde

Masks… we all wear them. They can be helpful or destructive, self-made or imposed upon us. They are denied and confessed; they can be used to reveal or to conceal. They can be cemented, nailed, glued, or hinged. They may be taped or painted directly onto one's face. Behind each one may lie recognized feelings and unfamiliar ones… feelings that may be suppressed, distorted, or protected.

The power of masks as a therapeutic tool, therefore, is enormous. They possess a tremendous potential for facilitating growth, understanding, and even, in the course of this, enjoyment. They may also serve as a powerful reminder of what we already know.

This discussion of masks is a segue between art and drama, at least historically, because drama (as well as dance) came from the art of mask making. Masks are an ancient form of expression used to celebrate earth forces and cycles, to communicate with the spiritual realm, and to thrust the wearer into a different persona and set of behaviors. By putting on a mask, the wearer suspends everyday reality and can dance, act, or sing about experiences outside of the tangible. Mask making can be found in most — perhaps all — cultures throughout the course of human history.

As a therapy technique, mask making with clients can be interesting and often illuminating. A mask in therapy is not a simple thing. Creating and wearing a mask can expose parts of ourselves that we are not usually willing to acknowledge in everyday life. A mask can also cover up who we really are at the moment and act as a protective shield from our true feelings. Masks also let clients try on different personas and free their imaginations. Therapists need to understand the many possibilities to work with masks effectively.

Mask Creation in a Therapeutic Context

- Always allow for self-description or self-disclosure.
- Showing examples can encourage or spark creativity as long as no comparisons are made.
- The leader is most effective when creating his/her own mask, too. Be conscious of what you are disclosing to the group.
- Once made, masks can be worn, interpreted, passed around, and traded. Other group members can contribute to understanding by expressing what they think a person is saying or trying to say, or by pointing out a person's patterns of expression.

We are drawn to masks because they remind us of faces and well-established research indicates that our brains are wired to respond to faces. In the book *Actual Minds, Possible Worlds,* Jerome Bruner (1986) asserts that universal aspects of the human experience lie in the seemingly unique experiences of an individual.

Creating a mask can also open the door to other modalities, such as drama and dance. Once the piece is created, encourage the maker to wear it and move in a way that is reflective of the mask. If a group of people have all made masks, there are even more possibilities for group members to interact with one another through their masks and movement.

Research

Using expressive art techniques in counseling is one way to allow clients to reflect on their concerns or problems in therapy. Trepal and Wester (2008) noted masks have been used throughout history in theater and counseling. In therapy, masks can be used as projective tools for clients to reflect their experiences. The study focused on clients' experiences in creating masks while working on their issues as survivors of sexual abuse. The researchers also provided recommendations for using masks with different populations.

The therapeutic use of masks adds to existing therapeutic approaches. Baptiste (1989) presented a creative way of using masks to change dysfunctional behaviors of families and increase therapeutic effectiveness. If used appropriately this technique can be an effective addition to family therapy for dysfunctional families.

Campbell et al. (2016) developed a randomized controlled study which was designed to determine if art therapy in conjunction with cognitive processing therapy (CPT) was more effective than cognitive processing therapy alone for reducing symptoms of combat posttraumatic stress disorder (PTSD). Veterans were randomized to receive either individual CPT or individual CPT with individual art therapy. On the PTSD Checklist — Military Version and the Beck Depression Inventory II (self-rating scales) scores improved with treatment in both groups. Art therapy in conjunction with CPT significantly improved trauma processing and veterans reported it to be an important part of their treatment. Art therapy provided healthy distancing, enhanced trauma recall, increased access to emotions, and led to a greater reduction in PTSD symptoms. The protocol for art therapy consisted of eight 75-minute sessions. The introductory session included the Art Therapy — Projective Imagery Assessment (Deaver & Bernier, 2014) and an interview with semi-structured interview questions. Session two included educational material about PTSD, goal setting, safety, symptoms, and triggers. Session three focused on creating a visual trauma narrative. Session four contained two elements: Mask making and mind mapping. Mask making assisted participants in identifying and expressing emotions that were difficult to address verbally. It also enabled them to explore both their inner feelings and how they present themselves to the world. Mind mapping included core emotions and the internal and external triggers that caused them. Session five compared the self before the trauma with the self in the present. Session six addressed grief and loss. Session seven constructed a new world view and self-concept. The final session focused on a post-intervention interview, a review of the trauma narrative, and creation of reflective art. All participants who received art therapy stated that they either recovered previously blocked memories or gained insights and realizations central to their healing process through art therapy. CPT alone was not as effective in recovering memories.

Also see the description of Kaimal's (2017) research later in this chapter (Masks as Therapy) for another demonstration of the efficacy of mask making.

Processes of Mask Creation

Many materials are appropriate for mask making. Visit a natural history museum to get an inkling of the possibilities for creating masks. Some of the materials that the group leader might want to have available for construction include:

- paper — all sorts, including construction and crepe paper
- craft materials — corrugated cardboard, cardboard tubes, fabrics, yarn
- decorative materials — sequins, beads, feathers, etc.
- art supplies — markers, paints, crayons, oil pastels
- ceramic supplies — if you have access to a kiln, wonderful masks can be shaped out of clay, fired, and glazed.
- face paints — an easy way to create masks, especially fun for children. For better results and easier clean up, use a good, water-based product like Aquarelle Caran D'Ache, which is applied with a brush.
- papier mâché materials (see process below)
- plaster gauze (see process below)

Papier Mâché

These masks are inexpensive and fairly easy to make. If the budget allows and/or the group is small, it is now possible to purchase paper pulp that mixes with water. A mask can then be formed by spreading this mixture over a blown-up balloon. This is a fast and easy medium for mask making. If the group is large or resources are limited, use the traditional newspaper and glue method, also known as papier mâché.

Materials

- Newspaper and newspaper strips
- masking tape
- wheat paste (for wallpapering) or common starch (watered down slightly)
- good latex balloons (flimsier balloons may burst while the mask is being made)
- paints (acrylics are preferable)
- gesso (optional)
- clear spray glossy finish (optional, unless there is a concern that the paints being used might flake or peel over time)

Procedure

1. Inflate a latex balloon to medium size. Don't overfill. Overfilling may cause the balloon to burst as the newspaper strips are laid down or may create too much surface area to work on.
2. Roll up a newspaper into the shape of a horseshoe. This will act as a cradle for the balloon. Tape this to the table and then tape the balloon gently to the horseshoe.
3. Cut or rip newspaper into 2" x 4-6" strips. Some strips will need to be shorter to fit contours like the nose area.
4. Make the liquid mixture. Follow directions on the package for wheat paste. Remember to ask if anyone has wheat allergies and to use rubber gloves to prevent a rash. If using starch, add a little water to thin it for easy use. Make sure there is good ventilation because the starch can have a strong smell.
5. Dip the strip of newspaper into the mixture and remove the excess. Work from top to bottom, crisscrossing layers for extra strength.
6. To build a nose or planes of face or forehead, roll newspaper pieces or paper towel pieces and tape them down with masking tape. This makes a temporary structure to place strips on until enough have been laid

down to hold additional strips in place. Tissue paper can also be used for an interesting surface texture over layers of newspaper.

7. Build a total of four or five layers for strength until the mask is about 1/8-1/4" thick.
8. Leave the mask undisturbed for several days until thoroughly dry and no longer cool to the touch.
9. Apply gesso, if desired. Gesso is a primer that covers the newspaper and creates a base for paint. One advantage of using gesso is that less paint is required to cover a mask.
10. Paint in desired colors. Make sure to wait for one coat to dry before painting over any spot with another color (e.g., painting eyes over the face color). Be patient — the results will be worth the wait. A heat tool or hair dryer can speed up the drying process.
11. When thoroughly dry, spray with acrylic gloss finish for durability and water resistance.
12. Finally, glue on any decorative items such as feathers, sequins, or beads.

Making a Life Mask Using Plaster Gauze

Those of us who are lucky enough to be or know a theater student, or to have contact with someone involved in doing special effects for movies, may have had the opportunity to have a latex life mask of their face made. It is an interesting experience, but not one for the claustrophobic. The whole idea of making life masks can be frightening for some people, not just for those suffering from claustrophobia, but also for individuals who have difficulty with touching or trust. By using plaster gauze, the potential for claustrophobic feelings can be dealt with by limiting the amount of surface covered by the plaster. Resolving touch or trust issues is more difficult — partners should be directed to be thoughtful and gentle in both touch and voice, and to stop if the process becomes uncomfortable for either of them.

Materials

- Plaster gauze (a material formerly used in making casts; made by Johnson and Johnson, it is also available in good craft stores)

- old clothes
- shower caps or hair pins to protect hair
- towels or newspaper
- bowls with water
- scissors
- Vaseline
- baby powder

Procedure

1. Make sure to wear old clothes.
2. Pair up with another person and take turns making the masks.
3. The person having the mask made should thoroughly cover his/her face (including any facial hair or hair lying close to the face) with Vaseline. This averts undesirable consequences such as pulling off eyebrow hairs as the mask is pulled off! Also pin back hair or use a shower cap to cover it.
4. The person then lies on a towel or a layer of newspapers. This makes the work easier for the partner but isn't strictly necessary. The person can sit in a chair or wheelchair if necessary.
5. The "sculptor" has cut a gauze roll into 2" by 3-4" strips and set them aside. S/he begins by dipping the strips into water and removing the excess. Don't leave the strips in the water, as this will remove all the plaster. Beginning from top to bottom, cover one entire area before moving to a new area. Crisscross for strength. Covering the eyes or mouth with plaster is *not* recommended. In order to cover the mouth, for example, it would be necessary to insert straws in the nose to facilitate breathing. This is not a pleasant or desirable experience.
6. Create a surface that is about 1/8-1/4" thick. The layers underneath will start to harden first. Feel with a finger to determine whether an area needs strengthening with more strips. Make any additions to the mask immediately after removing it and while it is still drying.
7. Let it dry once all the layers are applied. After about five minutes, ask the person under the mask to make some facial motions. If the mask begins to move away easily from the face it is time to gently remove the mask. Once removed, it is possible to remove the sticky feel of the

Vaseline from inside the mask by sprinkling baby powder onto the inner surface.

8. Some professionals like to blend the texture of the gauze by working a bit of plaster into the mask surface. Use some of the plaster that has fallen off the gauze for this purpose.
9. Paint and spray with acrylic gloss finish for protection.
10. Decorate with other items if desired.

Masks as Therapy

Kaimal (2017) reported on the use of masks to help armed service personnel work with creative arts therapists to heal the unseen wounds of war. Through art therapy sessions with experienced clinicians, service members (n = 370) were helped to externalize aspects of themselves they couldn't express in any other way. The therapy allowed them to share personal stories and narratives that connected and communicated with their clinicians, families, and comrades.

To see a mask is to see the impact of post-traumatic stress disorder (PTSD) and traumatic brain injury (TBI) and to understand how it impacts the service members' personal lives, relationships, and perceptions of their role in the world. For example, a mask with a lock on its mouth may be about the challenges of talking in the military and the universal challenges of sharing traumatic experiences. Another mask with a vise on its head may be about TBI and the pain and frustration for anyone with a traumatic brain injury. A mask with a question mark saying, "Why me?" is relevant to all challenged by the uncertainty of the future.

The masks created in therapy were reviewed by a research team, including staff from the National Intrepid Center of Excellence at the Walter Reed National Military Medical Center and Drexel University students and faculty with support from Creative Forces: NEA Military Healing Arts Network. They analyzed the visual elements and meanings associated with the masks made by service members. The research team spent over six months collecting the images and therapists' clinical notes and then uploading them to a database for analysis. The conclusion was that the masks expressed invisible wounds of war. The research team reported being moved by reading clinical notes and learning how they supported the visual imagery represented in the masks.

The research showed that the themes seen in the masks represent a spectrum of human experience. The many ways in which service members represented themselves followed a framework. "The masks represented the many different ways we interact with the world: as individuals depicting our subjective feelings and physical being, as partners and friends in relationships, as community members, and our role in society and our self as a life story that evolves over time. In each of these aspects the masks might represent the struggles of injury and loss of resilience" (Kaimal, 2017, p. 1).

In previous research Kaimal (2017) found that art therapy helps patients externalize and share experiences that they might be unable to express in any other way. In the new analysis researchers felt they knew the service members through their masks even though they never met. Each mask encapsulated a story and a warrior's journey. This is the unique contribution of art therapy: participants get to express and communicate their life stories in new dimensions and non-verbal ways. "The ability to say the unsayable is a powerful force for healing" (Kaimal, 2017, p. 2). Data sources included mask images and therapists notes over a five-year period. The data were coded and analyzed using grounded theory methods. Findings indicated that mask making offered visual representations of the self as it related to individual personhood, relationships, community, and society. Imagery themes referenced the injury, relational supports and losses, identity transitions and questions, cultural metaphors, existential reflections, and conflicted sense of self. The masks provided visual insights and an increased understanding of the experiences of service members, facilitating their recovery (Kaimal, 2017).

Inside/Outside Masks

What was found related to service people is true in other situations, too. Creative arts and support offer people with traumas a chance to break the silence. Masks made by women in a domestic violence support group show what a victim is really going through. The outside of the mask shows what a victim chooses to show the world. The inside shows inner feelings.

The purpose of this exercise is to create a mask that represents the faces that clients wear in different environments. The outside of the mask is decorated with words and images that represent how clients think the world sees them or how they present themselves. The inside of the mask reflects how they see themselves and what is hidden from the outside.

Participants may want to decorate one or two sides of a mask — they may even choose to do several. Many aspects of the self (internal vs. external, different personalities, ideal self) can be depicted in this way.

Mask Modalities

The following section groups suggestions for creating and using certain types of masks according to five different therapeutic issues (self-esteem, physical or body awareness, imagination and creativity, social skills, and rapport building). The research by Kaimal (2017) supports efficacy in each of the five therapeutic issues.

Every therapy group is different. These are only suggestions — there are a wide range of issues which can be explored using this medium. Within each category the group creates one of the types of masks and does one of the activities. The appropriateness of each activity will depend on the masks created.

Masks and activities are meant to be mixed and matched. These activities may be even further interchanged, and new ones added, as a therapist recognizes other applications and contexts for them. Read about theater games (Chapter 12) and refer back to masks to see if any of the ideas from that section can be applied. When possible, have the participants wear their masks during the activity. As stated previously, the mask is a vehicle for entering another reality and can enable the wearer to gain greater insight into the self.

Self-Esteem Masks

Masks

- How others see you or how you would like to be seen by a friend
- The person you would like to become

- A mask with two sides depicting the first two suggestions
- Your uniqueness and your strengths
- When you have felt your best
- What you like and dislike about yourself
- How you feel when you are frightened, happy, etc.
- An image from a dream
- Yourself as a child, adolescent, or adult
- Yourself as a child, adult, or parent (transactional analysis model)

Activities

- Introduce yourself in the present: "I am _______________," and name the areas of yourself that you want to strengthen (e.g., trust).
- Introduce yourself the way your best friend, family member, or other significant person in your life would.
- Answer this Orff Schulwerk rondo (see Chapter 15 for details of this technique):

  Masks can be happy, masks can be sad,
  What about your mask makes you glad?

- Fantasize that you just went to a Magic Shop and got more of some personal quality that you want. Introduce yourself and describe how that quality helps you in your life.
- Project the future: role-play meeting a friend or another client from your treatment program in one year and five years. Talk about your lives.
- Create a Symphony of Emotions theater game. Each participant produces a sound which relates the emotion that is portrayed on his/her mask. The leader orchestrates these sounds, by cueing the participants to start or stop, and lower or raise the volume or pace.
- Have a conversation with your mask. Give each sub-personality a name and a statement that would be typical for that part of yourself. You may ask other members of the group to portray each sub-personality.

Physical or Body Awareness Masks

Masks tend to be limited to the face and exclude the rest of the body. Use full-body tracing or tracings of specific body parts to create a mask that covers those parts. The larger masks invite a fuller understanding and a more holistic exploration of feelings.

Masks

- How a little creature living inside you might see you
- Yourself as a flower, sky, tree, stream, etc.
- Your most favorite or least favorite parts

Activities

- Interpret your mask through movement and/or sounds.
- If possible, tape or safety pin the body mask to your back so that it moves as you move. In motion it relates to others and takes on a life of its own.

Imagination and Creativity Masks

We can be or feel whatever we want — there is no limit to our imaginations. By encouraging participants to project themselves into new worlds and experiences they may be able to get in touch with and experience who or what they would like to be. This is the time to bring out the props: the hats, magic wands, and crystal balls — whatever helps to create the illusion and enhance the fantasy.

Masks

- Your favorite fantasy, comic, or storybook character
- What you would like to be like when you grow up, mature, are five years older, are ten years older, etc.
- Yourself in another age, past or future
- Yourself in heaven
- Yourself after your death
- Yourself as the happiest or most evil or wisest person in the world

Activities

- Be your hero or heroine. Identify qualities or behaviors you respect in them. Let this come through your actions in handling what you or the leader would consider difficult role-play situations.
- Make up a story about the mask you made.
- Use various masks (with two or three person groups) to create and stage a story or scene.
- Play Roving Reporter. Each group member becomes a character who moves, thinks, and speaks in a unique way. (See the "Radio and TV Exercise" in the *Theater Games* chapter to help direct the group in this.) Suggestions are taken for the setting — a school, an African plain, etc. The roving reporter (often the leader at first), circulates through the room, interviewing characters. Characters mill around until commanded to "freeze." The reporter picks a character and interviews him/her while the others listen.

Social Skills Masks

Social skills improve when we understand the world from another person's point of view. Masks let us take on the role of another person so we can learn his/her way of dealing with situations. Masks are also useful in letting us practice using a characteristic such as assertiveness that might currently be too difficult to use.

Masks

- People who experience varying degrees of comfort in social situations. A person's behavior might be talkative, shy, rude, vulnerable, happy, competitive, snobbish, etc.
- People of different cultures, races, or abilities/disabilities
- People in positions of authority, such as teachers, doctors, or police officers

Activities

- Create role-play situations for one another. Choose situations that would challenge and/or strengthen some quality in each person's character. The shy person may be challenged to stand up to a police officer's questions, for example. Choose real life situations.

- Create two- or three-character situations where clients can practice the following behaviors:
    - Giving appropriate greetings
    - Saying "no!"
    - Beginning a conversation
    - Sharing appreciation
- Try the experience of being someone else with his/her individual perspective and problems. This may help to bridge cultural and personal differences and promote empathy, respect, and/or insight into others. The group makes suggestions for role-play situations.

Rapport-Building Masks

Rapport building is important in making a group come together. These activities are designed to be done as a group project to allow the members of the group to get to know one another better.

Masks

- Create life masks.
- Each person in a small group (3-4 members) begins working on his/her own mask. After a certain amount of time, each person passes his/her mask to the person on the right. This continues until everyone receives his/her mask back.
- In small groups (3-4 people) each participant makes masks of the other group members.

Activities

- Create a mask mural.
- Exchange masks with a partner. Look at the mask, wear it, and experience what it feels like to have it on. Make a few statements that seem to fit and make up a movement to go with the mask. Return it to the owner. Discuss what happened.

- Mingle around the room, talking with different people about the process of creating your mask and what it represents.
- Pass each mask around the group. Each person may tell the group one thought about the mask.
- Place all masks in the middle of the floor. Each person chooses one and takes on the character of that mask, gives his/her interpretation of the mask, or creates an experience from the mask.
- Body Sculpting: One person wears a mask while his/her partner(s) sculpt or move him/her as a puppet. Remind the person acting as clay or a puppet to relax and let the partner(s) move him/her.

Resources

The National Endowment for the Arts Guide to Community-Engaged Research in the Arts and Health.

The NEA commissioned this guide from the cognitive neuroscientist Julene Johnson, PhD, and the arts consultant Jeff Chapline, New Art Horizons. It advises arts practitioners and biomedical or behavioral health researchers how to partner effectively in documenting and studying the contributions of community-based arts programs to positive health outcomes.

Creative Forces: National Endowment for the Arts Military Healing Arts Network. https://www.arts.gov/partnerships/creative-forces/research.

References

Baptiste, D. (1989). Using masks as therapeutic aids in family therapy. *Journal of Family Therapy, II*, 45-58.

Bruner, J. (1986). *Actual minds, possible worlds.* Cambridge, MA: Harvard University Press.

Campbell, M., Decker, K., Kru, K., & Deaver, S. (2016). Art therapy and cognitive processing therapy for combat-related PTSD: A randomized controlled trial. *Art Therapy, 33*(4), 169-177.

Dever, S. & Bernier, M. (2014). The art therapy-projective imagery assessment. In Handler, L. & Thomas, A. eds. *Drawings in assessment and psychotherapy: Research and application*. pp. 131-147. New York: Routledge.

Kaimal, G. (2017). Unmasking the trauma: A look at research on mask making as a creative arts therapy. National Endowment for the Arts, Art Works Blog (February 16, 2017).

Trepal, H. C. & Wester, K. L. (2008). The use of masks in counseling: Creating reflective space. *Journal of Clinical Activities Assignments & Handouts in Psychotherapy Practice, 2*:123-130.

11

Introduction to Theater Games and Drama Therapy

Many excellent therapeutic techniques have their origin in the theater. From theater games to psychodrama, clients enter a world of imagination and possibility that has relevance to behaviors —their own and other's — in the larger world beyond the stage.

Although the goals of the various drama therapies may be different, many of the techniques and processes of the drama group are the same across the board. The following is a broad outline for conducting drama therapy in a group. Details for each kind of group are in the following two chapters.

Levels of Therapies

- **Theater Games:** These are used to increase spontaneity and interaction within a group, and often form the basis for other group work.
- **Role-Playing:** Works on changing behaviors or introducing new ones. A problem-solving technique.

- **Sociodrama:** A group process that works on common problems, to help the group gain insights into behaviors that they all share.
- **Psychodrama:** Centers on one person's problems and aims to help that person reach a deeper understanding of his/her behavior and/or a resolution of emotional conflicts.

Common Objectives

These objectives are not all shared by every type of drama therapy, but there is considerable overlap. The objectives are to:

- **Increase interaction:** This is often done using theater games and improvisation to increase and develop trust. The emphasis is on group trust and group interaction.
- **Release and control emotions:** Often accomplished through theater games. The leader functions as director, steering the course of the dramatic action.
- **Change behavior:** Break behavioral and role patterns that are not constructive.
- **Find patterns:** Gain insight into familiar patterns and discover alternative patterns.
- **Explore conflicts:** Understand problematic processes and find different responses to them.
- **Increase spontaneity**.
- **Increase self-esteem and self-confidence**.
- **Create a safe space:** Provide a learning situation that is fun and reinforcing of positive behaviors.

Process

- Group warmups
- Pair warmups
- Improvisational scene, role-play, or a dramatic scene
- Declimaxing — Closure for entire group

General Guidelines

- Approach and begin at the current level of the clients. Don't force a greater dramatic intensity than they are ready to handle.
- Resistance and passivity are often seen in clients at the beginning of a session. They need to be addressed and worked through.
- Create structure. It increases the feelings of safety in the group.
- Remember the element of surprise to increase spontaneity.
- Exaggerating behavior — yours or a reflection of a group member's — can instill humor in a situation, *if* there is enough trust.
- Make sure each session is designed to promote success.

Warmup Exercises

The following exercises can be used with any drama group.

Essences

This activity can be done in verbal or written form. If done verbally, participants form a circle. Each participant has a chance to answer one of the following questions. Several questions may be asked in sequence. If the answers are written, each participant has a chance to read what s/he has written, or answers may be exchanged and discussed in pairs.

- If you could go anywhere in the world, where would you go?
- If you could be anyone (living or deceased), who would you be?
- If you won the lottery, what would you do? How would your life change?
- If you could invent something, what would it be?
- If you could live at any time in the past, present, or future, when would you choose?
- If you could discover something, what would it be?
- If you could win an award, what would it be for?

Personal

- If you could change your name, would you?
- If you could make a wish for yourself, what would it be?
- If you could receive the perfect present, what would it be?
- Plan your perfect day.
- Is there something you would like to hear from a friend or relative?
- Introduce yourself the way your best friend would.

Projective: Who We Are and How We See Others

Use questions such as these to ask about a person in the group. Describing yourself as a kind of thing can be a lot less threatening than describing yourself as a kind of person.

- If you were a ______, what kind would you be?
- If [name of a person] were a ________, what kind would s/he be?

Fill in the blanks with some of these objects.

- flower
- color
- movement
- piece of furniture
- sound
- weather
- ice cream
- fabric
- season
- food
- jewel
- holiday
- song
- smell
- animal
- movie

- mode of transportation
- perfume
- book
- landscape
- sport
- musical instrument

Interpersonal Exercises

- **Empty chair technique:** Details are in the Psychodrama section of Chapter 13, *Drama Therapy*.
- **Appreciations and resentments:** Feelings are expressed to group members.
- **For me:** Is there something you would like to hear from someone in this group?
- **For you:** Send a message to everyone in the group.

Suggestions for Agreements in the Group

To create an environment that is safe for emotional release and discovery, it is important to set up agreements with members of the group.

- Only one person talks at a time. Be respectful of others.
- Talk to someone, not about him/her. Don't treat someone as if s/he isn't present.
- Each person's pace is respected. We all open up, grow, and release at different rates.
- No one is forced to participate. The goal is to reinforce individual responsibility for participation, so that it can be carried over into other life situations.
- It is not acceptable to disrupt the group.
- Do not analyze.
- In sharing and giving feedback, respond subjectively with statements about your experience (e.g., How has the drama touched you? What have you experienced that related to ___'s experience?)

12

Theater Games and Improvisation

All the world's a stage,
and all the men and women in it merely players…
And one man in his time plays many parts,
His acts being seven ages…

— William Shakespeare

Shakespeare may have said it best: we are part of the ever-unfolding drama (or perhaps comedy) of life, which casts us in a variety of roles and situations. If we have a good life, we begin as small babies, charming our families. As children we cast ourselves as heroes, princesses and princes, animals, and characters out of our favorite books, TV shows, and movies. In adolescence and adulthood, we take on the roles of lovers, parents, workers, and friends. Then middle age and retirement present us with new roles: mentoring, grandparenting, and retirement. Good life or not, along the way we each develop our own script and a set of behaviors to help us play our part.

One of the goals of theater games is to help clients become aware of, and perhaps reflect on, the many roles they've played in their own lives.

If needed, theater games can help clients find new roles and rewrite scripts that have not served them well.

Most people would not classify themselves as actors in the sense of Hollywood or Broadway stars. But they need to be reminded that they had parts in challenging situations with a variety of personalities. Players in theater draw from their experiences in life and clients can, too.

Improvisation is the term for creating theater in the moment, drawing only on the techniques or resources at hand and without any preparation. It is "working without a net" — much like real life.

Theater games are the tools of improvisation, used for sharpening the skills of the players and for creating theater. They are exercises or techniques that have at their root the following beliefs and attributes:

- **Allow experimentation:** There is no right or wrong way to improvise.
- **Encourage spontaneity:** Theater games are first and foremost artifices against artificiality — structures designed to fool spontaneity into being. Through spontaneity we are re-formed into ourselves. We (re)discover our truer selves and a more authentic way of behaving. Spontaneity, the core element of theater games, is the moment of personal freedom when we are faced with a reality, see it, explore it, and act accordingly.
- **Involve problem solving and creative challenges:** For example, if a player is asked to become one of the cogs in an imaginary machine, s/he must first identify how s/he will sound and move and then how to fit with the other human parts of the machine.
- **Focus concentration:** A key element of drama and comedy — it enables the player to be present, open, and ready to react to and participate in the exploration and resolution of a situation.
- **Encourage intuitive responses:** These can only be made in the here and now, the immediate moment. A player learns to react to what is happening in the moment. It is almost impossible to plan ahead if there is no script and no way to know ahead of time how others will behave. This experience develops trust in self and affects overall self-esteem.
- **Understand learning:** People learn through experience and experiencing. No one teaches anyone anything unless they provide experiences.

- **Increase openness:** If the environment permits it, anyone can learn whatever s/he chooses to learn. If the individual permits it, the environment will teach him/her everything it has to teach.
- **Talent is not required:** Anyone can participate. "Talented behavior," according to Viola Spolin (1983), the originator of theater games, "may be simply a greater individual capacity for experiencing.... It is in the increasing of the individual capacity for experiencing that the untold potentiality of a personality can be evoked."

Research

Research shows that theater education provides developmental benefits. Walker (2014) hypothesized that a theater curriculum, utilizing the techniques of creative drama and theater games created by Viola Spolin, taught to students of the Stillwater Montessori School in kindergarten through fourth grade, would contribute to significant increases in children's self-esteem and empathy. Questionnaires regarding children' self-esteem and empathy were administered to children, parents, and teachers prior to and following the theater programming. Results were analyzed using repeated-measures ANOVA. There were several observable changes reported in the children's listening and nonverbal communication skills and their ability to give and receive praise. Individual progressions regarding involvement, self-esteem, and focus were also observed. Positive feedback from students and teachers indicated the theater programming had a beneficial effect.

Other therapeutic uses for theater games in improving educational results are reported in Bailey (2010).

Brazier (2016) reported that theater games related to drama therapy in prisons can have a positive impact on anger management and that increasing emotional awareness among young offenders can reduce the risk of them offending again.

Thompson (2000) reported on work following the ideas of Augusto Boal, a Brazilian theater director who described prisoners as "restricted in space, but free in time." Interactive theater, Boal said, creates free space where people can imagine and think about the past and the present, and invent the future instead of having to wait for it. Theater in prison, Boal believed, could lead to "a healthier and more creative lifestyle." Boal's concept of theater involved raising issues that needed solutions and he called on the audience to participate in finding the solutions. "We are all theater," said Boal.

Bissell (2016) reported on a program in a prison in Los Angles, California, where actor Tim Robbins worked with a group of men in a project called "The Actor's Gang." The work focused on their emotions — especially anger. Anger management classes involved trying out new emotions and responses in a safe place. Activities provided the opportunity to respond to a range of scenarios with different emotions. Prisoner participants developed new ways to react when confronted with anger. Feedback from participants said the program helped them change their lives and taught them that they can control their anger rather than their anger controlling them. In the words of one participant, "it allowed my past to empower me rather than define me." Robbins was impressed by the level of truth about emotions that participants shared. The study suggested a reduction in the number of infractions committed by inmates, and a potential drop in the rate of recidivism among those who took the course.

Further research on how drama therapy leads to positive changes in anger level is also provided in Reiss et al. (1998).

Preparing Therapists

One of the most difficult skills for therapists to acquire is the ability to lead improvisation. So much of therapy involves structured routines. Improvisation needs to be free flowing, but at the same time the therapist needs to guide clients to new understanding.

Toivanen, Komulainen, and Ruismaki (2011) conducted a study that looked at ways drama and improvisation could stimulate enjoyment and creativity in the educational process for both teachers/therapists and students/clients. The researchers reviewed studies from drama education and philosophy of education. Their review found that, though it is part of what they are taught in teacher education, student teachers have difficulty moving away from scripted teaching to lead interactive and creative experiences. According to Toivanen, Komulainen, and Ruismaki (2011), good teaching is based on confidence, interaction, and creative passion, which can be taught through drama and improvisational exercises such as verbal spontaneity games, role-playing, and physical movement. Most important for recreational therapists are drama activities and improvisational exercises which also train interaction skills.

Aspects of Spontaneity

In *Improvisation for the Theater*, Viola Spolin (1983) outlines seven aspects of spontaneity (elements which are connected to its development or its impact on behavior):

- **Games:** Games provide a form for inviting involvement and for encouraging the personal freedom necessary for genuine experience. Through engaging in play, a person is learning skills, having fun, relating to others, and feeling the freedom that makes him/her open to experiences. Ingenuity and inventiveness are encouraged and applauded. The person can reach the objective of the game in any manner or style s/he chooses, as long as s/he abides by the rules (freedom within structure). Any game worth playing is highly social and has a problem within it that needs solving. Learning is the result of solving the problem in an effective way.
- **Approval and disapproval:** The first step toward being able to play is feeling personal freedom and understanding that there is no right or wrong way to solve a problem. Looking for approval or disapproval in others is creatively paralyzing. With an emerging sense of self, the need for authoritarianism drops away and intuitive awareness emerges. Working through problems that arise, in subject matter or interpretation, allows them to be seen not as problems but as a means of increasing the knowledge of everyone in the group, including the facilitator.
- **Group expression:** Each person's energy, enthusiasm, and ideas are important to the success of the group improvisation. At the same time, each member must be a part of the group relationship. Through awareness exercises and heightened sensory receptors, the members become each other's arms, legs, and actions. Competition is not helpful;

cooperation is. The goal of these exercises is for players to be able to work interdependently with full individual participation.

- **Audience:** An audience is what makes performance meaningful. In improvisation the audience participates in the unfolding of theater. The player becomes freer with the understanding that the audience comes not to judge or encourage but, as a group, is there to share an experience with the actors. The actors and the audience are actually partnering in creation.
- **Theater techniques:** These are techniques of communicating. Achieving communication is more important than the methods used. Whatever the techniques, they are just tools to help sharpen awareness, thinking, and relating skills so that the individuals can respond to a variety of new situations and experiences.
- **Carrying the learning process into daily life:** In improvisation, there are no lines to learn, no characters to research. Through sharpening his/her sensory equipment the player can make direct, fresh contact with the environment, people, and objects in his/her world. The individual who develops a wider view of the world is richer in all aspects of life.
- **Physicalization:** This term describes the means by which material is presented to the player on a physical, non-verbal level as opposed to an intellectual or psychological approach. The experience is concrete and immediate. An important goal of theater games is to encourage freedom of physical expression, which opens the door for insight. The player experiences a more direct perception of the world — and a more open self in relation to it.

Viola Spolin's Theater Games

When facilitating or directing theater games it is helpful to set up space that invites participation. Players should be arranged so that they can be ready to join in at any time. This is accomplished by having everyone sit or stand in a semi-circle facing a center that is designated as on-stage. The facilitator/director takes part in the group.

Orientation Game

Description: Orientation is an important step in introducing improvisation to new players. It is the first step in learning to create reality (e.g., objects, feelings, situations) for the player and others.

Directions: One player goes on-stage, picks a simple activity, and begins doing it (e.g., painting a fence, raking leaves, cooking, sweeping the floor) without verbal or sound cues. Others come on stage one at a time and join in doing this activity. Players can join in even if they don't know initially what is going on. This is a good starting point for physicalization.

The activity may also be done with partners. When rapport has been established in the group, it's a great learning experience for one member (who has an idea) to take another member (who has no idea what is going on) to center stage and begin an activity. For example, the initiating player might begin the movement of combing and cutting hair. When the other player realizes what is being portrayed, s/he joins in and responds by being the client. Players are amazed to find that they can be engaged in an activity before they even know exactly what they are doing.

Variation: Players do an activity in pairs while other members guess the activity. Examples: tennis, volleyball, checkers, doing nails, cooking, hanging pictures, or watching TV, movies, or sports.

Observation Game

Description: Helps sharpen observation and concentration skills.

Directions: A dozen or more real objects are placed on a tray which is set in the center of the circle of players. After approximately 15 seconds, the tray is covered or removed. The players make individual lists (could also be done in pairs) of as many objects as they can remember. The lists are then compared to the tray of objects.

Involvement in 3s and 4s

Description: Players need to demonstrate cooperation in order to accomplish the task.

Directions: The group is divided into smaller groups of three or four. Each group agrees on an imaginary object which cannot be used without involving all of them. They are to participate in a joint action in which all move the same thing. The group's objective is to make the object seem visible to the audience. Examples of actions: rolling up a fishing net, pushing a stalled car, tugging a boat in or out of the water, taffy pulling.

How Old Am I?

Description: This exercise gives players an opportunity to explore their conceptions and possible stereotypes of age and allows them to put themselves in another person's place.

Directions: Facilitator/Director sets up a simple "Where," preferably a bus stop. A bench (chair, stool, etc.) is set up facing the audience. A player writes down an age on slip of paper and gives it to the director before going on stage. The player acts out this age while being in the established setting. If, for example, a bus stop is used, the player portraying a child might skip on stage chewing gum and then play with a yo-yo, fidget, and fumble for change. If the player is portraying an adult, s/he might walk briskly onstage carrying a briefcase, sit down and make notes, pace, and/or often look at a wristwatch. Props may be real or imaginary. The rest of the group guesses the player's age.

The Where Game

Description: Similar to orientation games, this helps focus the player on communicating a physical awareness of where the action is taking place. In *Where* games players learn to work in three environments: the immediate, the general, and the larger. The immediate environment is the area closest to us (e.g., the table at which we are eating and all the related objects). The general environment is the room in which the table is placed, with its doors, windows, and other aspects. The larger environment is the area beyond the room — outside the window — the birds, trees, and landscape.

Directions: A player goes on stage and shows us *Where* through his/her use of objects in the immediate and general environment. When another player thinks s/he knows *Where* the player is, s/he assumes a character (a *Who*), enters the *Where* and develops a relationship with the first player. Others join them, one at a time, in a similar fashion. Suggestions for environments include library, supermarket, airport, hospital, beach, art gallery, restaurant, and school.

Weather Exercise

Description: Sharpens the player's awareness of the environment and how it affects his/her body.

Directions: A player goes on stage and shows what kind of weather or climate s/he is experiencing. The other players try to guess the weather conditions — then a new player comes on stage. The group processes the activity asking questions such as: Did the weather envelop him/her? Did the player use his/her body to show us the weather? (e.g., heat — adjusting clothing that is sticking to the body; mopping sweat off face, taking off shoes). Did s/he focus on the weather or on a character? On the weather or a situation?

Word Game

Description: Similar to Charades.

Directions: Divide into teams. Each team selects a word that can be divided into syllables that also form individual words. (Words could be chosen ahead of time by the director and then picked out of a hat to facilitate the process.) For example, the word "industrial" divides into "inn," "dust," and "trial." The group tries to guess the words being enacted. Other word suggestions: window (win doe), planet (plan eat), carpool (car pool). Actor tries to convey the words to the rest of his/her team without speaking by using pantomime (gestures, movements, and facial expressions).

Variation: Use the standard Charades format with each person acting out a phrase such as a movie or song title without speaking.

Body Sculpting in Pairs

Description: Develops sensitivity to another person's character and increases spatial awareness.

Directions: Divide group into pairs. One person in each pair starts out as the sculptor and the other person as the clay. Take turns as sculptor arranging the partner's body to show his/her personality (or some aspect of it) as you perceive it.

Body Sculpting in Fours

Description: Sharpens clients' sense of touch and space awareness.

Directions: Form groups of four. One person is the sculptor and another person is the clay. The other two people close their eyes. The sculptor sculpts the clay into a statue. The two people with eyes closed then become the new sculptor and the new clay. *Keeping his/her eyes closed,* the new sculptor feels the statue and attempts to reproduce it using the person who has become the second piece of clay. Upon completion compare the sculptures.

Radio and TV Exercise — Roving Reporter

Description: The goals are to exercise the imagination, to think quickly, and to have a social experience.

Directions: The director asks for a suggestion of a place or situation (e.g., the Olympic Games, now or early days). The players are instructed to assume a character of any age or background (can be famous or an everyday person) and interact with the immediate environment of that place. The player who acts as the interviewer will freeze the action when an interview is going to take place by saying "freeze." This enables all the players to hear what is said during the interview. The Roving Reporter or interviewer circulates through the crowd until s/he interviews all the players.

Prop Round

Description: A good warmup activity which also helps develop creative thinking ability.

Direction: Players sit in a circle. A prop is passed around the circle and each player has to transform it from what it was originally intended to be into something new and different. For example, an empty toilet paper roll could be a telephone receiver or a bullhorn. An idea for use cannot be repeated. The other players in the circle must guess what the object is before it can be passed on. If a player cannot think of another use, he may simply pass the object on. Continue the activity around the circle until the players are having a difficult time thinking up new ideas.

Paper Bag Dramatics

Description: Exercises creativity and cooperation skills.

Directions: Divide players into small groups. Give each group a paper bag filled with five or six everyday objects. You may or may not give the groups the same objects. The task for each group is to incorporate their objects into a short skit.

The Three Wizards (also known as "Dr. Know it All")

Description: The goal of this activity is for players to work together to come up with an answer to any question.

Directions: Ask for three volunteers. Together they become "The Three Wizards" or Dr. Know it All and can answer any question asked. Each wizard (or part of the doctor) can only respond with one word at a time. If the first wizard begins the answer with "Because," the second wizard links his/her word to the first and the third wizard to the second. This panel of three must connect the words so that one complete statement is made in answering the question. For example, if the question asked is "Why is the earth round?", the dialogue might go as follows:

1st player: "Because…"
2nd player: "if…"
3rd player: "it…"
1st player: "wasn't…"
2nd player: "round…"
3rd player: "then…"
1st player: "it…"
2nd player: "couldn't…"
3rd player: "revolve…"
1st player: "around…"
2nd player: "the…"
3rd player: "sun."

The answer does not have to make sense as long as it is a complete statement. Ask group members to participate in questioning The Three Wizards. After some time, switch players and let others be The Three Wizards.

Let It All Hang Out

Description: Encourages players to get in touch with their inner feelings and express emotions.

Directions: Have everyone form a circle and face outward from the center. Name an emotion and ask players to react to it as if they were feeling that particular emotion at this particular time. Give them a while to play it out. Then go on to the next emotion.

Show Me How You Feel Game

Description: Players connect with their (relatively) simple emotions.

Directions: This is a pantomime game in which participants are asked in turn to silently (through facial expressions and body gestures) express how they might feel in one of the situations characterized below:

Show me how you feel…

- when your stomach hurts
- when the sun is shining
- when you are eating ice cream
- when the nurse gives you a shot
- when your arm hurts
- when you are outside playing
- when a parent who is not living with you makes a visit
- when you are allowed to leave the hospital

Symphony of Emotions in Music

Description: The goals are for people to work together, to express emotions, and to pay attention to the conductor.

Directions: This can be played two ways. One option is to divide the group into smaller groups and ask each group to choose an emotion and an accompanying sound. The other option is to use the entire group, asking each member to choose an emotion and an accompanying sound that describes the feeling. The facilitator acts as the conductor and creates a symphony. As the conductor points to each individual (or small group), the player(s) express the sound. After all individuals (or groups) have demonstrated their sounds, the conductor uses these sounds to create a symphony as if they were instruments in an orchestra. Everyone must pay close attention to the conductor in order to start and stop on cue, increase or decrease volume, or speed up and slow down the pace. Later the group can guess what emotions were being portrayed. After a demonstration, the facilitator asks for volunteers to take turns acting as conductor.

Additional Theater Games

Instant Replay

Description: A name game commonly used as an icebreaker with a new group.

Directions: Have players form one large circle. Each person will have an opportunity to introduce himself/herself to the rest of the group. Each player will choose a unique walk or movement which s/he will demonstrate by making the movement as s/he travels to the center of the circle. Once reaching the center of the circle s/he will introduce himself/herself by name and return to his/her original spot. Once the player has returned to his/her spot, the rest of the group will mimic his/her actions and his/her name. Each player in turn does a different movement until the turn comes back to the first player.

Walk My Walk

Description: This is a good activity for identifying characteristics of people and translating them into movements.

Directions: Have players stand in a circle with plenty of space in the middle. Discuss the many ways people walk and show a few examples. For instance, a spy might creep along on tiptoes while a fashion model walks with a studied, erect posture. Players select a role with a specific kind of walk. Some ideas are

- tightrope walker
- tired person
- astronaut on the moon
- window washer on a ledge
- body builder
- explorer at the North Pole
- infant learning to walk
- circus clown
- marching soldier
- ninety-year-old man

Each player walks across the circle several times as the group tries to guess his/her identity. When someone guesses correctly, the entire group imitates the walk and then forms into a circle again to view another walk.

Passing the Buck

Description: Another good warmup activity which helps the mind to wake up — the focus is on being creative and thinking fast.

Directions: Have everyone stand in a circle. The buck is any object that can be tossed easily from player to player — a glove, a beanbag, a Nerf ball, or rubber ball. Toss the buck to a player in the circle. The person catching the buck must begin to tell a story — something made up on the spot. This player (the one beginning the story) can start out with the familiar, "Once upon a time," or can start the story in any other way s/he chooses. The player holding the buck tosses it to another player who must catch it and continue the story. The story can take any form as long as there is an attempt to connect it to the last player's contribution. Players must not break the flow of the story no matter how fast the buck is passed. Those who have the buck must speak — if only a few words — before they can toss the buck to another player.

Who Started the Motion?

Description: Sharpens observational skills and awareness of others through the attempt to detect subtle changes in group's movements.

Directions: Players are seated in a circle. One player is sent from the room while the others select a leader to start the motion. With the group already in motion, the player is called back into the room. S/he stands in the center of the circle and tries to discover the leader, whose function it is to make a motion — tapping foot, nodding head, moving hands, etc. — and to change the motion whenever s/he wishes. The other players copy the leader's motions and try to keep the center player from guessing the leader's identity. Instruct players beforehand to stay closely in sync with the leader's motions and watch the leader using peripheral vision in order to better mask the leader's identity. When the center player discovers the leader, two other players are chosen to take their places.

Outright Lie

Description: Uses the imagination and humor. A good warmup activity.

Directions: Select a small object such as a key, a ring, a pencil, or scissors. Players should be seated in a circle and pass the object from person to person. As the object is passed around the room, each player must come up with an incredible story or fantasy to tell the rest of the group. For example, if a key is selected, the stories might sound like this: "This key unlocks a treasure worth more than Fort Knox, a treasure located at the bottom of the Mediterranean Sea." Or "This key saved the life of a man when it stopped a bullet while he was fighting in a war." After everyone has finished, ask the group members which lie they enjoyed the most.

Who (or "Who Am I?") Game

Description: This is an activity that helps players deal with an unknown situation and think on their feet.

Directions: Seat players in a circle. One player leaves the room. The remaining group decides on a profession or an identity for the person who left. One player (the informant) stands up. When the first person comes back into the room, the informant initiates a conversation with him/her. The informant relates to the returned player as if s/he had the profession or the identity that the group has chosen for him/her. The returned player must keep the conversation going and try to guess his/her own identity by the direction of the conversation. Everyone in the room knows his/her identity except this player. The questions and answers given in conversation by the informant shouldn't be too easy, but they should give clues to the returned player's identity. When the player guesses his/her profession, the audience applauds to show their acknowledgment and approval.

Talk Show

Description: A more advanced version of the "Who Game."

Directions: Two players leave the room in order to choose two famous characters to portray. Characters can be from real life or fiction, alive or dead, and should be familiar to all or most of the group members. It is usually helpful if the two have some common interest such as music, sports, or politics so that they can carry on a conversation. The two players then rejoin the group and begin to have a conversation such as two famous people meeting on a television talk show might have. Warn players not to give each other away with names. The other players (audience) try to guess who the two are by interviewing them. Group members who want to guess the two characters' identities do not call out their names but ask a question directly related to their identities. For example, if one of the guesses of famous people is George Washington, the question might be, "Do you get splinters from your wooden teeth?" If the guess is wrong and the player is not George Washington, s/he might answer, "I don't have to use wooden teeth since my teeth are all real." The audience continues to ask questions until many people seem to know the identities of the character. The leader asks the audience who the characters are and how they arrived at their conclusions. Usually the group agrees, but occasionally a character could be one of several people, which makes for an interesting discussion. The game ends when the group asks the characters to reveal their identities.

Mirrors

Description: Helps focus attention and teaches players to be both leaders and followers.

Directions: Divide the group into pairs. Have partners face each other. One player leads by making simple, slow movements which his/her partner mirrors — they then reverse roles. They may use props. After five minutes seat everyone in a circle. Select two players. They decide secretly who will be doing the mirroring. While looking at the mirroring person, the other player demonstrates a simple activity such as washing or dressing. The audience tries to determine who is the mirror and who is the leader. The better the players are at concentrating their attention on each other, the more in sync they will be, and the harder it will be for the audience to guess the mirror.

Ripples

Description: Resembles the wave done at sporting events.

Directions: Gather the group into a single line behind a person chosen to be the leader. The object of the game is for each group member to follow the movements of the person directly in front of him/her, rather than following the leader directly. The leader begins a motion that is passed down the line. If the leader raises his/her arm, the second person follows the leader, the third person follows the second, and so on down the line. The leader does not walk around the room but rather moves arms and legs, bends, leans, and so on, in place. After players have done this a few times, divide the group into two lines with two leaders facing each other. In this version the second leader mirrors the movements of the first leader, and the group members follow the movements as above. Tell the leaders when to switch roles. For the grand finale, divide players into four groups with four leaders facing each other in a big X pattern. Two leaders initiate moves while the other two leaders standing across from them follow (Leader C follows the movements of Leader A and Leader D follows Leader B, for instance). Their group members follow one another as before. This version can be accompanied by music to create spectacular dance performances.

Lip Sync

Description: A good activity for developing cooperation and teamwork.

Directions: Four people play at a time. Two are actors and two are dubbers. The rest of the group is the audience. The two actors decide on a real-life drama that includes two characters and a situation. For example:

- Two people on vacation when their car runs out of gas
- A person smoking a cigarette in a non-smoking area and a non-smoker
- A person in a restaurant who keeps changing his/her order and an impatient waiter
- A door-to-door sales representative trying to sell someone a kangaroo (or another unnecessary object)

The actors and the dubbers work out a very rough plot outline without actually deciding on the dialogue. The actors play out the performance in pantomime. Offstage (out of view), the dubbers fill in the words. As the performance progresses, the actors and dubbers eventually affect each other and spontaneous things begin to happen. Switch actors and dubbers frequently. Try to give everyone a chance to be an actor or dubber at least once.

Transformations

Description: Another team-building activity that requires cooperation without much time for discussion.

Directions: Divide the group into two teams. The object of the game is for players to form, as quickly as possible, into human representations of whatever you describe. Call out the name of an object. Team members must then arrange themselves into that shape. For example, if you say "helicopter," players must work out how they will link together into propellers, cockpit, and landing gear. Other ideas for transformations are suspension bridge, ship, cathedral, capitol dome, tree, waterfall, truck, bus, and skyscraper.

Real Life Drama

Description: Develops storytelling ability and sequencing (telling a story with a beginning, middle, and end).

Directions: Players sit in a circle on the floor and tell the most interesting, dramatic, or scary thing that has happened to them, such as: getting lost, playing in an exciting ball game, rescuing an ailing bird or animal, being in an accident, or riding in a parade. Set a one-minute time limit on each player's story. After everyone has told a story, divide the group into smaller groups of five or six. Each group selects several elements from each person's story that can be combined into a short skit. Encourage imaginative combinations, such as picking up a baby bird while crossing the goal line for the winning touchdown. Each group takes a turn to perform its skit for an audience of the other players.

City or Country

Description: This is done as a pantomime skit.

Directions: Divide the group into two or three teams. Pass out one (already prepared) situation card to each team. These situations can be located in either the city or the country. Examples include:

The City

- An older lady enters a crowded bus, makes her way to the back, and rides downtown.
- A fire breaks out in a school building and a teacher evacuates the frightened children.
- An all-night diner.

The Country

- An array of flowers growing in the garden.
- Giraffes feeding on lower branches of trees are joined by a friendly group of elephants.
- An approaching storm.

Each team has five minutes to determine who will do what in an impromptu skit depicting their situation. After five minutes each group performs for the others and the audience guesses what the situation was.

Laugh It Up

Description: Pure fun and a good icebreaker.

Directions: Divide the group into two teams. One side is heads and the other tails. The leader flips a coin and allows it to land on the floor. If the coin comes up heads, the heads team begins laughing, trying to make the opposite team laugh or smile. Teams must have eye contact with one another. There should be a time limit, perhaps three minutes. The tails team must hold firm, not laughing or smiling. If players do laugh, they must join the other team. Once all the tails people who laugh have joined the other side, and time is up, the coin is tossed once again. The game is over when everyone is on one side.

Pantomime

Description: Players try to convey a situation with pantomime (movements, gestures, facial expressions, etc.). No speaking is allowed. The audience must guess the situation from the pantomime. Everyone should have a turn acting out a situation. This can be played in teams keeping track of the time required to convey the situation. The following are examples of possible situations:

- Eating a banana
- Playing the violin
- Playing tennis
- Playing croquet
- Watching a tennis game
- Swatting a bothersome mosquito
- Walking a tightrope
- Juggling
- Putting on stockings
- A man shaving his beard
- Putting on a girdle

- Putting hair up in curlers
- Putting on lipstick
- Burping a baby
- Playing a trombone
- Conducting an orchestra
- Rowing a boat
- Paddling a canoe
- Doing the waltz
- Putting on nail polish
- Eating a watermelon at a picnic
- Typing on a typewriter
- Pitching a baseball
- Hanging clothes on a clothesline
- Milking a cow
- Policeman directing traffic
- Doing the hula
- Tying a necktie
- Washing clothes on a washboard
- Playing a harp
- Casting and catching a fish
- Shoveling snow
- Going to the dentist
- Putting a worm on a fishhook
- "Hear no evil, see no evil, speak no evil"
- Playing the bass drum, cymbals, triangle, etc.
- Voting in an election
- Threading a needle
- Making pancakes
- Getting ready to be married
- Hammering a nail into a stubborn piece of wood
- Listening to a dull minister in church
- Watching a horror movie
- Square dancing
- Toasting marshmallows over a campfire
- Playing in a craps game for a million dollars
- Doing a sailor's hornpipe

- Playing a piano dramatically in a concert

Group Hug

Description: A good-feelings group solidarity activity. Useful closure to a theater session.

Directions: Have the entire group stand in a circle holding hands. Have the group step back until arms are extended out fully. Have group walk to the center of the circle (slowly) never breaking grip with each other. Return the group to the larger circle (stepping back slowly). Then have everyone race to the center, not breaking the grip. Finally gather the group together, arms around each other (group hug) and have them share what they learned from the session.

References

Bailey, S. (2010). *Barrier-free theatre: Including everyone in theatre arts — in schools, recreation, and arts programs — regardless of (dis)ability*. Enumclaw, WA: Idyll Arbor.

Bissell, K. (2016). Actor's gang: How Tim Robbins has cut reoffending rates. *BBC News, Los Angeles* (14 March 2016). http://www.bbc.com/news/magazine-35786775.

Brazier, Y. (2016). Drama therapy: Unlocking the door to change. *Medical News Today* (30 March 2016). www.medicalnewstoday.com/articles/308452.php.

Reiss, D., Quayle, M., Brett, T., & Meux, C. (1998). Dramatherapy for mentally disordered offenders: Changes in levels of anger. *Criminal Behaviour and Mental Health.* 8(2):139-153. doi.org/10.1002/cbm.232.

Spolin, V. (1983). *Improvisation for the theater: A handbook of teaching and directing — revised edition*. Evanston, IL: Northwestern University Press.

Thompson, J. (2000). Critical citizenship: Boal, Brazil and theatre in prisons. *Annual Review of Critical Psychology, 2*:181-191.

Toivanen, T., Komulainen, K., & Ruismaki, H. (2011). Drama education and improvisation as a resource of teacher student's creativity. *Procedia Social and Behavioral Sciences 12*, 60-69. Department of Teacher Education, University of Helsinki, Finland.

Walker, S. (2014). It's not all just child's play: A psychological study on the potential benefits of theater programming with children. Honors College 198. https://digitalcommons.library.umaine.edu/honors/198

13

Drama Therapy

Drama therapy is a general term which encompasses three therapeutic techniques — Role-Playing, Sociodrama, and Psychodrama — all of which are based on the principle that acting out situations can induce behavioral and/or psychological change in a person. Drama, according to Webster's dictionary, is "a state, situation, or series of events involving interesting or intense conflict of forces." Drama is life in microcosm — action and reaction.

Therapists who choose to use the techniques of drama as a therapeutic modality should be aware of the purpose of each type, from problem-oriented role-playing to (potentially) emotionally charged psychodrama. This will enable them to engage their clients at an appropriate level of dramatic intensity.

Drama therapy, as a psychotherapeutic profession and academic discipline, draws from ancient ritual practices (Jones, 1996). It developed in the 1970s from theoretical foundations including theater, psychology, psychotherapy, anthropology, and play. A major influence is the concept of psychodrama developed by Jacob Moreno in the 1920s and 1930s as a method of group therapy based on encounter and enactment (Moreno, 1946). Professional associations were established in the UK in 1977 and the USA in 1979.

Drama therapy is defined by the National Association for Drama Therapy, USA (NADT) as "the intentional use of drama and/or theater processes to achieve therapeutic goals" (NADT, 2012). The NADT (2012) says that behavior change, skill building, emotional and physical integration, and personal growth can be achieved through drama therapy in prevention, intervention, and treatment settings. Drama therapists work in a wide variety of settings: schools, mental health, general health, social care settings, and prisons. Clients include children with autism, older people with dementia, adolescents who self-harm, people with histories of sexual or physical abuse, those suffering from mental illness, and women with post-natal depression (British Association of Dramatherapists, 2012).

Role-Playing

Role-playing evolved from psychodrama but is a less emotionally intense experience. It is a vehicle for assisting clients to replay upsetting interactions with friends or family members, to practice social skills or experiment with new behaviors, or to confront people with whom they are angry. Real life issues can be explored in a safe environment. Role-playing is problem oriented. One of its goals is to work out alternative and more effective approaches to identified problems. Another goal is to change behavior rather than to explore the psychodynamics of behavior (e.g., Why do I do this?). Since a primary aspect of this process is learning new behaviors, it is important for clients to receive feedback on the effectiveness of the behaviors practiced. Clients can continue to practice these behaviors until they are satisfied with them or until their anxiety is manageable.

Research

For clients with generalized anxiety disorder, therapists seek to gradually expose clients to anxiety provoking situations so they can apply and continue to build techniques to handle a variety of situations. The success experienced at each step helps to strengthen internal locus of control and self-confidence. Experiences may need to be therapeutically designed to allow gradual exposure. In general, being further away from actual involvement — talking about it, watching a video about it, or reading about it — is less stressful. Full participation in the actual event through role-playing or community integration is more stressful.

A study evaluated the two- and three-year outcomes of targeted, school-based drama group therapy in reducing behavioral symptoms as compared to the teaching of math and English (McArdle et al., 2011). This study indicated that drama group therapy can contribute to a rapid reduction in teacher-observed behavioral symptoms and that the gains are still evident after a year. The study concluded that school-based, small group interventions with different content are likely to share some effective components.

Guidelines for the Use of Role-Playing

Role-playing is effective:

- Whenever the therapist wants to allow group members to be able to see themselves as others see them
- When the group needs a change of pace from the activity or method currently being used to promote individual or group growth
- Especially with couples, siblings, co-workers, or for other relationships where problems in relating have developed
- As a good technique for enabling us to laugh at ourselves and get out of the "drama" of life and its ruts

Role-playing follows a sequence of events from creating a setting and designating a double through the actual role play to feedback from the rest of the group and closing activities, as described below.

The Setting

Chairs for the group are arranged in a circle. Depending on the nature of the role-play, one or more chairs may also be placed in the middle of the circle. Items such as foam sticks, batakas, or pillows may be available for clients who need to vent feelings.

Warmup: The Process of Selecting a Protagonist

From the standpoint of creating a positive learning experience, it is important to choose a group member who would benefit from assuming the role of protagonist. Evaluate information from the following warmup questions and considerations to help in making a choice.

Warmup questions for the group:

- You only have a landline and you want to talk to someone. Who would you call and what would you say?
- What person do you have unfinished business with?
- The empty chair is you. What do you think about when you see that empty chair and what do you have to say to it?

Considerations:

- Generally, the protagonist should be picked by the amount of emotional affect exhibited in the warmup.
- Avoid involving a reluctant protagonist.
- A protagonist who expresses a willingness to work should be considered.
- With an ongoing group you may choose to ask them who would like to work today and then have the group select from the situations offered or suggested.
- When in doubt, wait and be patient. Perhaps even extend the warmup period. There may be times when the whole session may become a warmup activity.

Purposes of the Action

- To stimulate change. If an individual experiences himself/herself acting in a spontaneous and creative manner in relation to others, and experiences others as accepting and giving, the person will tend to develop new perceptions of himself/herself and his/her universe. This can have a beneficial effect on all aspects of life. The spontaneity of the action disrupts old patterns of behavior and can create an appropriate response to a new situation or a new response to an old situation.

- To provide alternatives within the context of a life situation. Alternatives can be suggested by the therapist or the group.
- To allow the protagonist to play-act a situation in a non-threatening environment. A supportive, non-judgmental atmosphere is important.

Selection and Use of the Double

This is the first step to take after selecting a protagonist. A "double" is a person who takes on some aspect of personality or behavior for the protagonist. Determine who should play this role using one of the following methods:

- Ask the protagonist if s/he can choose someone in the group who knows him/her well enough to be able to help him/her.
- Ask the group if there is someone who identifies enough with the situation to serve as a double.

Roles of the Double

The double:

- may provide support or may be a mirror for the protagonist. S/he may also express thoughts and feelings the protagonist is unwilling to share.
- represents opposing viewpoints for the protagonist to consider
- takes cues from the director
- should try to imitate and try to get in touch with the feelings and thoughts of the protagonist
- speaks for the protagonist rather than for himself/herself

The protagonist may disagree with the double at any time. The director may need to check back with the protagonist throughout the action to make sure that s/he remembers that this is an option. More than one double may be used. The following offers a deeper look at two techniques used by a double.

Mirror by the Double

One of the purposes of the double is to project an image through which the protagonist can see himself/herself. For example, if the protagonist is expressing to a parent the fact that the parent never listens to what s/he says, the double may say, in the same intonation as the protagonist, "You never listen to what I say and how I feel!" This allows the protagonist to see and hear how the parent might perceive this statement. It adds another dimension, self-perception, to the reality of the situation.

Role Reversal in Role-Playing

Role reversal gives the protagonist the opportunity to see and feel what it's like to be in "someone else's shoes." It helps the protagonist to become aware of the perceptions and views other than his/her own. It also introduces another person (besides the protagonist) into the scene for the protagonist to relate to.

The Role-Play in Action

Any or all of these three techniques (double, mirror, and role reversal) may be used within the role-play period. The action may be set in the past, present, future, or in fantasy.

Sharing Reactions

This is the only time that the whole group may participate. They share how they identified with the protagonist in the action. No interpretations are allowed, but first-hand identifications and heartfelt responses are encouraged.

Closing

The closing is designed to fulfill two important functions:

- to provide support for the protagonist and thank him/her for his/her efforts
- to provide the group with the opportunity to share supportive feelings with each other (e.g., applause, verbalizing, a group hug)

Life Situations Adaptable for Role-Playing

Here are some ideas for role-playing. It is organized into two sections, the first containing general ideas for role-playing social skills, followed by a group of more specific situations.

Personal Relationships (Friends, Relatives, Neighbors)

Giving and receiving compliments:

- being told that you did a good job
- telling someone that you like the way…
- complimenting another person on his/her hair, clothing, style, etc.

Stating Feelings Directly

- finding something to be the focus of your life work and assuming your parent(s) disapprove
- anger towards someone who didn't keep a secret
- disappointment at a canceled date
- a friend continually being late
- stating fear about a situation
- needing more independence from family

Saying "NO!"

- to food not on your diet
- to an invitation
- to using drugs or alcohol
- to sexual involvement
- to a family gathering
- to someone smoking in your house
- to someone wanting to cheat off your exam

Asking For

- support
- help
- time to spend with someone
- confidentiality

Telling Someone about Your …

- lack of interest in a love relationship
- disappointment in a relationship
- job loss
- serious health situation
- serious financial situation
- issues with in-laws
- separation or divorce

Defining or Explaining to a Five-Year-Old

- the concept of "disability"
- the concept of "death"
- the concept of "divorce"
- the concept of "God"

Work-Related Issues

- Job interview
- Termination interview (initiated by you)
- Termination interview (initiated by your boss)
- Difficulties with co-workers and:
    - smoking
    - drinking
    - covering for them (e.g., their mistakes or absences)
    - competition for promotion
- Asking for assistance (feeling overworked)
- Dealing with authority figures (supervisor or boss)
- Dealing with social or sexual situations in the workplace
- Dealing with discrimination:
    - sexual
    - racial

- disability related
- social
- age
- professional advancement

Client/Therapist Relationships

Group members take on the roles required. Dealing with:

- "You are paid to care about us"
- Client flirting or asking for a phone number
- Motivating a client
- A member of another discipline questioning what you are doing with a client and the importance of your intervention

Risking Possible Rejection

- Your niece, nephew, son, daughter, or someone you love very much and to whom you always tell the truth, as you know it, wants to try out for a school play but is afraid s/he won't get the part.
- Your niece, nephew, son, daughter, or someone you love very much wants to have a birthday party. She wants to invite some new friends but is concerned that they might not come.

Being Spontaneous

- Your best friend in the world wins a trip to Mexico and wants you to go; it would mean missing one week of work or school.

Creating Balance in Your Life

- Last weekend you spent the whole time playing and having fun, then felt completely guilty for not studying or "accomplishing anything constructive." The weekend before that you spent the whole time studying, washing clothes, cleaning house, etc. and resented not doing anything fun. However, this weekend…

- You are studying for a test the next day that you must do well on. Your friend calls you up with extra tickets to a concert. You've been eager to go to it, but unable to get tickets. You are not prepared for the test. What do you do?

Confrontation

- Your co-worker is on drugs. You are always covering up for him/her because s/he is often late. Your boss knows that there is a problem but wants the co-workers to work it out between them. How do you confront this person? Also, this person denies his/her problem.

Acceptance and Assertion

- You are winning an award. It is a great honor. What is it for?
- Someone crowds in front of you at the store, grabs the last copy of a book out of your hands, or tries to talk you out of a purchase so that s/he can have it.
- Issues with authority and institutions, e.g., doctors or salespeople. For example, you have a feeling that you've been given too strong a prescription by your doctor.
- Disagreeing with a police officer (e.g., disputing whether you deserve a ticket).
- Being dissatisfied with:
    - a service done on your car
    - your landlord
- A person cuts ahead of you in line with two people ahead. The others don't say anything. Would you?
- You take yourself out to a nice restaurant. You feel that you deserve something nice and love going out to eat. It doesn't matter that you are alone. In fact, you're happy to have some private time. The waiter

seats you close to the kitchen at a small table where you are invisible to others. In addition, you are not receiving appropriate service.

- You've had a new roommate for the past three months. She is now five days late with the rent. She just recently became unemployed and she is also ill with some flu-like symptoms that have lasted a week. She has made no attempt to borrow the money and just assumes you'll cover her rent. You confront her on the issue, and she says she is too sick to talk about it. How do you react?
- Your boyfriend has recently started bringing up his old girlfriend's name. Although it seems harmless, you know that there is still a strong bond between them. What do you do?
- You have been making dinner for your friend/lover and s/he was expected at 7:30 p.m. The table is set. It is already 8 p.m. and your guest has not arrived. An hour later the person arrives. This is not the first time you have found yourself waiting for this person. What do you do?
- A child has a pet guinea pig which the mother insists must be kept caged. The child is caught having let the little animal out to run loose in his/her room. There is a scene between mother and child involving the idea of caging and not following through on an agreement.
- A young woman comes home from an exciting event (a party, a drama class, a dance class) and is behaving in a spirited, noisy way. Her home, however, is a quiet place where one person is studying and another is watching TV. It is clear that her excitement and animated behavior are not welcome.
- You told a friend a personally embarrassing secret and the next morning another friend calls to console you.
- You have had a crush on a good friend who has been unavailable for the past few years. S/he has recently broken up with his/her significant other. You are still interested. What do you do?
- Someone you are intimately involved with asks for personal details about your past. You have been burned before by being completely honest. How do you respond?
- You are invited to a party by a new friend you met in one of your classes. You don't know anyone else who is going to the party, which is on Friday night. You usually spend Friday nights at home, watching TV or studying. You tell your friend…

- A grown daughter is trying to care for her elderly mother at home. The mother is very dependent and demanding. The daughter has not had any relief from her duties in quite a long time. As she tries to relax with a book, the mother calls out two rooms away for companionship.
- Michael, aged 33, is going to LA to visit his parents who have been retired for a couple of years now. Since retirement his father has been drinking more than he used to. Both of his parents are strong followers of the Protestant work ethic and used to work long hours in their family-owned business. They sold the business at a profit in order to retire. When Michael arrives, his father has not returned yet from the golf club, so Michael decides to disclose his concerns to his mother. She becomes angry with Michael for implying that his father has some sort of a "problem." Their conversation ends when Michael's father enters, returning from having "a few with the boys at the club."
- John, aged 43, is married to Linda, aged 36. They have been married for four years and are both satisfied with their relationship. While they are having dinner, Linda announces that she is interested in having a child. Taken by surprise, John announces firmly that he has no interest in going through that with her. When they first married, Linda was wrapped up in her career and didn't think she wanted to have children. Now, as she hears her biological clock ticking, she has discovered that she has different feelings about the matter. Linda is disappointed in John's reaction; John is shocked and in a quandary at what he feels is Linda's change of heart.
- A divorced mother is at home cleaning on a Sunday afternoon. While picking up clothes off the floor in the room of her only daughter, who is aged 14½, she finds her daughter's diary lying open to a recent entry. She reads the diary and discovers that her daughter is experimenting with cocaine and alcohol. The mother becomes enraged and is also frightened. She herself is an alcoholic who has been sober and in recovery for five years. Her daughter is aware of this and used to go to Ala-Teen meetings but has lost interest and refused to go this last year.
- Your newly single mother is going out on a date and you don't like the man.
- A friend suggests going to the movies and out to dinner. S/he wants to see a horror film and eat Mexican food. You would rather see a

comedy and eat Chinese food, but every time you've gone out together, you've given in and have done what your friend wanted. This time however...

Additional Role-Play Situations

- Somebody cuts right in front of you on the highway and proceeds to drive ten miles an hour under the speed limit.
- You're at a party and your best friend is about to try cocaine.
- You're a babysitter. You're not supposed to have boyfriends over. Your boyfriend calls and wants to come over.
- You're at a very busy restaurant and the waitress is already impatient. She brings you a meal that looks good but isn't what you ordered. She's about to walk away.
- You're at a party and some nerd persists in asking you to dance. You've politely tried everything to give him the message. You're now a little irritated... here he comes again. What do you do?
- You're at a dinner party and you're not able to eat what's served.
- You have a potluck dinner, and everyone brings dessert.
- You're late for an exam. On your way to class you see some guy drop his little black book. He doesn't realize he's dropped it and keeps walking. He's about 100 yards away.
- Your neighbor plays loud music every Saturday morning at 8 a.m. You worked until 3 a.m. Friday night.
- You're at a wedding party and they're passing a jug of wine around the table as a ritual toast. The wine is coming your way when you notice that the guy next to you has a cold sore on his lip.
- You've arrived in town just two days before your best friend's wedding. You hate the bridesmaids' dresses she had raved about over the phone. They're the wrong fit and the wrong color.

Sociodrama

This is a form of dramatic enactment which aims at clarifying group themes rather than focusing on the problems of one individual. Although an individual may participate as the protagonist in the sociodrama, characterization is based on a type of person rather than on any one individual. Sociodrama borrows many of the techniques of psychodrama (see the next section), but the focus is always on creating or approximating real-life situations which concern the group as a whole. The goal of sociodrama is to help group members who share similar problems by exploring these problems together.

Research

Rousseau, et al. (2007) assessed the effects of a school drama therapy program for immigrant and refugee adolescents designed to prevent emotional and behavioral problems and to enhance school performance. This nine-week program involved 136 newcomers, ages 12-18, attending integration classes in a multiethnic school. Pretest and posttest data were collected from the students and their teachers. The self-report and teacher's forms of the *Strengths and Difficulties Questionnaire* (Goodman, 2001) were used to assess emotional and behavioral symptoms. At the end of the program, the adolescents in the experimental group reported lower mean levels of impairment than those in the control group, when baseline data were controlled for. Their performance in mathematics also increased significantly compared to that of their control peers. The findings suggest that sociodrama workshops have an impact on social adjustment of recently arrived immigrants and refugees. This program appears to be a promising sociodrama method of working preventively and in a non-stigmatizing manner with adolescents who have been exposed to diverse forms of adversity, including war and violence.

Sociodrama Situations

Examples of sociodrama include the enactment of such situations as:

- A youth in a transition home seeing his/her parents for the first time since leaving the home environment
- An alcoholic in a recovery program going to his/her first social event during recovery
- An adult in a support group confronting an abusive situation
- A group of residents in a nursing home confronting the nursing home administrator about a foul-mouthed aide
- A group of female co-workers approaching the personnel manager about a male co-worker who belittles them

Psychodrama

Psychodrama was developed by Jacob Moreno, MD, in the 1920s. The primary characteristic which distinguishes psychodrama from other forms of drama therapy is that it is an exploration of one individual's internal conflicts. It focuses on the intra-psychic (internal) rather than the social (external) dimension. In psychodrama, the individual who is the main character (the protagonist) explores a conflict through an enactment that enables him/her to watch and engage in an inner drama as it becomes visible and tangible. The psychodrama may shift among many facets of a protagonist's life — from his/her past to the present or future and back again.

This technique usually focuses on relatively deep emotional issues, such as childhood traumas or painful memories, in order to uncover the origins of unresolved internal conflicts. Psychodrama is a method of action which makes conflicts available to people in a safe setting. This permits them to examine relationships in the present or re-examine past relationships that they consider relevant to the present, and to experiment with possible changes for the future.

In view of these two goals (examining the past and experimenting with change), psychodrama is often a two-phase process. In the first phase — re-enacting — the core problem or frustration scene is acted out. Ideally the protagonist will experience catharsis (a profound emotion release) or fresh insight into a past problem in this phase. This is followed by the correcting or retraining phase. The protagonist corrects the negative scene by acting out a positive one that s/he delineates (Yablonsky, 1976).

Research

Yang and colleagues (2012) conducted a review of the literature prior to April 2011 related to psychosocial interventions and found support for the following interventions: cognitive behavior therapy; psychodrama; group sessions focused on psychosocial issues; strategy training for motor behavior; relaxation techniques; social skills training; and multi-disciplinary education programs that focused on activities of daily living, speech therapy, mobility, group relaxation training, and expert presentations on disease, diet, and medication. The authors concluded that, in spite of the methodological limitations, psychosocial interventions have the potential for improving depressive and anxiety outcomes among people with Parkinson's disease.

Ruddy and Dent-Brown's (2007) systematic review of drama therapy and psychodrama for inpatients with schizophrenia reported five studies. The reviewers had no conclusive findings about the harms or benefits of drama therapy for this client group. However, the review did include two studies with randomized control trials with Turkish school students who had high aggression levels (Karatas & Gokcakan, 2009). Findings of the study indicated significant effects, with group-based psychodrama appearing to reduce total aggression, anger, hostility, and indirect aggression scores. These effects were still measurable at a sixteen-week follow up.

Elements of Psychodrama

In psychodrama there is a ritualistic set of elements that help provide a structure for emotional release and discovery. These elements are the warmup, enactment and re-enactment, catharsis — movement — emotional insight, closure of individual drama, sharing integrative process, and closure of the group. When retraining immediately follows re-enacting, the warmup may be omitted and only a short closure may be necessary.

Warmup

Warmup techniques focus on spontaneity and interaction among group members in order to lessen inhibitions and prepare the group for the enactment. Group dynamics are revealed. (Who is included or excluded? Who identifies with whom?) The group experiences its own power, while the therapist balances the group needs against his/her own agenda for the group. During this period themes develop, and the choices of protagonist and audience are established.

Enactment and Re-enactment

Once the protagonist is chosen, s/he sets the scene and chooses roles for the enactment. The director now employs the techniques of psychodrama to begin the process. These techniques are meant to facilitate the protagonist's ability to experience feelings throughout the scene.

Catharsis — Movement — Emotional Insight

For Moreno, the concept of catharsis was an important aspect of psychodrama. The protagonist undergoes a self-purging and the audience witnesses and engages in an emotional experience. Psychodrama thus draws on the power of both the stage and religious ritual (Moreno in Emunah, 1994). The catharsis and emotional insight create a turning point that takes place near the closure of the enactment. Catharsis may involve regression in the service of the ego, but it is *not* an acting out to avoid a painful memory, it is a reprocessing of memory.

Closure of Individual Drama

The timing of closure is a therapeutic judgment. When the director feels that the drama is coming to a close, s/he may say, "How do you want to end this?" In addition to the protagonist, the director must also consider the group's investment in the enactment. At times, when a particular scene affects the group strongly, it may be difficult to continue the scene (e.g., themes of suicide, homicidal ideation, drug use). It is important to find out the group's feelings in order to determine what to do next. The director may say something like, "It looks like everyone felt strongly about what went on. Try finishing this sentence, 'What touched me was _________.'" The answers may give information for further work.

Sharing Integrative Process

This is the only time the whole group can participate by sharing how they felt. No interpretations are allowed — the group should also be discouraged from just saying what they saw the players doing. During the sharing statements following the enactment, the audience makes evident their identification with the protagonist. Most experience common or universal feelings about what took place. The director may check out impressions of the audience. For example, the director may ask a member of the audience, "You seemed tense during the scene. Did you feel tense? Did the scene have an impact on you?" The director will help the group identify the similarities and differences in group members' feelings and experiences. Through the sharing, the director tries to create opportunities to develop empathy and a trusting milieu.

Closure of Group

The closing of action provides support for the protagonist and thanks him/her for his/her efforts. It is also the time to give the group the opportunity to share supportive feelings with each other (e.g., applause, verbalizing, or group hug).

At closure the group may acknowledge that it will (in a new drama) further explore an area or examine a theme that emerged.

Techniques of Psychodrama

Warmup Techniques

These techniques facilitate spontaneity which helps lessen the emotional inhibition of group members. Thematic content is often obtained through warmups and may lead to the development of a psychodrama.

Magic Shop

Values are exchanged by barter. A hope, wish, aspiration, or personal quality is obtained by exchanging another personal quality for it. One after another, members of the group volunteer to enter the magic shop in quest of a dream, quality, or aspiration. The barter compels the subject to judge the relative value of the qualities and his/her desire for them. A written exchange may reinforce the interaction. The audience may be asked to assist the shopkeeper or to comment on the deal being arranged. A sample dialogue might be

Customer: "I would like to buy some time for myself."

Shopkeeper: "I have that over here in aisle two. What can you trade?"

Customer: "Well, I'll trade some ambition to get some time for myself."

Shopkeeper: "I thought you valued your ambition — that achieving was what made your life meaningful. Are you sure you are ready to give up your ambition?"

Customer: "I think that I am getting sick from not having time for myself. Maybe I can keep some of my ambition in this bottle until I need it and give the rest to you."

Empty Chair

Here the audience is told to imagine a person sitting in an empty chair which is before them. They are told to picture, for example, the person's dress, appearance, and posture. Each member then tells of the person that s/he projected to be in the chair. This frequently yields thematic content leading to a psychodrama.

One Wish

Group members are asked to state what they would wish for if a magic genie could grant them only one wish. For example, a client might wish for "fears and anxieties to melt away." This wish could lead to a psychodrama about what life would be like without fear and anxieties.

One Day to Relive

Group members are asked to choose one day that they would like to relive if they were given the opportunity to do so.

Who Would You Like to Be?

Group members are asked, "Who would you rather be?" This question, used in an enactment, might provide a good opportunity for role-play, enabling the protagonist to become the person s/he wishes to be.

Coloring Book

Members are asked to draw their own worlds, the imaginary materials being a crayon and blank pages. "What would you draw on the first page? On the second page?" and so on.

Non-Verbal Techniques

The group consents to interact with one another for a fixed period during which the use of words is forbidden. Members are encouraged to express anything they feel at the moment using movement of any body part(s) (e.g., hand gestures) as the mode of expression. They may use the physical setting (e.g., chairs) in any way but must respect the one rule — no words. Rich material develops as patterns of reaction come into relief against the background of silence.

Thematic Psychodrama Techniques

These techniques consist of thematic suggestions presented to the group. They are useful in group therapy situations to clarify and resolve interpersonal difficulties among group members.

Future Projection

The protagonist picks a future time and place and projects himself/herself there, enacting a situation that s/he thinks will come about, or one that may actually be expected to come about, e.g., an interview for a job, a pending marriage, or a birth. Future time techniques require that the protagonist imagines what life will be like "if."

Self-Realization

The protagonist enacts his/her hopes, plans, and aspirations as s/he wishes them to be, not as s/he expects them to be.

Dream Representation

The protagonist enacts a dream instead of telling it. In a discussion with the director, the protagonist describes the dream, then auxiliary egos are selected from the group to take parts in the dream as voices, objects, or persons. The protagonist takes the position s/he usually has when sleeping and then proceeds to enact the dream. In the retraining phase, the protagonist is told that s/he can change the dream in any way s/he wishes.

Hallucinatory Psychodrama

The protagonist enacts the hallucinations and delusions s/he is experiencing. S/he portrays the different aspects of the hallucination: the voices, sounds, or visions. Auxiliary egos may be called upon to enact the various hallucinatory phenomena so that the protagonist can interact with them and thereby put them to a reality test. The aim is to use enactment and interaction within the psychodrama to give the subject some control over his/her hallucinations.

Behind Your Back

Here the protagonist turns his/her back to the rest of the group. The group is told to imagine that the protagonist is not present. Each participant shares feelings towards the protagonist. This segment is followed by a discussion. The protagonist is then "brought back into the room" and the discussion continues.

Variation: Have the group turn its back on the protagonist, who then makes an honest statement about his/her feelings towards each group member.

Facilitative Techniques within a Psychodrama

Once a thematic structure has been established (see above), this group of techniques is aimed at facilitating catharsis, insight, and role perception within the psychodrama.

Double

In this technique the protagonist plays himself/herself. An auxiliary ego, usually a staff member, is asked to also represent the protagonist, e.g., to assume the same emotional and physical positions and therefore to assume the identity of the protagonist. The double then may express feelings, thoughts, opinions, and reactions which the protagonist cannot or will not voice himself/herself.

Multiple Double

The protagonist plays himself/herself, and several auxiliary egos play parts of the protagonist. This technique may aid in clarifying an issue or restructuring ambivalence about a person or situation and may facilitate catharsis.

Mirror for Expression

If a protagonist is inhibited to the point of immobilization so that s/he cannot represent himself/herself in word or action, an auxiliary ego may be chosen (by the protagonist or director) to be a "mirror" of the protagonist's movements and speech. Such a representation or mirroring would be under the direction of the protagonist who would inform, correct, or change the mirror's representation.

Role Reversal in Psychodrama

This technique has two major functions.

- Role reversal may occur during a scene in order to aid the auxiliary ego in accurately enacting the role assigned to him/her by the protagonist. Here, the reversal is of short duration but is long enough to provide clues to the auxiliary ego to create a more accurate representation of the role.

- Role reversal is especially useful in the learning or retraining phase of the process. Through reversal of roles, the protagonist is given the opportunity to experience the feelings of the "other" in an interpersonal situation. Moreno (1946) states, "the function of role reversal is to increase role perception."

Physical Elevation

In order to promote full expression of feelings toward an "other" (usually an authority figure) in a psychodrama scene, the protagonist can be physically elevated by standing on a chair, stool, or table to interact with the "other." Frequently, this produces authoritativeness on the part of the protagonist which can be difficult to attain using other techniques.

References

British Association of Dramatherapists. (2018). About dramatherapy. http://badth.org.uk/.

Emunah, R. (1994). *Acting for real: Drama therapy process, technique, and performance.* New York, NY: Brunner/Mazel Publisher.

Goodman, R. (2001). Psychometric properties of the Strengths and Difficulties Questionnaire (SDQ). *Journal of the American Academy of Child and Adolescent Psychiatry, 40*, 1337-1345.

Jones, P. (1996). *Drama as therapy: Theatre as living*. London: Routledge.

Karatas, Z. & Gokcakan, Z. (2009). The effect of group-based psychodrama therapy on decreasing the level of aggression in adolescents. *Turk Psikiyatri Dergisi, 20*(4), 1-9. Retrieved from www.turkpsikiyatri.com.

McArdle, P., Young, R., Quibell, T., Moseley, D., Johnson, R., & LeCouteur, A. (2011). Early intervention for at risk children: 3-year follow-up. *European Child & Adolescent Psychiatry, 20*(3), 111-120. Doi:10.1007/s00787-010-0148-y.

Moreno, J. L. (1946). *Psychodrama*. New York: Beacon House.

National Association for Drama Therapy (NADT). (2012). What is drama therapy? Retrieved October 2017 http://www.nadt.org/what-is-drama-therapy.html.

Porter, H. R. (2015). *Recreational therapy for specific diagnoses and conditions.* Enumclaw, WA: Idyll Arbor, Inc.

Rousseau, C., Benoit, M., Gauthier, M. F., Lacroix, L., Alain, N., Rojas, M. V., Moran, A., & Bourassa, D. (2007). Classroom drama therapy program for immigrant and refugee adolescents: A pilot study. *Clin Child Psychol Psychiatry. 12*(3), 451-65.

Ruddy, R. A. & Dent-Brown, K. (2007). Drama therapy for schizophrenia or schizophrenia-like illnesses. Cochrane Database of Systematic Reviews 2007, Issue 1. Art. No.: CD005378. DOI: 10.1002/14651858.CD005378.pub2.

Yang, S., Sajatovic, M., & Walter, B. L. (2012). Psychosocial interventions for depression and anxiety in Parkinson's disease. *Journal of Geriatric Psychiatry and Neurology, 25*(2), 113-121.

Yablonsky, L. 1976. *Psychodrama.* New York, NY: Basic Books, Inc.

14

Laughter and Clowning

Too often, when someone has an illness or disability, it is hard for that individual to look beyond the crisis and discomfort. This micro-focused vision produces an imbalance. Humor is often used to help the client achieve a balance again — a balance of recognizing all that is in his/her world, both the good and the bad. Laughter is an important component of wellness. This chapter will look at the difference between laughing with and laughing at someone and the treatment benefits of laughter.

One of the ways to promote laughter is with clowning activities. A clown is an entertainer who uses antics, jokes, and tricks to help produce a happy, lighthearted mood. If clowning is the activity, then smiles and laughter are the obvious signs of the desired outcome. The second part of the chapter will provide information on running clown activities as one of the ways to promote healthy laughter.

Laughter

Laughing with someone is based on mutual respect and caring for the other. Laughter develops empathy between groups, giving each a greater confidence. This brings individuals closer together, providing support and emotional nourishment through amusement. Healthy laughter breaks down emotional barriers instead of creating or reinforcing them. Some individuals (including clowns) may choose to make themselves the butt of their own jokes. This is done to bring joy and esteem to everyone, including the teller of the joke. The person who can laugh at himself/herself invites other people to laugh and feel more at ease.

Laughing at others tends to be based on contempt and insensitivity toward others. This type of laughter divides people and destroys confidence. This division excludes some people, offends others, and tends to reinforce negative stereotypes by singling out individuals or groups. When a person doesn't have a choice about being the butt of a joke, hurt feelings develop and grow, even if the teller of the sarcastic joke is the butt of the joke. This type of laughter is often abusive and chills any hope of developing a closer, open group.

Benefits of Laughter

There are many health benefits associated with laughter. Using laughter as part of a therapeutic intervention increases physical well-being, cognitive stimulation, feelings of social well-being, coping skills, and the individual's subjective well-being.

The physical act of laughing allows the individual to exercise his/her lungs and chest muscles. This, in turn, helps stimulate the circulatory system. It promotes better circulation and increases blood and oxygen flow to the brain. Laughter used on a regular basis relaxes muscles, lowers the pulse rate, and may even help lower blood pressure. Laughter also helps the individual cope with and control pain. Production of endorphins (the body's naturally occurring painkiller) increases. Laughter is a distraction from the pain. It is hard to hold strongly to anxiety, fear, tension, and/or anger when you are laughing.

Laughter also encourages the individual to cope with adversity, think flexibly, and achieve (and keep) mental health. Humor increases an individual's coping skills, reduces anger, and eases stressful situations. Somewhat tongue-in-cheek Konrad Lorenz (1963) observed, "Barking dogs may occasionally bite, but laughing men hardly ever shoot" (p. 285). Laughter is one of the primary defenses in the human repertoire for coping with and adapting to stress and trauma. Valiant (1977) conducted a study using a group of healthy men to identify mature coping mechanisms. Humor was one of the five coping mechanisms identified through his study.

Humor also helps social interactions. Humans are social creatures. Being close to others may produce tension, divide relationships, and require coping with antisocial acts by others. Humor provides one of the mechanisms for coping with the results of being close to others. Usually, joyful and humorous interactions between two individuals are indicators of a close and healthy relationship.

Research

There are many reasons why laughter makes us feel good and leads to better health. A summary article by David DiSalvo (2017) lists six benefits:

Laughter is a potent endorphin releaser. Manninen, Tuominen, Dunbar, et al. (2017) found direct neurophysiological support for endorphin release by using PET and the μ-opioid-receptor (MOR)-specific ligand [^{11}C]carfentanil to quantify laughter-induced endogenous opioid release in 12 healthy males. Studies in the same report also found increased pain thresholds as a result of laughter. A study by Mobbs et al. (2003) found a similar result: humor and laughter trigger the brain's reward centers.

Laughter contagiously forms social bonds. When someone starts laughing, others join in even when they are not sure why everyone else is laughing. As a result, social laughter creates a chain reaction throughout a group that results in endorphin release in the whole group. The spreading endorphin release promotes a sense of togetherness and safety (DiSalvo, 2017).

Laughter helps teach social communication. Not all laughter is the same. Joyous laughter, taunting laughter, and tickling laughter activate connections between different brain regions. Decoding the kind of laughter seems to foster understanding of the intentions of others and increases ability to decode social information in the environment (Wildgruber et al., 2013).

Laughter is central to positive relationships. Kurtz and Algoe (2015) recorded conversations between couples and found that global evaluations of relationship quality, closeness, and social support was positively associated with the proportion of the conversation spent laughing simultaneously with the romantic partner.

Laughter and antidepressants have a similar effect. Cha and Hong (2015) studied middle-aged women with varying levels of depression. They found that that serotonin activation through laughter therapy lessened depression and provided a possible method of depression control.

Laughter protects your heart. Laughter has an anti-inflammatory effect that protects blood vessels and heart muscles. This seems to be caused by lowering the body's stress response, which also lowers inflammation. One study by Miller and colleagues (2010) showed that laughter is linked to the healthy function of blood vessels. Stress negatively impacts the endothelium by causing vasoconstriction. During laughter, there is vasodilation with increased blood flow.

Laughter Activities

The benefits of laughter are so profound that every creative arts activity should include opportunities for joyous laughter. As you look at other activities in this book, think about how you can allow time and space for laughter in each of them.

In the second section of this chapter we will look at clowning as a way to bring about laughter. But first, we will look at the possibility that the laughter doesn't have to be genuine to be effective.

The Cancer Treatment Centers of America (2019) offer laughter therapy programs that include laughter-related exercises, including fake laughter and laughter greetings. Their program, known as Laughter Club, is based on laughter as a physical exercise, not on humor or jokes.

There have been studies showing that simulated laughter provides the same health benefits as real laughter, including the study by Greene, Morgan, Traywick, and Mingo (2017) on older adults and exercise.

Laughter yoga has a large set of exercises you can use. Since it's easier to understand how these work by actually seeing them, search for laughter yoga on YouTube and watch the videos available. One good one is "100

Laughter Yoga Exercises" by Madan Kataria (2013). Simulated laughter and laughter greetings can be used as warmup exercises before any session.

Clowning

Clowning offers a particular type of laughter therapy. Clowns have worked in hospital settings at least since the time of Hippocrates. Doctors of that era believed that mood influenced healing, and Hippocrates' hospital on the island of Kos had troupes of players and clowns. At the end of the nineteenth century the Fratellini Brothers (a famous clown trio) began the current practice of making occasional visits to hospitals, especially pediatric hospitals.

In 1986 Karen Ridd in Winnipeg and Michael Christensen in New York, began working with children in large urban pediatric hospitals. They were not aware of each other's work. Since that time clown doctors have become a part of the healthcare field as this new practice began to appear in more than a dozen countries around the world. Some of these are Theodora Foundation (Europe, South Africa, Hong Kong, and Belorussia), Le Rire Medecin (France), Die Clown Doktoren (Germany), Payasospital (Spain), Soccorso Clown (Italy), Clinic Clowns (Europe), Doctors of Joy (Brazil), Fools for Health (Canada). Each program is unique, but all value professionalism, regular training, and maintaining high standards (Otto, 2001).

Though initial work was focused on children, more recently clowning has moved outside the pediatric unit and beyond the hospital. This benefits patients, families, staff, and the community. In 2001, professional clowns started working with seniors in hospitals. The same year Hearts and Minds began their Elderflowers project for patients with dementia in nursing homes and senior centers in Scotland (Hearts & Minds, 2017; Killick, 2003). Services expanded to include people across the lifespan.

Most recently CliniClowns in the Netherlands developed web clowning. Patients and others can view the clowns on the CliniClowns website (http://www.cliniclowns.nl). By being on the web they can help more children. The website of clowns is visited by more than 200 children a week. Children meet the clowns via webcam, chat, and email.

Clown doctors work with clients, their families, and healthcare teams to promote wellness and to improve quality of life using music, movement, theater, magic, and puppetry. They have training on issues related to illness and disease. They can improvise and interact with their clients wherever healthcare is delivered.

Fools for Health currently delivers clown doctor programs at five hospitals and clown programs at five local long-term care facilities in Windsor, Essex, and the Chatham-Kent health regions in Canada. The organization began as a collaboration between Windsor Regional Hospital and the University of Windsor. Fools for Health keeps records of its work in order to document services and determine areas of improvement. It remains committed to "systematic and continuous research on factors that influence the efficacy of and limits to the roles and benefits of clowns working in the healthcare system and effects of the work on the clown doctors themselves." (Gervais, Warren, & Twohig, 2006)

In general, the research Fools for Health conducted over the last several years suggests the following:

- Smiles and laughter have the capacity to cross all barriers of age, gender, language, illness, and pain.
- No two patients, residents, or healthcare team members or units are the same.
- Patients, residents, nurses, and doctors are part of the community in which they live, and they are all interconnected. Each hospital is a focal point of the community, especially in a small rural community.
- Clown doctors are like mail carriers in a small village, they interact with all members of the village and spread smiles and create community in each room and ward throughout the hospital.
- Each facility should be considered a unique living organism and each clown doctor program needs to be designed to meet the unique properties of that facility.

Most specifically the Fools for Health research has shown that clown doctors help to do the following:

- They reset the clock or reframe perceptions of time for patients and staff. They are especially valuable in emergency waiting rooms and for patients waiting for surgery.
- They take the minds of patients and families off illness.
- They brighten the mood of nurses, doctors, and other healthcare staff.
- They reduce the anxiety of young children waiting for surgery.
- They act as a distraction during minor bedside procedures, such as inserting an intravenous drip or Ventolin treatment.
- They extend the range of motion for stroke and aphasia patients.
- They encourage patients with tracheotomies or aphasia to speak.
- They reduce the use of pain and antidepressant medication.
- They reduce the overall length of stay in the hospital.
- They increase staff morale.
- They reduce staff absenteeism.
- They increase satisfaction with rehabilitation programs (Warren & McAuslan 2002).

The Chatham-Kent Health Alliance's Annual Report 2005-2006 states that clown doctors "reduce stress and anxiety and improve clinical outcomes" (Chatham Kent Health Alliance, 2006, p. 22). Over the past few years clown-doctors have been involved in the process of hospital accreditations. Accreditors stated that clown doctors were one of the major reasons a rehabilitation program was given an excellent rating. They also said that clown-doctors were an example of "best practice" and recommended that other hospitals provide this service for adult patients as well as pediatric patients. Within five years clown-doctors became accepted as valuable members of a multidisciplinary healthcare team and are acknowledged as integral components of the healthcare delivery process.

As many nursing home and long-term care facility residents experience cognitive difficulties, such as dementia and Alzheimer's disease, medical clowns use laughter, music, storytelling, and reminiscence techniques to stimulate memory and cognitive functioning. Medical clowns try to improve the quality of life for seniors by engaging them in activities that help rejuvenate creative, expressive, and communication skills. They ask stimulating questions which motivate the resident to engage in conversations or interactions.

Fools for Health has coordinated medical clowns in six different assisted living homes across the Essex County region. Medical clowns have interacted with seniors and research has shown that they help seniors to connect with their immediate surroundings, recognize family members, remember the past, and improve cognitive functioning and communication skills, as reported in Down Memory Lane: Work with Seniors, funded by Ontario Trillium Foundation, 2008 (Dionigi, 2012).

An ethnographic study by Ramgard, Carlson, and Mangrio (2016), looked at interactions between medical clowns and residents with dementia to discover what medical clowns do. The study covered a ten-week period in two nursing homes. Descriptions of observations showed medical clowns interacted with residents by being aware of residents' unique life story and histories. The clowns used sensory triggers, encouragement, and culture to interact with each resident in their rooms. The clowns used objects in the daily environment that were meaningful for the resident and were aware of significant places and habits of their past. The clowns initiated joint interactions in common spaces in the nursing homes by using music, dance, and drama. Both verbal and non-verbal strategies used by the clowns affected social interaction. The strategies and encouraging way the clowns interacted with residents as individuals with objects of meaning to the residents is a model for how recreational therapists can improve communication in social activities in nursing home settings.

Research

Over thirty studies on various topics in medical clowning have been supported, published, and presented. Here are a few of the studies and their findings: Meiri et al. (2017) reported assistance of medical clowns improves the physical examinations of children aged two to six years. Ninety-three children participated and were randomly assigned to one of two groups: physical exam by a pediatrician in presence of caregivers vs. physical exam by pediatrician in presence of caregivers with assistance of a medical clown. Outcome measures consisted of the level of the child's discomfort, anxiety, and the quality of the examination. Duration of the exam was similar, but duration of discomfort was shorter in the clown groups than the control groups. In the medical clown groups, 94% of the pediatricians reported that the medical clown improved their ability to perform a complete physical examination. A trend of less hospitalization was noticed: 11.3% in medical clowning group vs. 18.3% in the control group $P<0.1$ but further study on this factor is needed.

A study by Dvory et al. (2016) addressed introducing an intervention by Dream Doctors (professional medical clowns) to avoid sedation in young children undergoing kidney imaging after urinary infection. Imaging requires that the patient lie perfectly still during the scan. Pediatricians often prescribe sedation to get quality results. When sedation is given, it requires medical observation and longer waits before the child can be safely discharged from the hospital. The Dream Doctors intervention included gaining the child's cooperation during the procedure. Each study was scored by a radionuclide physician to assess quality and interpretation. A total of 142 patients were studied over a 14-month period, ages was 1 to 4 years. Only five children (3.2%) required sedation compared with 100% before the study. Dream Doctors intervention was a good alternative to sedation.

Meiri et al. (2016) did a randomized controlled study of the effect of medical clowning on reducing pain, crying, and anxiety in 100 children aged 2-10 years old undergoing venous blood draws. The study compared the use of medical clowning in the process of venous blood drawing with two control groups: 1) local anesthetic cream (EMLA) applied prior to the procedure (active control) and 2) the procedure performed with neither clown nor EMLA (control group). It was hypothesized that a medical clown will reduce pain, crying, and anxiety in children having the procedure. Outcome measures consisted of the duration of the whole procedure, the duration of crying (measured by independent observers), subjective assessment of pain level (a validated scale), and anxiety level regarding future blood exams (by questionnaire). The duration of crying was shortest with clown and pain assessment was lowest with EMLA. Parental reporting of child's anxiety related to future blood tests was significantly lower with a clown present than in the control group or EMLA. The results support the use of medical clowns or similar support personnel while drawing blood in children.

Two research projects provide additional information about the use of clowns in healthcare.

- Fools for Health, What is the Value of a Smile? An Investigation of the Impact of Clown-doctors on the Lives of Patients, their Families, and the Healthcare Team in Windsor Hospitals, funded by SSHRC (Warren & McAuslan 2002).
- Down Memory Lane: Work with seniors on the work of familial clowns, funded by Ontario Trillium Foundation (Dionigi, 2012).

Clowning Activities

Clowning uses antics, jokes, and tricks to produce a happy, lighthearted mood. Smiles and laughter are the obvious signs of the desired outcome. The information for this section was furnished by Make*A*Circus of San Francisco, California, an organization which conducts clown therapy workshops for a wide variety of facilities.

The staff of Make*A*Circus generally use the following protocol when working with groups:

Meet with staff to prepare for the session

Topics of discussion include:

- Status of clients
- Staff availability
- Lessons to accomplish

Begin session by creating clear parameters to ensure safety

Within the safety parameters instill acceptance and appreciation for each other's work.

Warm up bodies and minds

- Explore within a safe environment.
- Begin the process of ensemble.
- Stimulate and support imagination and acceptance.
- Physically prepare the body and mind.
- Establish the process of "learning through imitation."
- Use clowning as a tool for assessment without embarrassing anyone.

Introduce and refine skills

- Learn to execute multi-step directions.
- Learn to work together in pairs.
- Continue to develop safe, controlled learning experiences.
- Develop specific fine and gross motor skills.

Allow all to experience the process

- Explore the ensemble process.
- Take risks.
- Support others.
- Stay within the rules of decorum.

Provide for a period of winding down and transition

- Relax.
- Redirect group focus to the next activity.

After class

Meet with staff to evaluate and plan the next session.

Clown Safety

Before starting an eight-to-ten-week session, the Make*A*Circus staff meet with agency staff in order to familiarize themselves with procedures and safety concerns of the individual facility. They then incorporate the agency's rules into the programming. They are there to support the agency and comply with staff decisions.

Basic Clowning Rules

There are three "NO" rules and three "YES" rules:

The "No's"

- NO sharp objects in pockets!
- NO teasing!

- NO flipping or tumbling without staff supervision!

The "YES's"

- YES…Listen!
- YES…Wait your turn!
- YES…Freeze like statues!

Extra Safety

On the day that they introduce "slaps and falls" they reintroduce the concept of the "Clown Oath."

I (clown name) promise never, never, never, never, never, never, never, ever, ever, never, ever, never, ever to hit or hurt another clown!

Hitting or hurting another clown is grounds for termination from the program.

Developing a Clown Program

Not all facilities will have access to clowns. In this section, Lisa De Vries, a recreational therapist in the Seattle area, tells how she started a clowning program to enhance her therapy program in a long-term care facility.

As a recreational therapist, I am always in search of new ways to meet the needs of my clients. In a conversation on the topic of new programs, a colleague suggested that I add clown visits to the program at my facility. It was successful with her patients. I began the search for a clown who would volunteer to come to the facility where I worked. That was a long and fruitless process. I entertained the idea of going to clown school, but my administrator was not willing to support the time or the money for the endeavor. That just left my staff and me to use our creativity to become clowns ourselves. We bought a book, found some costumes at a garage sale, practiced balloon animals, borrowed a popcorn maker, and the clowns were born.

Clowning is not an easy task. It takes a great deal of energy. People expect clowns to be funny and energetic. People expect clowns to make funny animals and dance to the music in their rooms and maybe even tell a joke. It was not easy, but we made ourselves up, so it was difficult for patients to identify who we were. We spent one afternoon a month at the facility visiting, making balloon animals, dancing, laughing, and even telling a joke or two. The results were amazing.

I saw patients in a long-term care center open their eyes wide, smile, laugh, and even speak, when those things were thought to be long gone for them. One patient lifted her head when I touched her, and she smiled and kissed my big red spongy nose. She let me hold her hand and dance with her in her chair. Patients where I worked looked forward to the visit of the clowns. We paid no attention to abilities or looks. We were the funny people who danced, laughed, and made a balloon animal for everyone.

The benefits of clowning are great for a variety of patients. With color alone the clowns can provide new and exciting sensory stimulation. The clowns are like pets and children in healthcare. We are accepting and we have no history of making the patient do something they do not wish to do. We have never hurt a patient. Clowns are things of happy memories. And clowns can help patients laugh. Often in healthcare, laughter is a forgotten commodity. Research has shown that part of physical health is mental health. Clowning is one way to improve mental health.

Not only is clowning beneficial to patients, it is beneficial to staff morale, family interaction and morale, and departmental recognition in your facility. Staff love to see the clowns come. I can recall a number of staff commenting on patient response to our visits as clowns. They comment on how the patients seem to perk up as we walk down the halls. They also enjoy some popcorn or a balloon animal. Families love to see their family member interact in a new way. It is a time to have fun together in what can be a bad situation. When the clowns began to visit, it increased the amount of discussion about the department among staff and administration. It also increased the amount to time that was spent with each patient, as we visited every patient on an individual basis in that afternoon.

The benefits of clowning can be transferred to other populations of patients. I happen to work with long-term care patients with a goal of sensory stimulation, social interaction, and increased quality of life. But clowns can work in rehabilitation, oncology, and general medical floors with some of the same goals and more. I have used my clowning skills to work with a rehabilitation patient on fine motor skills. He happened to be a clown in a local group. We made animals together after his stroke. It was beneficial for his fine motor skills, but it also engaged other patients on the unit who wanted to learn the skill or get an animal for a family member who would be visiting later.

As a recreational therapist, I have found that clowning has been one of the best therapy tools that I could ever have chosen to learn. It works with a variety of patients, it meets many different needs, and it makes the patient happy. It is far easier to refuse a therapist when it is time for treatment than it is to refuse a clown.

Cautions about Clowns

Clowns are not universally loved. Some people have strong negative reactions to clowns. Therapists providing clown programs need to give people who dislike clowns an easy way to avoid seeing them.

Children developmentally under the age of seven may have similar issues. In a hospital setting they may see twenty to thirty healthcare professionals a day related to their treatment. Many of these professionals will prod, poke, or otherwise cause pain while they are wearing funny blue cloth shoes, wearing masks which modify their faces, and big, baggy coats. Often young children do not distinguish between medical staff and clowns, quickly reacting with tears and screams when any adult dressed in strange clothes approaches. Therapists need to protect sensitive children from scary experiences when clowns are in the facility.

Any client who explores the world by mouthing objects is in danger when rubber balloons are present. Balloon tricks using rubber balloons should not be shared with them to eliminate the chance of inhaling and choking on broken balloon pieces.

Clowning Resources

Books

Bolton, R. (1982). *Circus in a suitcase*. Rowayton, CT: New Plays, Inc.

Burgess, H. (1990). *Circus techniques: Juggling, equilibristics, vaulting.* New York: Thomas Y. Crowell Co.

Cline, P. (1991). *Fools, clowns and jesters*. New York, NY: Simon & Schuster Children's.

Disher, M. W. 1979. *Clowns and pantomime*. Stratford, NH: Ayer Co.

Grock (Adrian Wettach). (1931). *Life's a lark*. Stratford, NH: Ayer Co.
Schechter, J. (1985). *Durov's pig: Clowns, politics and theatre*. New York, NY: Theatre Communications Group.
Towsen, J. (1976). *Clowns*. New York, NY: Hawthorn Books.

Websites

CliniClowns in the Netherlands developed web clowning. Patients and others can visit the website to view the clowns in action. Up to 2085 followers log in to see photos and videos of the clowns at work. www.cliniclowns.nl

Fools for Health: A charitable organization which uses the arts to promote health and wellbeing in hospitals, long-term care facilities, and seniors' residences. Clown-Doctors are specially trained professional artists who work in hospitals. They wear white lab coats and red noses and serve as an integral component of healthcare services. They provide information on services, impact, and research. www.foolsforhealth

Hearts & Minds: A Scottish arts-in-health charity founded in 1997. They work across Scotland using the performing arts to encourage communication, interaction, and laughter. The Clowndoctors Program started in 1999 and goes to hospitals, hospices, respite units, and special education schools across Scotland. The Elderflowers program began in 2001 and engages people living with dementia in assessment units, psychiatric wards, and long-term care environments. Their aim is to improve lives one smile at a time. Headings for Clowndoctors, Elderflowers, Workshops, and Impact provide further information for each category. www.heartsminds.org.uk

Kryolan (make up)
364 Blodgett Street
Cotati, CA 94931
415-863-9684
us.kryolan.com

Clown Antics (make up and juggling supplies)
16 Dalfonso Rd
Newburgh, NY 12550
734-454-6625

www.clownantics.com

Special Effect Supply
164 E. Center St.
North Salt Lake, UT 84054
801-936-9762
FAX: 801-298-9763
www.fxsupply.com

References

Cancer Treatment Centers of America. (2019). Mind-body medicine. https://www.cancercenter.com/integrative-care/mind-body-medicine.

Cha, M. Y. & Hong, H. S. (2015). Effect and path analysis of laughter therapy on serotonin, depression and quality of life in middle-aged women. *J Korean Acad Nurs 45*(2), 221-230.

Chatham Kent Health Alliance. (2006). Windsor Regional Hospital annual report, 2005-2006. www.wrh.on.ca.

CliniClowns Nederland. (2018). CliniClowns. https://www.cliniclowns.nl/.

Dionigi, A. (2012). Clowns in hospitals. In Gremigni, P, ed., *Humor and health promotion,* pp. 213-228. New York: Nova Science Publishers, Inc.

DiSalvo, D. (2017). Six science-based reasons why laughter is the best medicine. *Forbes* (5 Jun 2017). https://www.forbes.com/sites/daviddisalvo/2017/06/05/six-science-based-reasons-why-laughter-is-the-best-medicine/#1d81378c7f04.

Dvory, A., Goshen, Y., Ruimi, S., Bikoy, S., Halevy, R., & Koren, A. (2016). Dream Doctor intervention instead of sedation: Performing radionuclide scanning without sedation in young children: A study in 142 patients. *J Altern Complement Med. 22*(5), 408-12.

Gervais, N., Warren, B., & Twohig, P. (2006). "Nothing seems funny anymore": Studying burnout in clown-doctors. In Warren, B. (ed.) *Suffering the slings and arrows of outrageous fortune: International perspectives on stress, laughter and depression.* New York: Rodopi.

Greene, C. M., Morgan, J. C., Traywick, L. S., & Mingo, C. A. (2017). Evaluation of a laughter-based exercise program on health and self-efficacy for exercise. *The Gerontologist, 57*(6), 1051-1061.

Hearts & Minds. (2017). About us. http://www.heartsminds.org.uk/about-us/.

Kataria, M. (2013). 100 laughter yoga exercises video. https://www.youtube.com/watch?v=Fq4kTZuLops.

Killick J. (2003). Funny and sad and friendly: A drama project in Scotland. *Journal of Dementia Care 11*(1), 24-26.

Kurtz, L. E. & Algoe, S. B. (2015). Putting laughter in context: Shared laughter as behavioral indicator of relationship well-being. *Personal Relationships 22*(4), 573-590.

Lorenz, K. (1963). *On aggression.* New York, NY: Harcourt, Brace and World.

Manninen, S., Tuominen, L., Dunbar, R. I., Karjalainen, T., Hirvonen, J., Arponen, E., Hari, R., Jääskeläinen, I. P., Sams, M., & Nummenmaa, L. (2017). Social laughter triggers endogenous opioid release in humans. *Journal of Neuroscience 37*(25), 6125-6131.

Meiri, N., Ankri, A., Hamad-Saied, M., Konopnicki, M., & Pillar, G. (2016). The effect of medical clowning on reducing pain, crying and anxiety in children aged 2-10 years old undergoing venous blood drawing — a randomized controlled study. *European Journal of Pediatrics 175*(3), 373-379.

Meiri, N., Ankri, A., Ziadan, F., Nahmias, I., Konopnicki, M., Schnapp, Z., Itzhak Sagi, O., Hamad-Saied, M., & Pillar, G. (2017). Assistance of medical clowning improves the physical examinations of children aged 2-6 years. *Isr Med Assoc J. 19*(12), 786-791.

Miller, M., Mangano, C. C., Beach, V., Kop, W. J., & Vogel, R. A. (2010). Divergent effects of joyful and anxiety-provoking music on endothelial vasoreactivity. *Psychosom Med 72*, 354-356.

Mobbs, D., Greicius, M. D., Abdel-Azim, E., Menon, V., & Reiss, A. L. (2003). Humor modulates the mesolimbic reward centers, *Neuron, 40*, 1041-1048.

Otto B. K. (2001). *Fools are everywhere. The court jester around the world.* Chicago: University of Chicago Press.

Ramgard, M., Carlson, E., & Mangrio, E. (2016). Strategies for diversity: Medical clowns in dementia care — an ethnographic study. *BMC Geriatrics, 16*, 152.

Valiant. G. E. (1977). *Adaptation to life.* Boston, MA: Little, Brown.

Warren, B. and McAuslan, P. (2002). What is the value of a smile? An investigation of the role of clown doctors working on an in-patient rehabilitation unit. https://artshealthnetwork.ca/sites/default/files/what_is_value_of_a_smile_2002.pdf.

Wildgruber D., Szameitat D. P., Ethofer T., Brück C., Alter K., Grodd W., et al. (2013). Different types of laughter modulate connectivity within distinct parts of the laughter perception network. *PloS ONE 8*(5), e63441. https://doi.org/10.1371/journal.pone.0063441.

15

Music

Music expresses that which cannot be said and on which it is impossible to be silent.

— Victor Hugo

Music has always been a part of people's lives. Music is used for communication, personal expression, understanding, enjoyment, socialization, and relaxation. "Music can provide friendship, make you laugh when you are down, console you when you are lonely, and even comfort you when you are sick" (Madsen & Kuhn, 1994, p. 11). The power of music on human behavior has been described as magical, supernatural, mythical, and, according to Congreve in 1697, having the "charms to soothe the savage beast, to soften rocks, or bend a knotted oak" (as quoted in Hanser, 1999, p. 1).

Music therapy is defined as "the use of music to achieve non-music goals and address a person's development in cognitive, behavioral, physical, emotional, social, and communications domains" (Adamek & Darrow, 2005, p. 103). Music therapy blends well with other creative arts therapies, such as dance, art, and drama. The American Music Therapy Association supports music for all and applauds the efforts of individuals who share their music-making and time. They say the more music the better! (American Music Therapy Association, 2017).

Therapists of all kinds can use music to help clients from many different populations in a variety of settings, and music can be used in both individual and group sessions. Therapy sessions may be designed to promote wellness, manage stress, alleviate pain, express feelings, enhance memory, improve communication, and promote physical rehabilitation (American Music Therapy Association, 2017).

Using music as therapy dates to ancient times with the works of Plato and indigenous medicine men and medicine women, as well as the musical treatises of Pythagoras (Heller 1987). "When World War II veterans filled hospitals beyond capacities, musicians involved in hospital work became aware of the need for knowledge and understanding of the psychopathologies experienced by war victims … [and saw] an imperative to offer service of a therapeutic nature through music" (Barksdale, 2003, p. 4). In 1944 the first academic music-therapy training program was started at Michigan State University, and 1950 saw the beginning of music therapy as a profession (Barksdale, 2003).

Research

Music can be beneficial in many therapeutic settings. It is a motivational stimulus that can involve multimodal networks in the brain that may aid nonmusical therapeutic learning. As Thaut and McIntosh (2014) wrote, "[T]he brain that engages in music is changed by engaging in music" (p. 106). Thaut & McIntosh (2014) reviewed many evidence-based research studies for motor, cognitive, and speech and language intervention techniques in stroke rehabilitation.

Motor Skills

Motor skills and music have been the subject of numerous studies. Chong, Han, and Kim (2017) investigated subacute stroke patients. Their study examined the effects of keyboard playing on hand dexterity. Seventeen patients participated in twelve 30-minute keyboard sessions over a six-week period. They used a Yamaha P-85 keyboard connected with a Musical Instrument Digital Interface (MIDI) for pre-, mid-, and posttest data collection. Subjects were asked to repeat a keystroke using an individual finger, play a three- or five-note pattern sequentially, play more than two keys at a time using certain fingers, and play a melody using a fingered number sheet. The overall hand function scores showed significant differences between pre- and posttest interventions ($p<.05$). Tip pinch (measured by Jamar dynamometer) and hand dexterity, as measured by Box and Block (BBT) and Jebsen-Taylor Hand Function Tests (JHFT), showed the most significant effect sizes (0.785 for tip pinch test and 0.840 for BBT). This research demonstrates great potential for keyboard playing as a therapeutic intervention.

Certain musical characteristics can influence a client's response to a therapy situation. Particular musical elements were chosen by cardiac rehabilitation patients to support walking-based therapy in research by Clark, Baker, and Taylor (2016). Twenty-seven adults (age 60 and older) selected music to support their walking therapy during a six-month period. Using the Structural Model of Music Analysis, patients identified seven characteristics of preferred music for walking: duple meter, consistent rhythm, a major key, a rounded melodic shape, predictable harmonies, changes in volume, and passages of tension and release. There was no preferred music tempo (speed).

Walking was also part of gait and balance research conducted by Bykowska and colleagues (2016). Thirty persons diagnosed with Parkinson's disease were part of an experimental group who attended music therapy sessions four times a week during a four-week period. The twenty-five members of the control group were asked to remain active (walking) throughout the same time period. Music therapy sessions were 45-minutes in length and included warmup exercises to increase the range of motion. Daily life movements (sitting to standing and vice-versa, lying to sitting and vice-versa, reaching in front, back, above, and below, stepping up and down) were analyzed by Optoelectrical 3D Movement Analysis System, System BTS Smart for gait, and Computerized Dynamic Posturography CQ Stab for stability. Rhythmic music, percussion instruments, and a metronome were used as a cue for fluency to initiate and continue the movement activities. The experimental group demonstrated significant improvement in the majority of the spatiotemporal gait parameters compared to the control group. Substantial differences were also found in stability tests with eyes closed, suggesting that the use of rhythmic music may improve the patient's ability to perform daily life activities.

Sensory-Integration Skills

Patients with Parkinson's disease (PD) need therapy to help with speaking, breathing, and swallowing. Stegemöller et al. (2017) examined the effects of a group-singing intervention as a treatment option for improving voice, respiration, and swallowing. Twenty persons with PD were interviewed four to six months following their singing intervention in this qualitative study. Group singing sessions occurred once a week over an eight-week period and included vocal exercises of:

- lip buzzing with high, medium, and low pitches
- glissandos (vocal slides between pitches)
- singing a pitch, then increasing or decreasing the volume
- articulation exercises (singing a five-step scale using "mee, meh, my, moh, moo" and then changing the beginning consonant to t, d, s, and k)
- group singing of familiar songs — *You Are My Sunshine* and *Mairzy Doats*.

Participants noted improvements in their speaking and breathing ability, but the overall benefit was the involvement in the group — fun and engaging — suggesting this involvement as a positive impact on their lives.

Sharda and colleagues (2015) investigated brain response to music versus speech stimuli with 22 children (ages 6-16) at different ends of the autism spectrum. They used 30 spoken words, 30 sung words, and 15 piano tones. Their study found that, during the sung-word experience, these 22 children activated bilateral temporal brain networks similar to 22 typically developing children in the control group. This illustrated the ability of singing to overcome the speech deficits across varying levels of the autism spectrum.

Cognitive Skills

Cognitive abilities can also be affected by music. In a nursery-rhyme-reciting study, Bolduc and Lefebvre (2012) divided 100 kindergarteners into four conditions to measure phonological and musical processing. The four groups conditions used (a) music — singing to known melodies, playing pitched and nonpitched instruments, (b) language — using syllables, rhymes, and phonetic tasks similar to the nursery rhyme studied, (c) combined music and language, and (d) passive listening — control group. Children in the experimental groups met 40 minutes a week over a ten-week period while children in the control group listened to recordings of the same nursery rhymes daily for 15 minutes. Results showed significantly improved phonological awareness and invented spelling skills at posttest. Only the two music conditions significantly enhanced verbal memory tasks. Complimenting a nursery rhyme with musical activities could increase phonological processing skills.

Additional research studies by Flaugnacco et al. (2015) and Bonacina et al. (2015) found that rhythm can enhance the reading and phonological abilities of children with dyslexia.

Social/Emotional Skills

Music affects emotions, and music therapy has helped relax patients about to receive medical treatments. Gooding, Yinger, and Iocono (2016) developed music therapy interventions to help reduce preoperative anxiety with 103 patients, ages two to nine. Interventions included singing, instrument playing, musical games, songwriting, and lyric analysis. Sessions lasted from three to 34 minutes. Children tended to demonstrate low levels of distress during the preoperative music therapy treatment and, afterwards, improvement in their ability to express emotion, an indicator of anxiety reduction. Parents reported that their child's distress level was better when receiving music therapy treatment than it had been during past medical experiences.

Youth indicated that music therapy sessions were helpful for reducing anxiety and improving mood and interactions with others in research by Preyde, Berends, Parehk, and Heintzman (2017). They conducted a study with 72 youth (mean age 14.8) at a child and adolescent mental health unit. Music therapy sessions were offered once per week for one hour over six months. Sessions included a warmup (such as a musical game) followed by activities such as song-singing, lyric analysis, and improvisation, and ending with group drumming or relaxation intervention.

Music in Therapy

According to music therapist Suzanne B. Hanser (1999), the benefits of music therapy are available to "almost anyone who is willing to try it" (p. 43). Brunk and Coleman (2000) identified several questions to assist in finding the best candidates:

- Is the person motivated to begin or finish discussions through music?
- Is music a favored activity where attention remains more focused than with non-musical tasks?
- Would another form of communication benefit this person?
- Does the person initiate activities that use music or instruments at school or at home?
- Does the person retain information presented in a song better than information presented without a song?

Active music making and music listening have the potential to affect one's health. Darrow and Segall (2015) provide ideas on how to use music to promote better physical, nutritional, and social/emotional health for students with (and without) disabilities. The ultimate goal? Healthy adults.

According to Barksdale (2003), the goals and objectives that a therapist can address in a music therapy session include:

- **Motor skills:** gross and fine motor, eye-hand coordination, and orientation in space
- **Communication skills:** auditory perception, vocal expression, verbal expression, nonverbal expression, and auditory memory. Therapist Maegan Morrow helped Congresswoman Gabrielle Giffords recover her speech after the latter suffered a gunshot wound to her brain. Morrow sang "Happy Birthday" while playing guitar and would wait for Giffords to speak the word "you" at the end of every stanza. By layering the words on top of the melody and rhythm, Morrow enabled Giffords' brain to regain language (National Arts Policy Roundtable, 2013).
- **Sensory integration skills:** visual perception, tactile and kinesthetic perception and discrimination, touch memory, body awareness, body image, and relaxation

- **Cognitive skills:** sequencing; categorizing; classifying vocabulary; problem solving; basic concepts of letters, numbers, etc.; using imagination; and independent musical leisure skills
- **Social/emotional skills:** self-awareness, increased self-esteem, awareness of others, empathy, turn-taking, sharing, positive peer interaction, respect for peers, acceptable avenues for freedom of expression, and participation in a fun experience. An example of this goal is shown in a study by Cunningham (2014), who investigated the role of music in the lives of those affected by the Holocaust — before, during, and after their capture. One theme that emerged from the survivors is that music served many functions and was "a form of national pride, a way to preserve sanity, a source of gratification, a method of survival, and a mode of ritual" (p. 69).

One piece of music can cause several reactions (depression, excitement, pain, arousal from sleep). Therapists should be familiar with a wide repertoire of music in order to select appealing music for their clients (Standley, 1996).

Modalities

Creative music activities involve the client in making decisions about the choice of instruments or sounds. Sound stories (using instruments for sound effects or characters in a story) or building a sound-maker are possible creative music activities. Cooper (2010) states that "songs and stories have a strong relationship to each other, to family and cultural traditions. Children (and adults) of all ages can be engaged through songs and stories, have behaviors and moods affected, and creativity inspired" (p. 24).

Singing alone and with others is a form of interaction. Echo songs, call-and-response songs, songs that use repetition in words and music, short note ranges, and songs with actions or movement may help improve participation in singing (Birkenshaw-Fleming, 1993).

Listening is an activity that may take many forms in a therapy setting. Clients may sing with a recording and then discuss the meaning of the song and how the song relates to them. Clients can also listen to a song and identify musical elements (instruments heard, patterns, tempo, dynamics, contour, texture, pitch, and emotion) (Barksdale, 2003).

Instrument playing is also a highly motivating activity. German composer Carl Orff and his student, Gunild Keetman, developed an approach to build musicianship through singing, playing percussion instruments, movement, speech, and drama. This approach is multisensory and creative, making it complementary to a therapy setting. Orff Music Therapy adopts this idea of creative music making and makes use of the Orff instruments (xylophones and metallophones) that were designed for use in the Orff Schulwerk (schoolwork) approach (Orff, 1974).

Pitched (melodic) and non-pitched instruments may be used during therapy sessions. Both categories of instruments have five characteristics that relate to how they can be used in therapy sessions (Orff, 1974):

- **Surface texture:** wood, metal, skin
- **Hardness:** wood and metal are harder than skin or string
- **Weight:** wood is lighter than metal
- **Elasticity:** tension on skin and string instruments
- **Vibration:** metal vibrates more strongly than wood

Instruments are made in different sizes and shapes and may be played with the hands or a beater. Instruments provide aural, visual, tactile, and kinesthetic sensory stimulation. The following considerations will help the therapist decide which instrument is best for a particular client:

- Determine if instruments are played one-handed (castanets, jingle bells) or two-handed (triangle, boomwhacker).
- Consider the size of the target, a bass drum provides a larger target than a woodblock.
- Find appropriate complexity, striking one resonator bell is easier that finding the correct note on a xylophone.

Some instruments may need adaptations for clients who need an alternative way for holding or playing instruments. Consider the following when looking for appropriate adaptations (McDowell, 2010).

- Insert mallets, strikers, or small handles through a foam or rubber ball for easier gripping.

- Attach mallets or small instruments to hands or gloves with Velcro.
- Use baby teething rings or rubber doorstops to strum guitars or autoharps if the client lacks a pincer grip.
- Restring guitars or ukuleles, if client requires, so s/he may strum with the left hand and chord with the right hand.
- Tape soprano recorder holes closed to allow clients with missing fingers to play.
- Tape or clamp instruments to desks or music stands for clients to strike.
- Use magnetic tape to attach lightweight bells or other small instruments to metal surfaces.
- Place a drawer gripper on desks to prevent instruments from sliding off.
- Have one person hold an instrument while a client with limited mobility strikes it.
- Have a client hold a mallet in his/her mouth to strike an instrument.
- Strap simple rhythm instruments to a hand or foot for striking.

Movement Adaptations

Music almost always causes movement — tapping a toe, clapping, or dancing. Whether the movement is structured or free, locomotor or non-locomotor, some adaptations may need to be made. Such adaptations might include the following (McDowell, 2010).

- Create a large space for activities, including spaces large enough to accommodate wheelchairs, walkers, and crutches.
- Perform patterned dances in a space large enough and open enough so non-ambulatory clients can dance in their chairs.
- Use a standing table or walker for support for movement activities.
- Use music with a tempo that clients can manage.
- Assign an ambulatory partner to dance with a non-ambulatory client.
- Help client move by walking next to him/her while supporting with a hand or elbow if needed.
- Use partners for dancing.
- Use hula-hoops, ropes tied in circles, or parachutes for circle dances.

- Ensure a comfortable room temperature and adequate ventilation.
- Make clients aware of the room arrangement.
- Have a client move a mobile part of his/her body: open and close his/her mouth to the beat, click the rhythm pattern with his/her tongue, sway to the beat, lift legs up and down to the beat.
- Have a client nod his/her head instead of taking steps for a dance pattern.
- Have a client walk using hands in the air.
- Keep chairs, tables, and instruments in the same place.
- Talk through movements for dances or instrument playing.
- Guide individual movements in personal space in time with the music.

Music Session Basics

If the therapist determines that music would be beneficial, s/he must gain rapport with the client or group within the first session. S/he must also learn more about his/her clients' past, present problems, and their responsiveness to music (Hanser, 1999). Following the therapist's initial assessment, goals can be developed in motor development; cognitive ability; communication and speech; and social, emotional, and spiritual abilities (Tucker, 2017).

Therapy sessions usually meet at least once a week for 30-60 minutes and may be held at home or a facility. Because clients differ in their abilities, it is impossible for a therapist to use exactly the same session outline for everyone. There are similarities, though. Barksdale (2003) suggests the following activities as a basis for most sessions:

- Greeting song or activity to focus the client's attention. In a group session this provides opportunities for interaction with others.
- Musical activity, such as singing, chanting, instrument playing, listening, moving, and creating.
- Closing activity to practice certain skills or review what occurred during the session.

The same greeting song is used in every session, although movement or instruments may be added. The greeting song can be sung, spoken, rapped, or signed. Examples of greeting and closing songs include:

- Lynn Kleiner's Music Box (www.lynnkleinersmusicbox.com) (Kleiner, 2018)
    - Come through in a Hurry
    - Funga Alafia
    - Make New Friends (see next page)
    - See You Later, Alligator
    - Sing Your Way Home
    - Tideo (Time for Music)
- *Kids Can Listen, Kids Can Move* (Kleiner, 2003).
    - Come My Friends, p. 33
    - Good-bye, Now, and Thank You (see next page)
    - Making Music (see next page)

The following ideas will increase the effectiveness of music therapy sessions (McDowell, 2010).

- Keep the room neat and free of clutter.
- Seat client near the equipment s/he will be using that day.
- Distribute instruments one at a time rather than all at once.
- Model correct ways to hold mallets or other instruments and correct playing technique.
- Minimize distractions.
- Place instruments under chairs when finished or collect them immediately by instrument type.
- Remove an instrument from a client who is not respecting it.

The therapist using music must be well prepared for each session. Plan for each session but also have a backup plan in case of an unexpected occurrence. Here are a few more helpful tips (McDowell, 2010).

- Having visual schedule of activities may make clients more comfortable.
- Begin and end each session with the same songs, chants, greetings, or activities.
- Vary the activities between moving and sitting.
- Hide props and instruments until the moment you use them.

Make New Friends

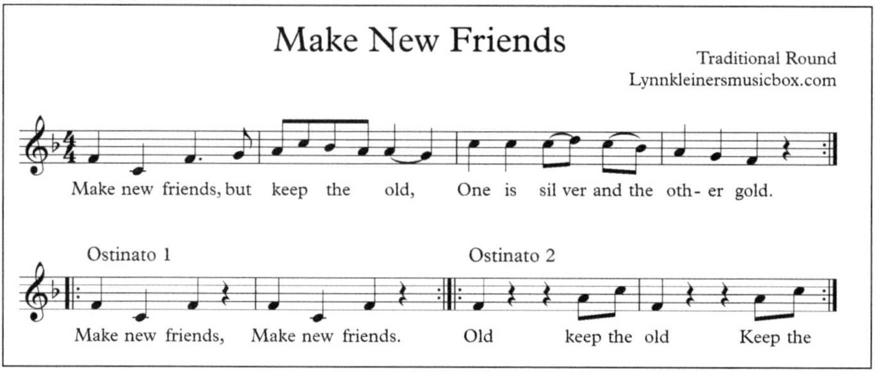
Make New Friends
Traditional Round
Lynnkleinersmusicbox.com
Make new friends, but keep the old, One is sil ver and the oth- er gold.
Ostinato 1
Make new friends, Make new friends.
Ostinato 2
Old keep the old Keep the

Good-bye, Now, and Thank You

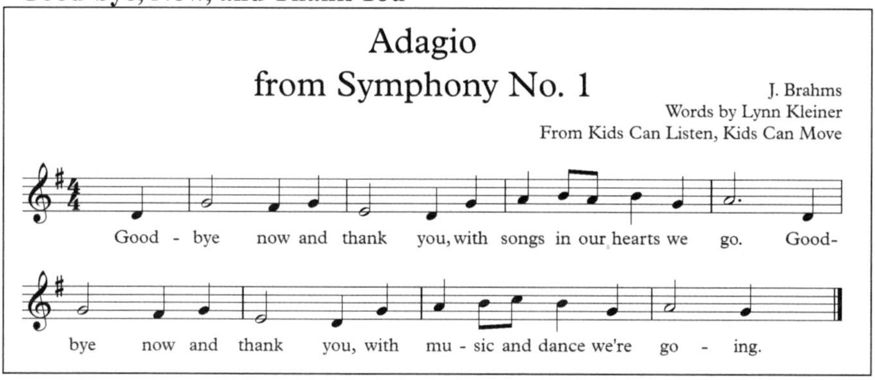
Adagio
from Symphony No. 1
J. Brahms
Words by Lynn Kleiner
From Kids Can Listen, Kids Can Move
Good - bye now and thank you, with songs in our hearts we go. Good-
bye now and thank you, with mu - sic and dance we're go - ing.

Making Music

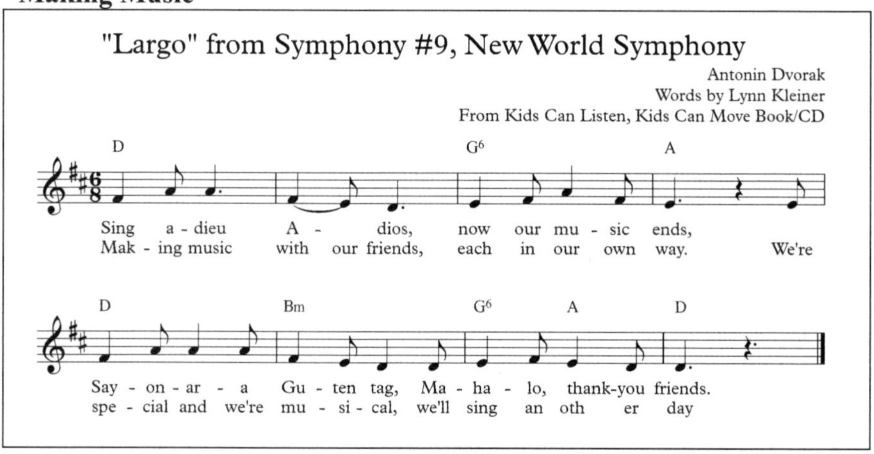
"Largo" from Symphony #9, New World Symphony
Antonin Dvorak
Words by Lynn Kleiner
From Kids Can Listen, Kids Can Move Book/CD
D G6 A
Sing a - dieu A - dios, now our mu - sic ends,
Mak - ing music with our friends, each in our own way. We're
D Bm G6 A D
Say - on - ar - a Gu - ten tag, Ma - ha - lo, thank-you friends.
spe - cial and we're mu - si - cal, we'll sing an oth er day

Permission from Lynn Kleiner, Music Rhapsody

Music Session Plans

There are many possible plans for a therapy session using music. Some possibilities are described below, but therapists need to create plans that work for the clients who are in their group.

Therapists may use music in several different ways during a session.

- Therapists may have music playing in the background as a way to begin a session. The music may encourage people to talk or begin a discussion.
- Music could also be used as a contingency (reward).
- Music can be part of an activity (singing, dancing and movement, playing instruments, discussion, or listening)
- Music could serve as a cue for an action or behavior. For example, rhythmic cuing for a motor behavior (walking). The stride width, length, and evenness of steps improve as the music's tempo is increased.

Kelley Pujol (2017), licensed music therapist, has developed two basic therapy session outlines for use with her clients, one for children and one for adults. They each have an opening segment to bring the group together, a segment of activities for a therapeutic purpose, and a closing segment that signals the end of the group and prepares the clients to go back into the world.

Children's Music Therapy Plan 1

- Hello song
- Warmup: vocal exercises and movements
- Instrument play: orchestration (choosing or arranging instruments, sound stories with a book)
- Songs that teach concepts
- Game or another fun activity
- Good-bye song

Adult's Music Therapy Plan 1

- Hello song and check-in
- Lyric analysis: using the words to a song to encourage meaningful discussion. Why do you like this song? What does it mean to you? What do you think of when you hear it?
- Positive coping strategies: anticipation, social support from others, deriving meaning from a stressful experience, humor, adequate nutrition, exercise, sleep, and physical exercise
- Relaxation — deep breathing, guided imagery, massage
- Good-bye song

The following therapy plans suggest more specific activities for a particular group of children or adults. They show the activity with the therapy goals for that portion of the session.

Children's Music Therapy Plan 2

Materials

- Melodic curve visuals
- Step bells
- Boomwhackers
- "Rockin' Scale" song
- Pictures of skylines and mountains
- Egg shakers

Activity

- Hello Song: "Welcome to Music" from the *Musicplay for Kindergarten Music Program* Teacher's Edition (Gagne, 2003).
  - Orient clients to session
  - Speech/language skills
  - Group participation
- Warmup: Read the following two stories while clients act them out using colored scarves.

"You're playing with a kite. It's going up, up, up. It's getting away! You let go of the string. Then you jump up to catch it again. Too late! The kite has crashed to the ground. You bend down to find where it's flown and broken. You kneel down beside your poor broken kite."

"You're a bird flying in the sky. You're going higher and higher, up to the stars. Suddenly you see a nice fat fish in the water below. You swoop down low over the water and catch the fish."

What types of motions occurred during these two stories? Like kites and birds, music can also move up and down.

- o Locomotor movement
- o Creativity

- Instrument Play: Present clients with various visuals of melodic curves. They will vocalize and/or use egg shakers to illustrate note direction while listening to the therapist play up/down/repeat patterns on step bells to illustrate the shape.
    - o Vocal development
    - o Auditory discrimination
    - o Non-locomotor movement
- Songs that teach concepts: Sing "Rockin' Scale" while playing the step bells. Ask the group which way the notes moved — up, down, or stayed the same (repeat). Echo-sing each phrase, add the body scale as movement, or use hand bells, step bells, or Boomwhackers to accompany the song.
    - o Locomotor movement
    - o Pitch-matching
    - o Singing
    - o Speech/language skills
- Game or another fun activity: Show pictures of skylines or mountains and have clients compose a sound piece using instruments to illustrate the contour.
    - o Auditory discrimination

- Fine motor skills with instrument playing
- Creativity

- Good-bye Song: "Making Music" from *Kids Can Listen, Kids Can Move*, p. 37.
  - Announce end of session
  - Speech/language skills
  - Group participation

Adult's Music Therapy Plan 2

Materials

- Recordings of songs
- United States and world maps

Activity

- Hello Song: "Make New Friends" from Music Box.
- Lyric analysis: Listen to Nat "King" Cole's "Route 66" or Johnny Cash singing "I've Been Everywhere Man" and write down or remember the names of three cities mentioned in the songs. Listen to the song several times. What is this song about? (traveling, having fun) What was the importance of these words? (They are cities you would pass while traveling by car, plane, or boat). Locate some cities on a map.
  - Fine motor skills
  - Eye-hand coordination (for writing)
  - Verbal expression
  - Auditory memory
  - Turn-taking
  - Sharing
  - Positive peer interactions
- Listen to a different version of either song, perhaps Natalie Cole singing "Route 66" and Hank Snow's version of "I've Been Everywhere Man." What differences do you hear? (voices, instruments, tempo/speed). Which version do you like best and why?

- Verbal expression
- Auditory memory
- Turn-taking
- Sharing
- Positive peer interactions

- Positive coping strategies related to traveling.
  - Anticipation of traveling
  - Social support for change based on the abilities of performers to change song
- Relaxation: deep breathing, guided imagery. Which of the cities mentioned would you like to visit and why? What would it be like to live there?
  - Visualization of the future
  - Ability to make changes
- Good-bye song: "Goodbye, Now, and Thank You" from *Kids Can Listen, Kids Can Move*, p. 36

Orff Schulwerk Rondos

Carl Orff created this technique in Germany during the 1920s. By the end of World War II, it had made its way to the United States. Schulwerk literally translated means "schoolwork" and was originally created to teach schoolchildren the fundamentals of music and creative expression. Clinically, Orff is a group process that respects individuality, provides an outlet for self-expression and creativity, and ensures success for the participant.

In Orff, participants learn the power of creativity as it affects other members of the group. The activities are based on making a response in imitation of the model. This design develops the echo form or question-answer form. Leadership is passed around the circle and a sense of group ensemble starts to build.

Use the rondos below to work on concepts of rhythm and group interaction. Some, especially the interpersonal game rondos, provide non-threatening ways to express feelings that might be hard to express in normal conversation.

Name Game Rondos

Name game (clap clap)
Name game (clap clap)
Let's play (clap clap)
A name game (clap clap)

Name game, name game,
What's your name?
And what's your game?

One hand says, "How do you do?"
The other says, "Who are you?"

If a fruit for a name
You had to take,
What kind of choice
Would you make?

Names go up *(use hand motions to indicate up and down)*,
Names go down.
Play the way
Your name sounds.

Interpersonal Game Rondos

Music, music in the air.
Make some music
A friend can share.
(pick an instrument and play it, then next person chooses an instrument to play with him/her)

Anyone can be any shape they want to be.
Anyone can be any shape they want to be.
Big, tall, short, small,
Anyone can be any shape they want to be.

What can you be?
I've got my face.
I've got my hat.
I've got my body under that.
How do I seem? How do I feel?
Look at me and see what's real.

Great big people
Stamp around,
Little tiny people
Touch the ground.

Tambourines, bells,
Triangles, and a gong.
Now it's your turn
To make up a song.

It's late at night
And I'm as hungry as can be.
When I get to the kitchen,
What do I see?

If wishes and dreams
Could come true,
This is what
I'd wish for you.

Rhythms are fun,
Rhythms are free
Can you make
A rhythm for me?

You are you.
If you were me,
What would you do?

Whispers are nice,
Whispers are fun.
Pass one along.
How far will it run?

Magic blob,
What can it be?
Make it into something
Then pass it to me.

Look out the window,
See the sky
What do you feel?
What would you do
If you could fly?

When you feel low,
Know what you can do?
Just say goodbye
To whatever's bugging you
What's got you?

Tee shirts and jeans,
Tee shirts and jeans,
What else do you wear
Besides Tee shirts and jeans?

The witch has an itch.
The witch has an itch.
Where, oh where,
Is the witch's itch?

Alike and different,
Alike and different,
We are both,

Alike and different.

Hey shadow, ho shadow,
Show us what you do.
Hey shadow, ho shadow,
Show us what you do.
We'll do the same as you.

Icka becca soda cracker,
What a silly sound.
Icka becca soda cracker,
Get up and move around.

Rondos with Props

Prop: shoe
Listen carefully to the shoe.
Tell us what it says to you!

Prop: ball
Wall, ball,
Where do you fall?

Prop: box
What's in the box,
What's in the box?
Sweat socks, goldilocks,
What's in the box?

Prop: broom
This is my broom
To sweep away
The things I don't like
In myself today.

Prop: magnet
This is my magnet
To bring to me
The things I like
And want to be.

Prop: pillow
Pillow, pillow
Stuffed with love,
Release in me
My adventurous dove.

Prop: paper cup
Look what I found,
It's small and round.
Before I lose it
I'll show you how to use it.

Prop: bubbles
Bubbles, bubbles
In the air.
Blow some bubbles
We all can share.

Prop: top
Spin, spin, spin till it stops.
When it stops,
I'll be on top.
(Group says: on top of what?)

Prop: wrapped box with bow
Boxes, boxes
Tied with bows.
Show me how
Your present goes.

Prop: mask (blank paper plate)
This is my mask.
My mask makes me glad.
I like my mask
Because it's _________.

Prop: wall made of cardboard
This is a wall, this is a wall.
How can we get over it?
How can we get over it?
Once and for all?
Answer:
This is a wall, this is a wall.
We can use a ladder
Once and for all.

Prop: stick, like a wand
(Everyone helps to choose one animal. Touch person with "wand.")
You are (name of animal, e.g., baboon)
A baboon, a baboon.
What do you do, baboon?
What do you do?

Prop: tambourine
This is a tambourine,
A tambourine, a tambourine.
This is a tambourine
What else could it be for?

Prop: key and tambourine
(Two people, person A and person B)
A: I'm the musical lock.
B: I'm the musical key.
A: To open the lock
You must do the same as me.
(B imitates simple rhythms played by A on tambourine.

B then "opens" lock and chant is repeated with next person.)

Prop: assorted hats
Each participant chooses a hat, puts it on, and takes on the role that the hat suggests (cowboy hat, police hat, veiled lady's hat, army hat, baseball cap, etc.). Participant may then be interviewed by an "on the street reporter" as the group chants:
S/he walks right over
Pats the hat on his/her head.
Walk up to the microphone
And this is what s/he said…

Projective Game Rondos

Who's that tapping at my window?
Who's that tapping at the door?
It's my __________ tapping at the window,
And my __________ tapping at the door.

When I was a little girl (boy), little girl, little girl
When I was a little girl, _____ years old
(tell something that happened, for example)
My ice cream cone fell on the floor, *(repeat line)*
My ice cream cone fell on the floor.
Bless My Soul.
(positive resolution)
My grandpa got another one, another one, *(repeat line)*
My grandpa got another one, another one.
Bless My Soul.

Tok-a-dee *(hit knees twice)* Ko-dee *(clap hands twice)*
(Snap fingers on left hand twice and look to left then snap fingers on right hand twice and look to right.)
Tok-a-dee Ko-dee
Tok-a-dee Ko-dee

(Snap fingers on left hand twice and look to left then snap fingers on right hand twice and look to right.)
After you have established a rhythm, say the name of the person to your left and right as you snap your fingers. This process continues around the circle of participants. The tempo may be sped up or slowed down.

Additional Activities Using Music

The following activities range from those imposing the least amount of structure to those with the most structure:

Total Group Effort

Everyone begins playing the Orff Schulwerk instruments. The leader listens, finds a steady beat, and plays it. The group repeats the pattern set up by the leader.

Play How You Feel and Title It

This activity may be done individually, in a group with each person taking a turn, or as a group. Express a feeling using the rhythm, volume, and/or pace of the music.

For a directed activity, play Louis Armstrong singing "What a Wonderful World" while showing the pages of the illustrated book *What a Wonderful World* (Bryan, 1995). Hand out lyric sheets and pencils to everyone and have them list five things that make them happy. Fill in the words to the song from the clients' lists and sing the new version of the song.

Letting Go of Something

Players imagine something that they are trying to let go of. It could be, for example, a worry, an angry feeling, or a troubling thought. Individuals in the group play to express this letting go experience.

For a directed activity, participants listen to the lyrics of "Release Me" as recorded by Ray Price (1954) or Wilson Phillips (1990). They imagine something that they are trying to let go of and play an instrument, create a new verse to the song, or both to the express this letting go experience.

Conversations between People

Two group members have a conversation using their instruments. You may add a third person (limit to three people so the observers can still follow the "conversation").

One example might be two group members having a conversation using scat singing. Fred Flintstone and Scooby Doo used scat words "Yabba-dabba-doo" and "Scooby-scooby doo." Create a scatting conversation — possible conversations include going to an amusement park, meeting a new or old friend, taking a driving exam, needing to borrow some money, trying to get someone to do something. Listen to some scat singers for examples (Bobby McFerrin, Ella Fitzgerald, Mel Tormé, Sarah Vaughan). A list of scat syllables is included at the end of this chapter.

Creating a Musical Sound Story

Divide the group into several small groups. Each group decides on a story or event to present using instruments or vocal sounds to represent characters or action words in the story. Story examples include: *What If the Zebras Lost Their Stripes?* By John Reitano (1998) and *The Crayon Box That Talked* by Shane DeRolf (1997). Participants may write the word and the instrument on a chart to help them remember when to play as the story is being read or told. The narrator also serves as conductor of the group.

Creating a Musical Score

Divide the group into several small groups. Each group decides on symbols (which are then cut out of colored construction paper) for each of the musical instruments available to them. On a large piece of butcher paper, they place the symbols and notes to create a musical score. Each person chooses an instrument, identifies the symbol that represents his/her instrument, and plays the notes. One member needs to be the conductor.

Exploration

Sitting in a circle, the leader begins by playing a one-beat sound. Others follow. Then the leader changes to two beats. See if the group can follow. Start gently, gradually become more aggressive, then gentle again... building to faster, fastest, then slowing down, to closure.

For more capable groups, the leader begins by playing a four-beat pattern on an instrument (drum). The group then echoes back that pattern. The role of being the leader is passed around the circle until everyone has a turn. The activity begins again, only this time the leader plays a rhythm pattern, and chooses someone to play an answer to that pattern. Continue until everyone has a turn. Instrument sounds may be loud or soft, high or low, growing slow to fast and vice-versa, growing soft to loud and vice-versa.

Rain

Group members sit in a circle, facing the center. Members close their eyes, pausing for a moment or two of quiet while getting ready to repeat the sound the person on his/her right will be making. All members keep their eyes closed and the rainstorm gets underway as the leader rubs his/her palms together, back and forth in a circular movement. The person to his/her left joins in, and then the next person to the left, and the next person, continuing around the circle until everyone is rubbing palms and listening to the drizzling rain building in intensity. When the leader hears the drizzling sound being made by the person on his/her right, s/he starts snapping his/her fingers. One by one around the circle, finger snapping replaces palm rubbing and the sprinkling rain turns into a steady patter. When the snapping action has been picked up by everyone, the leader switches to hand clapping, then progresses to slapping thighs and finally stomping feet. Then the storm subsides, in reverse of the way it grew moving from foot stomping to thigh slapping, hand clapping, finger snapping, and back to palm rubbing. If the group is having trouble hearing the changes, members can alert neighbors with a gentle nudge each time their movement switches from one action to the next.

Activities Using Music for Specific Purposes

Hillier, Greher, Poto, and Dougherty (2012) list these additional music activities, which were particularly beneficial in promoting self-esteem:

- Lyric analysis of songs helps young adults identify and express current feelings.
- Songwriting activities provide an outlet for expression and produce a sense of pride with the finished product. Songs may be recorded and shared to increase socialization.
- Group music activities build positive experiences and relationships.
- Learning to play an instrument develops a leisure skill.

For the unique needs of military service members and veterans, Darden Smith founded the program "Songwriting with Soldiers," which pairs professional songwriters with wounded soldiers to help those men and women release pent-up emotions (National Arts Policy Roundtable, 2013).

Scat Syllables

One-Syllable Scat

Doo, Boo, Shoo, Loo
Bay, Day, Way
Skwee, Dwee, Bwee
Bop, Wop
Bip, Zip

Two-Syllable Scat

Doo-ba
Bee-bop
Shoo-bee, Shoo-ba
Did-dle

Three-Syllable Scat

Dag-a-da

Dig-i-dy
Shoo-ba-day
Oo-ba-da

From the Teacher Training Institute, American Jazz Museum, Kansas City, MO. June 22-24, 2000. Rene Boyer Alexander, clinician.

Resources

The following articles, books, and websites provide information on songs that are appropriate for specific client groups.

Cevasco, A. M. & Vanweelden, K. (2010). An analysis of songbook series for older adult populations. *Music Therapy Perspectives, 28*(1), 37-78. Doi: 10.1093/mtp/28.1.37.

Cevasco-Trootter, A. M., Vanweelden, K., & Bula, J. A. (2014). Music therapists' perception of top ten popular songs (1960s) for three subpopulations of older adults. *Music Therapy Perspectives, 32*(11), 165-176. Doi: 10.1093/mtp/miu028.

Dalton, T. A. & Krout, R. E. (2006). The grief song-writing process with bereaved adolescents: An integrated grief model and music therapy protocol. *Music Therapy Perspectives*, *24*(2), 94-107. https://doi.org/10.1093/mtp/24.2.94.

Gardstrom, S. C. & Hiller, J. (2010). Song discussion as music psychotherapy. *Music Therapy Perspectives, 28*(2), 147-156. Doi: 10.1093/mtp/28.2.147.

Gibbons, A. C. (1977). *Popular music preferences of elderly people.* In Standley, J. M. & Prickett, C. A. (1994). *Research in music therapy: A tradition of excellence*, pp. 716-725. Silver Spring, MD: American Music Therapy Association.

Kleiner, L. (2017). Music box (Children) https:www.lynnkleinersmusicbox.com.

Moore, R. S., Staum, M. J., & Brotons, M. (1992). Music preferences of the elderly: Repertoire, vocal ranges, tempos, and accompaniments for singing. In Standley, J. M. & Prickett, C. A. (1994). *Research in music therapy: A tradition of excellence*, pp. 738-755. Silver Spring, MD: American Music Therapy Association.

Prickett, C. A. & Moore, R. S. (1991). The use of music to aid memory of Alzheimer's patients. In Standley, J. M. & Prickett, C. A. (1994). *Research in music therapy: A tradition of excellence.* pp. 765-775. Silver Spring, MD: American Music Therapy Association.

Standley, J. M. (1991). *Music techniques in therapy, counseling, and special education.* Appendix: Discography by counseling topic, pp. 155-161. St. Louis, MO: MMB Music, Inc.

VanWeelden, D. & Cevasco, A. M. (2007). Repertoire recommendations by music therapists for geriatric clients during singing activities. *Music Therapy Perspectives, 25*(1), 4-12. https://doi.org/10.1093/mtp/25.1.4.

Yinger, O. S. & Springer, D. G. (2016). Analyzing recommended songs for older adult populations through linguistic and musical inquiry. *Music Therapy Perspectives, 34*(1), 116-125. Doi: 10.1093/mtp/miu028.

References

Adamek, M. S. & Darrow, A. A. (2005). *Music in special education*. Silver Spring, MD: American Music Therapy Association.

American Music Therapy Association. (2017). www.musictherapy.org.

Barksdale, A. L. (2003). *Music therapy and leisure for persons with disabilities*. Champaign, IL: Sagamore Publishing, Inc.

Birkenshaw-Fleming, L. (1993). *Music for all: Teaching music to people with special needs*. Toronto: Gordon V. Thompson Music.

Bolduc, J. & Lefebvre, P. (2012). Using nursery rhymes to foster phonological and musical processing skills in kindergarteners. *Creative Education, 3*(4), 495-502. http://dx.doi.org/10.4236/cd.2012.34075.

Bonacina, S., Cancer, A., Lanzi, P. L., Lorusso, M. L., & Antonietti, A. (2015). Improving reading skills in students with dyslexia: The efficacy of a sublexical training with rhythmic background. *Frontiers in Psychology 6,* 1510. Doi: 10.3389/fpsyg.2015.01510.

Brunk, B. K. & Coleman, K. A. (2000). Development of a special education music therapy assessment process. In Adamek, M. S. & Darrow, A. A. (2005). *Music in special education.* Silver Spring, MD: American Music Therapy Association.

Bryan, A. (1995). *What a wonderful world.* New York: Macmillan.

Bykowska, A. A., Krezatek, P., Mirek, E., Bujas, P., & Marchewka, A. (2016). Neurologic music therapy training for mobility and stability rehabilitation with Parkinson's disease — A pilot study. *Frontiers in Human Neuroscience*, *9*, 1-12. Doi: 10.3389/fnhum.2015.00710.

Chong, H. J., Han, S. J., & Kim, S. J. (2017). Keyboard playing as a hand exercise for patients with subacute stroke. *Music Therapy Perspectives*, *35*(2), 144-150. Doi:10.1093/mtp/miw023.

Clark, I. N., Baker, F. A., & Taylor, N. F. (2016). Older adults' music listening preferences to support physical activity following cardiac rehabilitation. *Journal of Music Therapy, 53*(4), 364-397. Doi: 10.1093/jmt/thw009.

Cooper, S. (2010). Lighting up the brain with songs and stories. *General Music Today, 23*(2), 24-30.

Cunningham, D. A. (2014). Musical meaning in the lives of those affected by the Holocaust: Implications for music education. *Update, 33*(1), 65-72.

Darrow, A. A. (2014). Promoting social and emotional growth of students with disabilities. *General Music Today, 28*(1), 29-32. Doi: 10.1177/1048371314541955.

Darrow, A. A. & Segall, L. (2015). Students with disabilities: Using music to promote health and wellness. *General Music Today, 29*(1), 34-37.

DeRolf, S. (1997). *The crayon box that talked.* New York: Random House.

Flaugnacco, E., Lopez, L., Terribill, C., Montico, M., Zoia, S., & Schön, D. (2015). Music training increases phonological awareness and reading skills in developmental dyslexia: A randomized control trial. *PloS ONE*, *10*(9), e0138715. https://doi.org/10.1371/journal.pone.0138715.

Gagne, D. (2003). *Musicplay for kindergarten music program, teacher's edition.* Red Deer, AB: Themes & Variations.

Gooding, L. F., Yinger, O. S., & Iocono, J. (2016). Preoperative music therapy for pediatric ambulatory surgery patients: A retrospective case series. *Music Therapy Perspectives, 34*(2), 191-199. Doi: 10.1093/mtp/miv031.

Hanser, S. B. (1999). *The new music therapist's handbook* (2nd ed.). Boston: Berklee Press.
Heller, G. N. (1987). Ideas, initiatives, and implementation: Music therapy in America, 1789-1848. In Standley, J. M. & Prickett, C. A. (1994). *Research in music therapy: A tradition of excellence*, pp. 714-725. Silver Spring, MD: American Music Therapy Association.
Hillier, A., Greher, G., Poto, N., & Dougherty, M. (2012). Positive outcomes following participation in a music intervention for adolescents and young adults on the autism spectrum. *Psychology of Music, 40*, 201-215.
Kleiner, L. (1998). *Kids make music, babies make music too!* Miami, FL: Warner Brothers Publications.
Kleiner, L. (2003). *Kids can listen, kids can move!* Miami, FL: Warner Brothers Publications.
Kleiner, L. (2018). Music box. https:www.lynnkleinersmusicbox.com.
Madsen, C. K. & Kuhn, T. L. (1994). *Contemporary music education* (2nd ed.). Raleigh, NC: Contemporary Publishing Company.
McCaffrey, R. (2008). Music listening: Its effects in creating a healing environment. *Journal Psych Nursing Mental Health Services. 46*(10), 39-44.
McDowell, C. J. (2010). An adaptation tool kit for teaching music. *TEACHING Exceptional Children Plus, 6*(3) Article 3. Retrieved from http://escholarship.bc.edu/education/tecplus/vol6/iss3/art3.
National Arts Policy Roundtable. (2013). Arts and healing: Body, mind, and community, the 2013 report and recommendations. Retrieved January 15, 2018 from: www.americansforthearts.org.
Orff, C. (1974). *The Orff music therapy*. New York: Schott Music Corporation.
Reitano, J. (1998). *What if the zebras lost their stripes?* New York: Paulist Press.
Preyde, M., Berends, A., Parehk, S., & Heintzman, J. (2017). Adolescents' evaluation of music therapy in an inpatient psychiatric unit: A quality improvement project. *Music Therapy Perspectives, 35*(1), 58-62. Doi: 10.1093/mtp/miv008.
Prickett, C. A. & Moore, R. S. (1991). *The use of music to aid memory of Alzheimer's patients*. In Standley, J. M. & Prickett, C. A. (1994). *Research in music therapy: A tradition of excellence*, pp. 765-775. Silver Spring, MD: American Music Therapy Association.
Pujol, K. J. (2017). Personal interview, University Autism Center. Cape Girardeau, MO. June 26, 2017.
Sharda, M., Midah, R., Malik, S., Mukerji, S., & Singh, N. C. (2015). Fronto-temporal connectivity is preserved during sung but not spoken word listening, across the autism spectrum. *Autism Research, 8*(2), 174-186. https://doi.org/10.1002/aur.1437.
Standley, J. M. (1996). *Seminar in music therapy*. Class lecture notes, fall semester. Tallahassee, FL: Florida State University.
Stegemöller, E. L., Hurt, T. R., O'Connor, M. C., Camp, R. D., Green, C. W., Pattee, J. C., & Williams, E. K. (2017). Experiences of person with Parkinson's disease engaged in group therapeutic singing. *Journal of Music Therapy, 54*(4), 405-431. Doi: 10.1093/jmt/thx012.
Thaut, M. & McIntosh, G. C. (2014). Neurologic music therapy in stroke rehabilitation. *Current Physical Medicine and Rehabilitation Reports, 2*(2), 106-113. https://doi.org/10.1007/s40141-014-0049-y.
Tucker, J. (2017). Services. Retrieved from: http://www.accessmusictherapy.com

16

Dance and Movement

Two separate areas of work have come out of using dance and movement in therapy settings: dance/movement therapy and creative movement. These two modalities are not, despite the similarity of their names, interchangeable. Dance/movement therapy is much more concerned with the psychological implications of movement on and by the client. Movement exploration is just that: an exploration of the possibilities of movement through space. This chapter is divided into two parts, one for each of the modalities.

Dance/Movement Therapy

Dance/movement therapy is defined by the American Dance Therapy Association (ADTA) as "the psychotherapeutic use of movement as a process that furthers the emotional, social, cognitive, and physical integration of an individual." (Brooke, 2006 p. 95) Thus dance/movement therapy causes changes in feelings, cognition, physical functioning, and behavior (Levy, 2005).

History

Dance/movement therapy began in 1942, during the healthcare crisis of World War II, when disabled veterans returned home. Marian Chace, a former Denishawn modern dancer and teacher, was a volunteer at St. Elizabeth's Hospital in Washington, DC, in a program then called "dance for communication." (Chaiklin, 1975) At the request of DC area psychiatrists, Chace began experimenting with dance and music therapy for psychiatric patients who had been considered too disturbed to participate in group activities.

A nonverbal approach was needed, and dance/movement therapy met that need (Stuart, 2001). Her training in the Denishawn School of Dancing and Related Arts, founded by Ruth St. Denis and Ted Shawn, led to some of her most effective techniques. One was "music visualization," a process that communicates specific qualities of music through movement, including assigning each dancer an instrument of the orchestra and asking them to move when that instrument played. Chace worked individually with her participants at first, but their responses often led to cohesive group activities, such as a set of dancers representing a whole orchestra, demonstrating that the patients were capable of being in a group.

Chace's contributions to dance/movement therapy included: therapeutic movement relationships, ongoing verbal narration as a form of reflecting on the group and the individual process, rhythmic movement as an organizing and clarifying force, and dance as a cohesive group process (Levy, 2005).

Goals of Dance/Movement Therapy

Dance/movement is a statement of emotion expressed through movement (Warren, 2008). Therapists who focus on dance/movement as therapy seek to correlate cognitive processes, emotions, and movement. The primary goal of dance/movement therapy is to assist clients in achieving a greater degree of body integration and awareness. Within this broad goal are three sets of goals which have different levels of importance for a given client population.

Emotional: Movement also releases emotion. Through dance/movement therapy, clients may find a structure that will help them express overwhelming emotions, such as anger, fear, and sadness. Dance/movement can enable them to work through conflict, tension, and distortion (as in the case of those suffering from dyssynchrony, fragmentation, or catatonia). An increase in the ability to express oneself may correlate with an increased range of physical motion.

Physical: Dance/movement exercises help clients control impulsive, random behaviors, such as manic ritualistic movement. A client can learn to better integrate a range of movements, from spontaneous to coordinated (coming from either extreme, the infantile and impulsive or the mechanical). For individuals with physical challenges (e.g., cerebral palsy) dance/movement may help the client gain control over muscle spasms as part of a creative and relaxed experience. Dance/movement therapy improves the accuracy of the perception of body image and self (e.g., for patients with eating disorders).

Social: Clients interact and share with others in a way that is nonverbal (through movement — as in the responding and relating through "group rhythm") and verbal (imagery). Dance/movement offers clients, especially more withdrawn individuals, a unique way to develop relationships with others and with their environment.

As recreational therapists, it is our responsibility to match each client's movement capabilities with music experiences and movement activities that offer success, challenges, independence, and opportunities for creative expression and interaction.

Research in Dance/Movement Therapy

Results from the First International Research Colloquium on Dance/Movement Therapy in Hanover, Germany, in 2004 found the following: Dance/movement therapy treatment for oncological patients reduced depression and anxiety (Mannheim & Weiss, 2006). For fibromyalgia patients it reduced pain and increased energy (Bojner Horwitz, 2004). For persons suffering from stress and psychological strain it reduced stress and increased quality of life (Brauninger, 2005).

The Second International Research Colloquium in Dance Therapy was held in Germany in 2006. Thirty-nine researchers from 14 countries world-wide presented efficacy studies which supported dance/movement therapy treatment for depressed patients, persons suffering from schizophrenia, and parent-child interaction (Koch, 2006). Results of this research and other findings are compiled in *Advances in Dance/Movement Therapy Theoretical Perspectives and Empirical Findings* (Koch & Brauninger, 2006).

Koch, Kunz, Lykou, and Cruz (2014) studied the effects of dance/movement therapy and dance on health-related psychological outcomes using a meta-analysis of the last twenty years of research findings with twenty-three evidence-based primary studies on fifteen populations (N=1078). Results showed that dance/movement therapy and dance are effective for increasing quality of life and decreasing clinical symptoms of depression and anxiety. The results also demonstrate consistent effects for improvement of well-being, affect, mood, and body image.

Shanahan, Morris, Bhriain, and Saunders (2015) studied dance for people with Parkinson's disease. They found thirteen studies that provided information on the frequency, intensity, duration, and type of dance used in the program. The evidence suggests that two one-hour dance classes per week over ten to thirteen weeks had beneficial effects on endurance, motor impairment, and balance for individuals with Parkinson's disease.

Assessment/Observation

Every movement in dance/movement therapy is seen as *adaptive* (a coping mechanism) and *expressive* (reflective of the individual). The following aspects and ranges of movement are observed, evaluated, and worked with in dance/movement therapy:

- use of effort and presence
- shape of actions (away or toward body)
- use of body planes (vertical, horizontal, sagittal)
- attitudes toward space (direct to indirect)
- time (ranging from quick to sustained)
- force (strength to lightness)

- movement into space (directional and shaping motions)
- relationships between gesture (isolated body part) and posture (the activation of many parts in relation to each other)

Dance/Movement Therapy in Practice

Many methods are used to help clients develop an accurate, strong, and delineated sense of their body. Therapists using dance as therapy lead groups that teach interaction through touch, the exploration of movement fundamentals, and props that broaden and embellish movement dynamics. Fundamentals are basic movement actions of body parts. Dynamics include the force of the movement and the tension or lack of tension in body parts.

In this section, we will look at several of these methods including the Chace technique, Orff Schulwerk, Canner techniques, Levy techniques, and other dance/movement group ideas.

Chace Technique

Marian Chace developed techniques to accomplish the emotional, physical, and social goals of dance/movement therapy (Chace, Chaiklin, Sandel, & Ohn, 1993). She described how to kinesthetically perceive, reflect, and react to clients' emotional expressions through the therapist's own body movement and voice tone in a "therapeutic movement relationship." By taking the clients' nonverbal communications and helping to broaden, expand, clarify, and include them, Chace's techniques meet the client where s/he is. Chace's techniques say to clients through music and movement activity, I understand you, I hear you, and it's okay. The concept of the teacher/therapist involving herself in a movement relationship or interaction with the client/student as a way of reflecting a deep emotional acceptance and communication is Chace's contribution to dance therapy and to therapists in their first interactions with a special-needs student or client.

The following activity descriptions show how the Chace Technique can be implemented.

Copying Exercise

This exercise demonstrates the components identified above and can be utilized by recreational therapists. The exercise works on group cohesion and following a leader. When working with a group with diverse physical abilities, participants may need to modify certain movements. The focus should be on staying in the rhythm or flow of the movement rather than copying the exact action.

The group stands or sits in a circle. The therapist starts a repetitive action, such as patting legs. The group copies the action as closely as possible. When everyone is synchronized, the leader calls, "Change." The person to the left becomes the new leader. The new leader changes the action, to something like patting shoulders, and continues repeating the action until the group is in synchrony. Then the current leader calls, "Change." Leadership passes to the left. The exercise continues until everyone has had a chance to be a leader.

It is helpful to begin this exercise in silence to focus on the rhythm (or steady beat) of the movements. When the group has grasped this idea, then music may be added. This exercise allows individuals to create their own movement ideas yet work towards group cohesiveness. The creative movement/music dances created in this way are every bit as fun and fascinating as choreography (Warren, 2008).

Chace Movement Therapy Session

The following outline is a form that Marian Chace used to guide her movement therapy sessions (Chaiklin, 1975). The format enhanced interaction, communication, and expression by movement activity. Each session had a beginning (warmup), middle (theme development), and end (closure). Many of the elements may be used by recreational therapists for music/movement sessions.

Warmup

- Initial contacts: In these steps the therapist/teacher is reflecting the students' movements and guiding them to new movement actions until a movement dialogue — back and forth initiation of movement actions — occurs between the therapist/teacher and student.

- Mirroring: participant copies the therapist's movement.
- Clarifying and expanding the movement repertoire: changing levels, body parts
- Movement elicitation and movement dialogue
- Group development — gradual formation of a circle
- Group rhythmic expression/physical warmup: Rhythm or moving on a beat provides organization and meaningful dance action and helps modify behaviors of hyperactivity, hypoactivity, bizarre gestures, and mannerisms.

Theme Development

- With a client's non-verbal communications as a starting point, Chace used movement, verbalization, imagery, and various theme-oriented actions to lead the client into a deeper exploration. For example, if the therapist observes rigidities in a client's arms and back and realizes the client needs to express anger or release tension, the therapist can add a chopping motion or a swinging motion to release tension.
- Picking up on nonverbal clues
- Broadening, extending, and clarifying actions (and intensions)
- Use of verbalization and imagery
- Various other theme-oriented possibilities (role-playing, group themes)

Closure

- Being in a circle, sitting or standing
- Communal movement: everyone moving the same way
- Possible discussion and sharing of feelings

Chace stressed structuring a supportive closure that allowed clients to leave with satisfaction. When forming a circle, holding hands and swinging could be a communal movement to focus on being part of a group. Or it could be everyone coming together in a large swoop down and then raising their hands high in the center.

Orff Schulwerk

Orff Schulwerk is based on things children like to do: sing, chant, clap, dance, and keep a beat. Carl Orff believed in allowing children to play. "Since the beginning of time, children have not liked to study. They would much rather play, and if you have their interests at heart, you will let them learn while they play; they will find that what they have mastered is child's play" (Estrella, 2019). Lessons are presented with an element of play, which helps children learn at their own level of understanding. But most teens and adults like to do the same things children do — and they often are not fond of study. So, Orff's ideas can be applied to almost any therapy group.

The Orff Schulwerk process asks clients to think and work creatively with others. Creative movement activity helps explore another dimension of Orff, where the human body is the client's instrument. In an Orff group, the therapist may act as a conductor who gives cues to her orchestra, just as a dance therapist does to her clients. If the therapist selects a song, some clients may be chosen as instrumentalists. Some of the group may sing along. Some clients may keep the beat, moving various body parts, while others may step to the rhythm. Parts may or may not be notated, but if they are notated, the therapist and clients can design a diagram of the notes, steps, and movement actions.

Many examples of Orff exercises were presented in the Music chapter. They can be used as the basis for dance exercises for a group that is divided into various roles, as described above.

Canner Techniques

The dance/movement therapist Norma Canner shared Carl Orff's philosophy. "Experience first then intellectualize" (American Orff-Schulwerk Association, 2019). "Elemental music is never just music. It's bound up with movement, dance, and speech, and so it is a form of music in which one must participate, in which one is involved not as a listener but as a co-performer" (Estrella, 2019).

In the 1950s and 1960s, when the institutionalization of children with disabilities was under scrutiny, Norma Canner brought those children dance, music, and the spirit of play. Canner was an innovator of early intervention and dance/movement programs for children with physical, visual, cognitive, and multiple disabilities as well as children without disabilities (Bushey Theater, 1998).

As a pioneer in dance therapy with children, Canner developed and utilized a sensory-based approach. Rather than work on skills development from only a functional perspective — the traditional approach — Canner facilitated movement-based experiences that motivated children to be active through the medium of play. "Play is essential to the growing brain, play stimulates development of the cerebellum, which coordinates movement, and the frontal lobe, which regulates decision making and impulse control" (Keats, 2014).

Canner's (1968) groundbreaking book, *...and a time to dance* was one of the earliest books on creative movement methods for children with disabilities. Photos in the book show the children's positive responses to guided creative movement experiences.

Deborah Stuart, one of the authors of this text, studied dance/movement therapy with Norma Canner through the Harvard University Summer Dance Therapy Program (1982-1986). Together, Canner and Stuart designed creative movement sessions for children who were blind, visually impaired, and deaf-blind attending Perkins Institute for the Blind in Watertown, Massachusetts. They used dance and creative-movement guided sessions which incorporated musical instruments and sound to increase mobility, movement range, confidence, and social interactions. At the same time, they chose activities to expand the children's sensory awareness and spatial concepts. For the deaf-blind children, they explored vibrations of instruments and ways bodies can move.

They began with a warmup, which consisted of making a circle. Canner and Stuart moved inside the circle to partner with each student in hand-to-hand mirroring activities. Theme development activities included identifying body parts and exploring how they can move, as well as rhythm activities such as stepping to the beat. For children with hearing impairments, they used instruments with vibration, such as drums and triangles. Finger cymbals were used with children who were deaf and blind. A sighted assistant coordinated coactive body-to-body movements with each child who was deaf and blind. Stretch material was used for partner activity and large group circle movement activity. Each session finished by holding hands in a circle and reaching forward to touch one another.

Professor Canner's methods with children are documented in the film, *A Time to Dance: The Life and Works of Norma Canner* (Klebanoff, 1998). The photographer and film producer, Harriet Klebanoff, showed Canner's approach with a girl described as withdrawn, who removed herself from group social interactions. In the movie, Canner offers the girl a piece of cloth to touch, then returns to the group. But periodically Canner comes back to her. She moves closer and touches the girl on the face and arms with the cloth. Over a fifteen-minute period, Canner encourages the girl's participation with verbal prompts, glances, and use of the cloth, until the girl joins the group by engaging with another girl. Klebanoff describes this as quite remarkable as no one had expected this child would do more than sit outside the group, withdrawn within herself. The clip demonstrates how to offer an invitation to dance or to interact with the group.

Perhaps these words from Norma Canner provide the best insight into her vision and career:

> Dance therapy in my view, is really about spontaneous, creative movement and about experiencing oneself from a feeling place rather than an intellectual one. When we are moving spontaneously, we come closer to our primal selves and that is nurturing and healing. We use the language of movement to access deep emotions and early memories without censoring them. The focus is to go somewhere where you leave off your usual movements to find the ones that are just there. It is not to do more or less, it's just what happens — it's in your whole body, in your cells. This way of working brings you back to a time when you didn't have to think that you would have to learn to dance in order to move. Think of yourself as movement, you are the movement, the dance is in you and always has been. (Canner, 2001 personal communication cited in Levy, 2005).

While Canner worked primarily with children, her techniques can be modified to work with any therapy group. The first priority of therapists using dance is to establish trust and empathy. When clients play together, there is an element of trust. The therapist creates a safe environment by starting at the client's developmental level. By mirroring a client's movement or responding to and working from the client's movements, the therapist guides clients to explore other movement possibilities and become more confident in their bodies.

A key theme of therapists using dance is to guide structure. Appropriate structure provides protective boundaries for clients yet allows them to express themselves. Some therapists use games or mirror movements; others may teach techniques, as described in Marian Chace's work. The goal is to learn the social skills required to be part of a group along with mobility, movement range, and confidence.

Levy Techniques

The following dance/music movement therapy techniques are an excerpt from an outline identified by Fran Levy (2005) and published in *Dance/Movement Therapy: A Healing Art.*

The dance/movement therapy techniques may be used by dance therapists, Orff music educators, recreational therapists, and others to guide creative music movement experiences.

Dance Therapy Outline

Warmup and body awareness techniques:

- Articulation of body parts (e.g., rotations and swings, how each part can move)
- Rhythmic movements, explorations and games (moving on a beat)
- Repetitive movements (repeated movements)
- Education in the rudiments of movement (Laban efforts, glide, press, slash, flick, wring, punch, dab)
- Introduction to basic dance steps (folk, social, etc.)
- Use of props (hoops, scarves, percussion instruments, etc.)
- Relaxation and breathing techniques
- Exploring tension fluctuation and extremes (tension release)
- Exploring contrasting movement themes (extremes and gradations)
- Body awareness techniques

- Postural explorations (alignment of body, use of spine)
- Music as a facilitator of movement and background support

The therapeutic interaction with the therapist includes the therapist:

- Mirroring and reflecting clients' feelings back to them through a dance/movement interaction
- Reacting and responding through movement to clients' needs and non-verbal communications
- Engaging in playful movement dialogues as in the creation of games, fantasies, and dramatic movement interactions
- Verbally narrating and reflecting the conscious and unconscious thoughts and feelings of clients during the dance/movement process
- Empathizing, observing, listening, and teaching body movement and guiding the client

Music and rhythm are designed to:

- Help organize clients' thoughts and feelings into expressive actions
- Support and encourage self-expression
- Facilitate improvisation
- Reflect clients' moods and needs
- Facilitate rhythmical action and expression
- Motivate and activate
- Create emotional responses
- Modulate emotions and activity levels

More Dance/Movement Activities.

The following activities offer more ways to use dance/movement therapy in a therapy setting.

Body Warmup

Group members are asked, "Where in your body do you store stress?" Members then organize themselves in a line according to where they store it, beginning with those who feel stress in the head area and ending at the feet. Form a circle staying in the same order. Starting from the top (the head or neck), each person demonstrates an exercise that s/he does to relax that part of the body. Everyone then tries out the motion. This process continues around the circle until each person has had a turn. This is very effective when done non-verbally.

Dance Cards

One card is given to each group member. On each card is an image of a person, animal, or object. The leader starts the music and invites participants to interpret the image using movement. Group members exchange cards as part of the activity.

Sound and Motion Pass

Group members form a circle allowing distance between themselves for movement. One participant (the "leader") creates a motion and sound and "passes" them to the person on his/her right. The motion and sound are then imitated by this person and passed on, until they return to the original leader. A second leader then chooses a motion and sound and the process is repeated.

Hand-on-Hand

Two partners face one another and decide on who is "leader" and who is "follower." The leader's hands are upturned; the follower's hands are placed, turned downward, on top of the leader's. The leader moves his/her hands in any direction in a gentle rhythm and the follower responds accordingly. This activity is like "Mirroring" except physical touch is included.

Scarf Dance

The group forms a circle. Each participant holds colored fabric, ribbon, or crepe paper in each hand. Each person in turn uses the strips to make a movement such as arm circling, jumping over strips, or twirling.

As each person shows his/her version of the dance, everyone else imitates the movement.

Walking/Moving with a Partner

The group is divided into partners. One person (A) leads the other person (B) around the room. At first B is passive and trusting and moves as directed. Then B begins to offer some resistance. Finally, B very actively resists A's attempts at moving him/her. Reverse roles and then discuss what occurred.

Movement Through ...

Using your imagination, move through:

- honey
- water
- sand
- air
- daisies in a field
- lime Jell-O
- jungle underbrush
- clouds
- a large bubble gum bubble
- a deep pocket full of odds and ends

Eye Contact

Standing or sitting in a circle, each participant tries to make eye contact with another person. When the contact has been acknowledged by a given signal (pointing or a nod of the head, for instance), the two switch places as quickly as possible. This exercise facilitates eye contact with little threat (in the context of the game) and helps increase observational skills.

Exploration of Trust and Support

Group members stand in large circle holding hands. They pull away from each other while maintaining balance. They lean in. They lean to the right and to the left. They lean on one another.

Alphabet Movement

Moving through the alphabet from A to Z — using animals or object names that start with each consecutive letter. A dance or movement is made up for each. For example, "Move like an 'A'…alligator, 'B'…ball, 'C'…caterpillar." Encourage dancers to call out suggestions for each letter.

The "Land of S" Action Verbs

Group members move to the "S" action verbs, e.g., sliding, skipping, slumping, sauntering, strolling, striking, strutting, stomping, slithering, snapping, smashing. Leader or group members can call out suggestions.

Moving to Opposites

These activities help group members explore ways of moving and the use of space. The leader can ask for movement suggestions from the group.

- open — closed
- near — far
- high — low
- wide — narrow
- large — small
- straight — slanted
- heavy — light
- linear — curved

Moving to Divergent Emotions

Exploring these contradictory emotions will produce a wide range of movements. The leader can ask for suggestions from the group to build a longer list of emotional opposites.

- love — hate
- knowledge — ignorance
- lost — found
- happy — sad

Footprints

The leader creates footprints out of heavy, colored paper or vinyl and creates a pattern for the dancers to follow. (Make sure that the clients don't slip — tape the footprints onto the floor well!)

Complementary Stretching

In pairs, dancers engage in various exercises using each other's weight, strength, and balance to stretch. Be careful not to overstretch and cause injuries.

Mirroring in Groups of Four

Mirroring may begin with partners taking turns being leader or follower, then reversing roles. Pairs then move into groups of four. In these groups, one member is the leader and three are followers. The leader's goal now is to pick up on movements made by the other three members of the group. Can group members find a balance between who is "leading" and who is "following"?

Create a Dance

In groups of four, participants create a dance (given about five minutes to make it up) and then perform it for the entire group.

Contact Improvisation

Pairs explore movement together — a good activity for "staying in the moment." The group divides into partners. Pairs are then given the following instructions: Keep your eyes open, be alert; look for opportunities to support your partner (e.g., move in underneath them), but don't give or take weight without listening for and feeling the agreement of your partner's body. Let each movement evolve from mutual agreement rather than letting an image in your own mind dictate what happens next. Mutual trust is based on "uncompromising attention." *(Exposed to Gravity Project)*

Circle Walk

The group forms a large circle. Begin the activity by facing forward with left sides toward center of the circle. Count together and walk, one step to each count; 1, 2, 3, 4, 5, 6, 7, 8, 9, 10, 11, 12, 13, 14, 15, 16. On the count of 16 turn to face the opposite direction and count and step 1 to 15. You have subtracted one step. On the count of 15 turn again and count and step 1 to 14. Continue to the end of counting.

You Can Tell How I Feel by the Way that I ________

Group members takes turns using their creativity to express emotions through movement and/or facial expressions. Each person demonstrates how s/he feels while the other members look on. The leader can ask for more suggestions for expression.

- walk
- skip
- hop
- smile
- wiggle
- stomp
- scream
- spin

Example: You can tell how I feel by the way that I walk.

This chant is one that either the group or the dancer can do while s/he demonstrates in movement how s/he feels:

the way that I (walk)
the way that I (walk)
You can tell how I feel by the way that I (walk)
walk
walk
walk

Think of Someone Who Moves the Way You'd Like To

Group members imitate the style of someone they admire. Each person performs (e.g., a walk, gestures, body language) while others in the group observe.

Letting Go and Holding On

Group members are asked to react physically to the question: "How would you look if you were letting go of __________ and moving towards ________."

Example:

"How would you look if you were letting go of *fear* (hunching shoulders, hands in front of face) and moving towards *trust* (standing straight, opening up)?"

Other possibilities: anger, sadness, pain.

Suggesting Movements and Varying Them

The leader suggests a series of movements for group members to make and then varies them — a spatial exploration exercise. The leader might, for example, suggest making a pantomime movement of painting a fence. S/he could then call out suggestions for modifying the painting motion: faster, slower, smaller, larger, higher, lower, rougher, smoother.

Movement Map

Each member of the group draws a map of his/her movement path. For example, the map may show "3 hops, 4 slides, and a turn, then change directions, and so on." S/he dances it, then finds a partner and they guide one other through their maps.

Body Talk

Every participant makes two cards — one with a single emotion and another card with a single body part. The emotions cards are put into one hat and the body parts are put into another. Participants take turns drawing a card from each hat (one emotion, one body part). Using only the body part indicated on the card, the participant displays the emotion found on the second card. The rest of the participants guess the emotion and body part.

Elbow Tag

The leader divides the group into sets of three. The "center" person links elbows with the two on either side of him/her. One group is designated "it." One person in the "it" group receives a "marker," such as a scarf. This threesome then separates to act as three separate individuals.

Action: The person with the marker tries to tag either of the two free runners. If a free runner is tagged, s/he is given the marker and the other person becomes a free runner. The two free runners each try to join elbows with some other threesome. When a threesome becomes a foursome, the fourth person (the person on the opposite end from the former free runner) becomes a free runner. The threesomes move as units around the area trying to avoid free runners.

Object: Try not to become "it."

Back to Back

The leader divides the group into pairs. Each pair first sits on the ground, back to back. Participants then bend their knees, pulling them up to their chests, keeping their feet on the ground. The leader instructs each pair to hook their elbows together. Working together and using the combined strength of their backs, each pair tries to stand up together. This may be a new and difficult experience for some participants. Also, having slippery socks (no shoes) or a slippery floor might create an added difficulty. The leader stresses working together and using combined strength — then the task can be done fairly easily.

Writing Your Name with an Imaginary Pen

The leader suggests a part of the body, then asks the participant to pretend to hold an imaginary pen with that body part and to write his/her name using as much space as necessary. For example, the leader might say, "Write your name using your head."

Closure for Music Groups

Each member of the group creates and uses a gesture (small movement, e.g., tipping hat) as their personal sign off at the end of a session.

Movement Exploration

This section looks at movement exploration as a direct expression of self through the body. Movement exploration includes analyzing human movement capability, expressing oneself, learning concepts, reducing anxiety, communicating, designing goal-directed movement, and using imagination.

Movement exploration, long an accepted part of elementary education, is a set of progressive problem-solving experiences designed to teach a person to control body movements and improve physical skills (Deighton, 1971). The basis of movement exploration lies in exploring fundamental patterns of physical activity — both locomotor (e.g., running, skipping, walking) and non-locomotor (e.g., bending, pushing, pulling). This exploration is important to children and adults, but especially important in improving the physical and perceptual abilities of people with disabilities.

Today, people of all ages can benefit from creative movement. A person's physical, mental, social, and emotional needs may be addressed through developing therapeutic movement activities. Movement and music can provide opportunities for participants to express themselves physically and emotionally where perhaps they cannot verbally. The participants, according to their needs and how their bodies can move, may structure creative movement and music experiences according to their choices and decisions.

Movement exploration activities can be structured for a wide variety of populations. Inclusive sessions can be designed for those with and without disabilities (Stuart, 2016). A basic movement chart (Stuart, 2006) can be used to guide creative movement experiences, by exploring what, where, and how we can move, and then finding new ways of moving.

Goals of Movement Exploration

These goals are the basic learning units of movement exploration. They are often taught in the following progression:

Safety: This should be the first item covered in a lesson or set of activities. When a whistle is blown, participants must learn to stop, look, and listen.

Body Image and Spatial Awareness: A very important aspect of movement exploration is learning about the body. What are the parts of the body? How do they move and in how many different ways? How can they be used in skilled activities and how can they be used in combinations with other body parts? How does your body fit into the environment around it? How do you move through the environment avoiding obstacles and maneuvering safely?

Self-Confidence, Self-Assurance, and Solving Challenges: The challenges in question may include going to greater heights, maneuvering over a narrow surface or a broad expanse, covering unstable ground, or even traveling safely at high speed. The theory is that people take their success in meeting challenges in these activities and generalize it to other activities.

Visual Focus and Balance: These two abilities are considered together because of the influence of balance on focus. Balance is, in and of itself, fundamental to almost all motor tasks: sitting, kneeling, standing, walking — even sleeping on one side. Most learning tasks require visual focus, the ability to focus on a something and maintain the connection. If balance is poor, a person's field of vision may shift frequently in an attempt to maintain some kind of balance.

Strength and Endurance: Both strength and endurance are basic to successful movement, health, and safety. For example: strength is needed to pull yourself to safety from a dangerous situation, while endurance is critical to performing throughout an active day, with energy to spare for engaging in special play time after work or in case of emergency.

Hand-Eye Coordination: Good hand-eye coordination enables a person to be a part of the action in games, especially ball games. Hand-eye coordination is also important in reading, writing, and most creative endeavors.

The basic learning units of movement exploration address or improve mobility, balance, walking gait, fall prevention, sequencing, attention span, quality of life, social interaction, and self-expression.

Specific diagnoses may have their own set of goals for movement exploration. For example, Keus et al. (2007) recommended the following key components of an exercise program for individuals with Parkinson's disease.

- Cueing strategies to improve and initiate gait
- Cognitive movement strategies to improve transfers
- Exercise to improve balance
- Training of joint and muscle power to improve physical capacity

Research in Movement Exploration

There have been many studies on the benefits of movement exploration for Parkinson's disease (PD). PD is a progressive neurodegenerative movement disorder often causing impaired balance, difficulty walking, falls, and reduced quality of life.

A National Institute of Health literature review by Earhart (2009) summarized 73 research studies and found the following:

- Falls are a major concern for individuals with Parkinson's disease. People with PD are 3.2 times more likely than those without PD to sustain a hip fracture when falling (Melton et al., 2006).

- Reduced functional mobility can contribute to withdrawal from activities, social isolation, osteoporosis, and muscle weakness (Bloem, 2001).
- Axial impairment, which includes gait and balance problems, has been identified as a major influence on health-related quality of life (Muslimovic, 2008). Other major influences on quality of life issues are psychological adjustment to PD, depression, and impaired cognition.

According to the NIH review by Earhart (2009), the following benefits were found for movement exploration and related therapy techniques.

- Increased balance as measured by Berg Scale of Balance
- Decreased falls
- Increased mobility
- Improved gait and ability to initiate walking with rhythmic cadence
- Increased sequencing
- Increased attention span
- Increased self-expression and quality of life

Evidence also suggests that individuals with higher levels of regular physical activity are at lower risk for developing Parkinson's disease. (Thacker et al., 2008)

An early study examined benefits of dance therapy for individuals with traumatic brain injury and stroke. Berrol, Ooi, and Katz (1997) described improvements in balance, gait, and cognitive performance with a twice-weekly, five-month intervention.

Other benefits of creative movement and dance noted in research studies include improved coordination, balance, and functional ability in following directions and sequencing, interacting with peers, and developing friendships (Garcaro, 2011; Lopez-Ortiza et al., 2012; Sterba, 2006). Youth experienced better identity, pride, and belonging. (Kunstler & Stavola Daly, 2010).

In studies by Overby et al. (2005) youth with and without disabilities were able to learn educational concepts through structured creative movement adventures from the book *Interdisciplinary Learning through Dance: 101 Moventures*. Concepts, such as the hydrosphere, were better understood through participation in creative movement activity. For assessment materials for community engagement see Overby (2015).

Anne Green Gilbert (2000) the author of *Teaching the Three R's through Movement Experience*, found her third-grade students, with and without disabilities, had greatly improved scores on spelling tests after sessions in body spelling. The children took a new interest in math after making up problems with their bodies. There also was an atmosphere of cooperation and understanding of the revolutions of the planets after moving around the classroom in the solar system they had created. The children reported that creative problem solving through movement was "interesting" and "fun."

Movement Exploration in Practice

Stuart (2006) created a basic movement chart that describes types of movements that can be taught in a therapy session.

Where Can You Move?

- **Self-space:** the immediate area surrounding the body
- **General space:** the area surrounding the body, with outside boundaries
- **Directions:** forward, backward, two sides, up, and down
- **Levels:** high, medium, and low
- **Change shapes:** curved, twisted, straight and angular, straight and wide, straight and narrow
- **Ranges:** relationship of one's body to space. How much space is used? How close are body parts? Large, medium, small. Near to, far from.
- **Planes:** horizontal, vertical, diagonal
- **Pathways on the floor or in the air:** straight, curved, zigzag
- **Relationship to another person:** near to, far from, meeting, parting, facing, side-by-side shadowing, mirroring, leading, following

What Can You Move?

- **Different body parts:** head, neck, shoulders, chest, waist, stomach, hips, legs, arms, back, spine, upper arm, elbow, lower arm, wrist, fingers, thumb, hands, toes, feet, heels, ankles, shins, knees, thighs
- **Body surfaces:** front, back, sides
- **Relationships of body parts:**
    - Near to each other: curled, bent
    - Far from each other: stretched
    - Rotation of one part

How Do You Move?

- **Force:** strong, medium, light
- **Qualities of force:** sudden, explosive, sustained, smooth, swinging
- **Creating force:** quick starts; held balances; sustained, powerful movements
- **Absorbing force:** Sudden stops on-balance, gradual absorption ("give")
- **Weight transfer:** step-like action, rocking, rolling
- **Balancing:** active stillness, center of gravity, weight on different body parts or different number of body parts
- **Movement sequence:** series of movements, one following the other smoothly, with a beginning and end; a logical whole

Find a New Way of Moving

The four elements of movement are space, force, time, and flow.

- **Space:** the where of dance
    - Levels: low, middle, high
    - Pathways.
- **Force:** produced by muscle tension, firm to light
- **Time:** speed of movement, quick to slow. Rhythmic movements are in an ordered time structure. A pulse beat creates a rhythmic structure with even, equal time intervals.

- **Flow:** actions joined together smoothly, blending the preparations, actions, and recoveries
    - o Bound flow: controlled, careful, on-balance, can stop at any time, restraining
    - o Free flow: ongoing smoothness and fluidity

Movement exploration activities can teach clients about any of these aspects of movement using the Stuart's movement chart. For example, clients who are rehabbing from a stroke could work on force and time aspects using the Change Shapes part of Where, the Different Body Parts part of What, and the Creating Force part of How.

Laban Techniques

More ideas about how to use movement exploration come out of the work of Rudolf Laban (1879-1958). He was a modern dancer and a pioneer in movement education who contributed to many fields through his work in movement analysis. Laban believed that knowledge of movement would lead to increased information about people's behavior. His work is of interest to music and movement educators and professionals who use movement for therapeutic purposes. Laban inspired people to discover the natural movement capabilities of their bodies and to communicate the emotion from which the movement originated. Instead of prescribed steps and positions, Laban taught "movement in all its possibilities and varieties." Movements could be simple or complex, natural or symbolic, and free or controlled.

Laban's pedagogical strategies were based on the theory that all movement, regardless of its function, shares common elements that can be analyzed. His basic notation system, kinetography and labanotation, is widely used to describe direction, body part, weight transference, and duration of movement. Therapists most often use his qualitative analysis of movement: how movement is performed and how effort can be analyzed in terms of its components of space, weight, time, and flow. The system is based on a simple grid used to describe effort.

Laban thought of weight as light or strong and flow (or control) as free or bound (Laban, 1963). Laban noticed people tend to limit their range of movement by using habitually preferred motions while rarely or never employing others. He concluded people could benefit from training designed to expand their range of movements.

Possible applications of Laban's principles include:

- structured or guided movement experiences to develop body control
- movement experiences to communicate emotion and expressiveness
- opportunities to explore the elements of motion inherent in both music and movement (e.g. tension-relaxation, strong-weak, flow-motionless, and expansion-contraction)

Laban's original sixteen basic movement themes can be applied to design movement sessions that address:

- awareness of the body
- awareness of resistance to weight and time
- awareness of space
- awareness of flow of the weight of the body in space and time
- adaptation to partners
- instrumental use of the limbs
- awareness of isolated actions
- occupational rhythms
- shapes of movement
- combinations of eight basic effort actions
- space orientation
- shapes and efforts using different parts of the body
- elevation from the ground
- awakening of group feeling
- group formations
- expressive qualities or moods of movement

Approaches to designing movement sessions include questioning; sequencing; use of Laban movement themes; and basic movement questions of what, where, and how body parts can move. Movement actions are categorized by body, rhythm and time, space, and force. Participants gain better understanding of ways the human body can move.

If clients are unable to respond to verbal directions, the therapist can guide them with visual and verbal prompts and physical interactions.

Musical excerpts may also help participants respond. Concepts taken from a movement analysis chart combined with music concepts can guide creative movement and music experiences with therapeutic objectives.

The sequencing example shown below is one of many possibilities for using Laban's methodology.

Sequencing

Therapists can teach sequencing of actions using this procedure.

- Decide on a subject or concept (curricular, social, or interpretive) that can be reinforced through movement concepts, such as shape, time, energy, space, etc. A possible concept is open vs. closed.
- Discuss the properties or qualities of the subject with the participants, making a list of these properties. The list should be adjectives and not nouns.
- Select three tasks to sequence from the list (e.g., shapes or designs, long movements, short movements, axial or locomotor).
- Develop each task separately, instructing the participants to recall their inventions. Encourage a new spatial level or direction for each task.
- Put the tasks in an order, if they are not already in a sequence.
- Develop smooth transitions from one task to another.
- Rehearse the three tasks as a smooth sequence.
- Add accompaniment: vocals, instruments, or recorded music.
- Watch each other's compositions in smaller groups.
- Evaluate and appreciate the design, balance, expression, interpretation of assignment, and achievement.

To build the session progressively, participants can work in twos or threes. Participants can expand the movement experience to include more tasks. They can also use a movement chart to add contrast and variation to the creative experiences.

The following sequencing activity was designed by McDowell and Stuart (2016).

Sequencing: A Methodology for Movement Lessons

This sequence is a guideline for designing a music and movement lesson, using the poem "From the Sea" (author unknown). The focus is on physically expressing the words of the poem. The words may also be accompanied by classroom instruments. The sequence can be performed by a group or an individual. Students design one movement action for words in the poem. Suggested examples for some of the words are

- Ocean — arms broadly expanding to outstretched arms (ocean drum)
- Timeless — arms push forward until fingertips extend reaching to the future (flexatone)
- Sand — hands rub together making a shushing sound (sand blocks)
- Pebble — fingertips extend and rotate around each other (play circles on a hand drum using fingertips)
- Island — arms and body lean forward drifting to the floor (glockenspiel)
- Pearl — cupped hands open to reveal the pearl, like an oyster opening (triangle)

The poem (shown in bold) is read and accompanied by the movements for the words in the poem. The art for this kind of sequencing is creating movements for the appropriate number of words.

From the Sea

Ocean — arms broadly expanding to outstretched arms (ocean drum)
Timeless, tireless — arms push forward until fingertips extend reaching to the future (flexatone)
Frolicking, rollicking, rolling
Waves

Sand — hand rub together making a shushing sound (sand blocks)
Tiny grains,
Clinging, crunching, bunching
Specks

Pebble — fingertips extend and rotate around each other (play circles on a hand drum using fingertips)
Worn, smooth,

Crashing, tumbling, churning
Endurance

Island	arms and body lean forward drifting to the floor (glockenspiel)

Quiet, secluded
Isolating, renewing, rejuvenating
Retreat

Pearl	cupped hands open to reveal the pearl, like an oyster opening (triangle)

Iridescent gem,
Smoothing, polishing, refining
Cache

Movement Exploration Activities

There are many other kinds of movement exploration activities. Some examples are shown here. They can be adapted for many kinds of therapy groups. Each activity in this series is formulated as a set of directions which can be given to a group by a leader or therapist.

Individual Activities

Body Parts to the Floor

Find a way to touch different numbers of body parts to the floor. (The leader calls out how many: 1, 2, 3, etc.)

Finding a Space

Find a place in the room — a place you feel drawn to.

- Find three points of the space that will help you "find your way home" to that place (e.g., a mark on the floor or wall).
- Pretend you have a paint brush and decorate your space.

Begin to move through your space.

- How slowly can you move?
- How gently? softly?
- How low can you move?
- How high can you move?
- Can you find a middle height for moving?

How can you form the first letter of your name while staying in your space?

- Print your first name within your space.
- Can you use the top half of your body to form your name?
- Can you use the lower part?
- Can you write your name using your whole body?

Leave your "home base" and begin to meet your neighbors and see your neighborhood.

Walking the Line

Walk a line on the floor. (The leader can make a line with masking tape or use a pattern in the floor).

More Movement Practice

Move as if you are moving through space now — without music. How small can you be? (Make a sound that goes with it, if you can). How light and feathery can you be? How proud? How large? Do a silly walk. Walk as if you are very heavy, as if on a planet where you weigh more than you do on earth. Feel the weight of your steps.

Pair Activities

Body Parts Game

Call out two body parts. Group members find a partner and touch these two parts together (e.g., one partner's nose to the other's elbow). Participants are asked to find a new partner for each new challenge. Examples:

- nose to elbow

- knee to elbow
- shoulder to shoulder
- hand to back
- hand to foot
- chin to ear

If possible, ask group members to call out two (appropriate) body parts.

Pattern Walk

Using a large piece of paper and a crayon, each person draws a pattern, walks it, and then leads his/her partner through the pattern. The pattern can, for example, consist of varying step sizes, turns, twist, circles, and gaps.

Bubbles

Remind the group of what happens when a bubble comes in contact with other bubbles — they can become a bubble cluster! With your partner begin moving around the room, bumping into other pairs to become groups of 4, 8, 16.

Mirroring Movement

Find a partner and mirror each other's moves. See how many ways you can challenge yourselves with tests of your balance and visual focus.

Group Activities

Touch Blue Game

Start the game by reminding everyone to be gentle and appropriate in their touching. One person is designated as "it." Ask everyone except "it" to get into the position of "touch blue" (touch someone who is wearing blue). The "it" person calls out a series of other colors ("touch red," "touch black") for participants to locate and touch. At some point, the person who is "it" calls "touch blue" and everyone must rush to find blue before "it" tags him/her. The one who is tagged becomes "it."

Animal House

This activity will use total imagination. First set the scene:

- Ask everyone to think of an animal that they wish to be for this session and how they might imitate this animal's movements.
- Encourage the group to use facial expressions, to walk, crawl, and/or make sounds to show what animals they are imitating.
- Tell the group that the theme will be set in the jungle.

Then set everything in motion by speaking to the group and giving them the following instructions: "As the group moves around on the mats, each of you will encounter other creatures and must decide what you will do as you approach other animals. Will you run, or snarl, or just look curious? Will you fly away or swim? How do you react to being in the jungle? Are you scared or do you rule the jungle? Are you large or small? Two-legged or four? Are you loud or quiet? Continue moving among the group until you have found a position among the rest of the group that shows what animal you are and who you might hang out with."

Animals

- The group forms a circle.
- Each member chooses a favorite animal s/he wishes to act out.
- The leader begins by imitating his/her favorite animal. S/he travels towards any person in the group and greets that person as his/her animal would greet any other animal.
- The person being greeted should respond in her animal character and then approach another member in the group.
- Continue until all members have had a chance to demonstrate an animal.

The Human Seesaw

- Divide into two groups and form two lines facing one another.
- Group One goes from a standing position to the floor in a way specified by the leader (e.g., quickly, slowly, like a cat).
- Then Group One moves from the floor to a standing position while Group Two goes from standing to the floor in specified ways.
- The groups continue to take turns, moving up and down like a seesaw.
- This up and down activity may continue until all ways have been explored.

The ways of getting up and down may be designated by the leader, or group members may make suggestions. Each group may also be given a list of ways to get up and down and may choose from the list.

Ways to go down:

- in awe or worship
- formally and gracefully
- as a melting snowman (or woman — would she melt differently?)
- slipping on something slick
- after losing a long-distance race
- after winning a long-distance race
- to tie a child's shoelace

Ways to get up:

- waking up after sleeping on the floor
- someone you love has come into the room
- like a child who is caught somewhere s/he's not supposed to be
- you heard a loud crash outside
- you smell smoke
- a dancer on stage

Activities Using Equipment

Ball Movement Activities

- Show how quietly you can come up, get a ball, and, without touching each other, go back to your space.
- How many body parts can you bounce the ball with?
- How many times can you bounce the ball in one minute?
- How many times can you throw the ball up and catch it in one minute?
- Choose a partner — you should each have a ball. Toss one of the balls back and forth; start close and slowly increase the distance.
- How many ways can you throw the ball to each other?
- Introduce the second ball and find way(s) to keep the balls moving in opposite directions.
- How quickly can you return the balls without touching each other?

Hula-Hoop Activities

Individual Activities

- Show how tall you can be as you come up to get your hula-hoop. Holding your hoop, how high can you stretch?
- Can you hold a hoop above your head and drop it so that it hits the ground without touching your body?
- Can you spin a hoop and keep it going like an eggbeater?
- Can you jump in and out of the hoop while holding on to one part?
- Being careful not to bump into anyone, can you roll your hoop in a straight line and keep it from falling over?
- Can you change direction? Right? Left?
- How fast can you roll your hoop?
- How slowly can you roll your hoop?
- Can you roll your hoop on the floor so that it will roll back to you?

Pair Activities

- Can you exchange hoops with a partner by rolling them back and forth?

- Can you create a rhythm? How fast? How slow?
- Who can jump into a hoop held by your partner? Now, let your partner try.
- Your partner is going to hold two hoops in different positions. Can you go through both hoops? Let your partner try.
- Can you and your partner exchange hoops by throwing and catching them at the same time? Can you catch a hoop that has been thrown by your partner on your arm?

Musical Hoops — Non-Eliminative

Hoops are laid on the floor — at first there is one for everyone. The game begins with each person standing in his/her own hoop. The music starts, everyone steps out of the hoop and one or two hoops are removed by the leader. Everyone begins moving through the hoops. When the music stops, everyone must stand inside a hoop. Some people will end up sharing a hoop. The elimination of hoops continues in each round, and each time more people must double or triple up inside the hoops. At the end the entire group is squeezed into one or two hoops. There is a lot of physical contact and laughter.

Creating Obstacle Courses

Divide people into groups of three or four. Each group creates an obstacle course using the hula-hoops and themselves as challenges to be gotten around. Then take turns trying out each other's creations.

Collecting the Hoops

1. Line up. Each person gets a hoop and puts it on his/her right arm.
2. Everybody then puts his/her left arm through someone else's hoop and holds hands, until everyone is joined together in a circle, with hands joined and each hoop between two people and over their arms.
3. One person is the end of the line; his/her right hand is not joined.

4. S/he will get "buried" by all the hoops. Starting to the right, the hoops are transferred by each person all the way around the circle, over people's bodies until they all get to him/her.
5. This is done with everyone *holding hands* with the person next to him/her.

Parachute Activities

Roll the parachute inward to form a sturdy handle.

- How far back can you stand, still holding the parachute?
- How far overhead can you stretch? How low to the ground?
- How can we make waves using the parachute?
- Can you run in a circle holding the parachute extended overhead with the right hand?
- Show how you would raise the chute overhead, then release it and re-grasp it while it is floating in space.

Organizations

The organizations described below are defining dance for people with disabilities. They are valuable resources for additional ideas on how to expand the range of clients who can participate in your programs.

Dance for Parkinson's Disease

Dance for PD offers dance classes for people with Parkinson's disease in Brooklyn, New York, and through its network of partners and associates in more than 100 other communities in 11 countries around the world. In Dance for PD classes, participants are empowered to explore movement and music in ways that are refreshing, enjoyable, stimulating, and creative. Through an ongoing non-profit collaboration between the Mark Morris Dance Group and the Brooklyn Parkinson's Group, the Dance for PD program also provides teacher training and encourages relationships among other organizations so that classes based on their model are widely available. They found 10 reasons why people benefit from Dance for PD (Westheimer, 2008).

- Dance develops flexibility and instills confidence.
- Dance is first and foremost a stimulating mental activity that connects mind to body.
- Dance breaks isolation.
- Dance invokes imagery in the service of graceful movement.
- Dance focuses attention on eyes, ears, and touch as tools to assist in movement and balance.
- Dance increases awareness of where all parts of the body are in space.
- Dance tells stories.
- Dance sparks creativity.
- The basis of dance is rhythm.
- The essence of dance is joy.

The website www.danceforpd.org lists all affiliated classes in the U.S. and abroad, class schedules, addresses, contact information, and video clips of classes.

Dancing Wheels

Professional Flair, Inc. is a nonprofit arts/disability organization established in 1989 as the parent company of Dancing Wheels, an integrated professional company of dancers with and without disabilities. The mission of Professional Flair/Dancing Wheels is to educate, integrate, and employ people with and without disabilities in the arts through outreach activities, public performances, and advocacy. The company provides classes, lectures, performances, and main stage concerts throughout the United States and internationally, reaching over 120,000 people annually.

As a role model for inclusion, Dancing Wheels published the nation's first physically integrated dance training manual and DVD in 2012. To date, university and college dance departments have not offered degrees in dance to wheelchair dancers because they did not have a way to measure their capabilities and achievements. The manual and DVD are a first step toward an accreditation program.

Dancing Wheels Summer Dance Workshops are intensive dance workshops open to dancers, educators, health professionals, and dance enthusiast with and without disabilities, who wish to learn the Dancing Wheels technique based on traditional modern dance techniques. Under

the direction of President and Founding Artistic Director Mary Verdi-Fletcher, workshops include dance technique, composition, improvisation, and reparatory. The School of Dancing Wheels, 3615 Euclid Ave., 3rd floor, Cleveland, OH 44115. www.dancingwheels.org.
Email: proflair1@aol.com. Phone 216-432-0306.

Dance Therapy Resources

Organization

American Dance Therapy Association (ADTA)
10632 Little Patuxent Parkway, Suite 108
Columbia, MD 21044
phone: 410-997-4040
fax: 410-997-4048

Film

A time to dance: The life and work of Norma Canner. Feature-length documentary film produced by Bushy Theater, Inc., Sommerville, MA: 1998. To order *A Time to Dance* visit www.btifilms.com.

Websites

American Orff-Schulwerk Association (www.aosa.org)
Dance for Parkinson's Disease (www.danceforpd.org).

References

American Orff-Schulwerk Association. (2019). www.aosa.org.

Berrol, C. F., Ooi, W. L., & Katz, S. S. (1997). Dance/movement therapy with older adults who have sustained a neurological insult: A demonstration project. *Amer J Dance Ther. 19*(2), 135-160.

Bloem, B. R., Grimbergen, Y. A., Cramer, M., Willemsen, M., & Zinderman, A. H. (2001). Prospective assessment of falls in Parkinson's disease. *J Neurol. 248*(11), 950-958.

Bojner Horwitz, E. (2004). Dance/movement therapy in fibromyalgia patients: Aspects and consequences of verbal, visual and hormonal analyses. University of Uppsala, 2004. Google scholar.

Brauninger, I. (2005). *Tanztherapie. Verbesserung der Lebensqualität und Stressbewältigung. [Dance therapy. Improvement of quality of life and coping].* Weinheim, Germany: Beltz Verlag.

Brooke, S. (2006). *Creative arts therapy manual.* Springfield IL: Charles C. Thomas.

Bushey Theater. (1998). *A time to dance.* Medford, MA: Bushey Theater.

Canner, N. (1968). *...and a time to dance.* Boston, MA: Beacon Press.

Chace, M., Chaiklin, S., Sandel, S., & Ohn, A. (eds.). (1993). *Foundations of dance/movement therapy: The life and work of Marian Chace.* Columbia, MD: American Dance Therapy Association.

Chaiklin, H., ed. (1975). *Marian Chace: Her papers.* Columbia, MD: American Dance Therapy Association.

Deighton, L. C. (Editor-in-Chief). (1971). *Encyclopedia of education.* New York: MacMillan.

Earhart, G. M. (2009). Dance as therapy for individuals with Parkinson disease. *Eur J Phys Rehabilitation Medicine 45*(2), 231-238.

Estrella, E. (2019). The Orff approach to music education for children. www.thoughtco.com/the-orff-approach-2456422.

Garcaro, D. C. (2011). Influence of dance therapy on the functional mobility of children with spastic hemiparetic cerebral palsy. *Motricidad, 7*(3), 3.

Gilbert, A. (2000). *Teaching the three R's through movement experience.* Seattle, WA: University of Washington Press.

Keats, J. (2014). Twenty things you didn't know about play. *Discover*, July/August 2014.

Keus, S. H., Bleom, B. R., Hendriks, E. J., Bredero-Cohn A. V., & Munneke, M. (2007). Practice Recommendations Development Group evidence-based analysis of physical therapy in Parkinson's disease with recommendations for practice and research. *Mov Disord. 22*(4), 451-460.

Klebanoff, H. (1998). *A time to dance: The life and works of Norma Canner.* Sommerville, MA: Bushy Theater, Inc.

Koch, S. (2006). Report from 2nd International Research Colloquium in Dance Therapy, Pforzheim, Germany. *Body Movement and Dance in Psychotherapy 1*(2), 161-163.

Koch, S. & Brauninger, I., eds. (2006). *Advances in dance/movement therapy. Theoretical perspectives and empirical findings.* Springfield, IL: Charles C. Thomas.

Koch, S. & Brauninger, I. (2005). International dance/movement therapy research: Theory, methods, and empirical findings. *American Journal of Dance Therapy 27*(1), 37-46.

Koch, S., Kunz, T., Lykou, S., & Cruz, R. (2014). Effects of dance/movement therapy and dance on health-related psychological outcomes: A meta-analysis. *Arts in Psychotherapy 41*(1), 46-64.

Kunstler, R. & Stavola Daly, F. (2010). *Therapeutic recreation leadership and programming.* Champaign, IL: Human Kinetics.

Laban, R. (1948). *Modern educational dance.* London: Macdonald & Evans Ltd.

Laban, R. (1963). *Modern educational dance.* (revised by Lisa Ullman). London: Macdonald & Evans Ltd.

Levy, F. (1995). *Dance and other expressive art therapies.* New York: Routledge.

Levy, F. (2005). *Dance/movement therapy: A healing art.* Reston, Virginia: American Alliance for Health, Physical Education, Recreation, and Dance.

Lopez-Ortiza, C., Gladdena, K., Deona, L., Schmidt, J., Girolami, G., & Gaebler-Spira, D. (2012). Dance program for physical rehabilitation and participation in children with cerebral palsy. *Arts & Health, 4*(1), 39-54.

Mannheim, E. & Weis, J. (2006). D/MT with cancer inpatients. Evaluation of process and outcome parameters In Koch, S. & Brauninger, I., eds. *Advances in dance/movement therapy: Theoretical perspectives and empirical findings.* Springfield, IL: Charles C. Thomas.

McDowell, C. & Stuart, D. (2016). Sequencing: A methodology for movement lessons, music and movement as a therapeutic tool. Midwest Symposium on Therapeutic Recreation, St. Louis, MO.

Melton, L. J., III, Leibson, C. L., Achenbach, S. J., Bower, J. H., Maraganore, D. M., Ober, A. L., & Rocca, W. A. (2006). Fracture risk after the diagnosis of Parkinson's disease. *Mov Disord. 21*(9), 1361-1367.

Muslimovic, D. (2008). CARPA Study Group determinants of disability and quality of life in mild to moderate Parkinson disease. *Neurology 70*, 2241-2247.

Overby, L. (2015). *Public scholarship in dance: Teaching, choreography, research, service and assessment for community engagement.* Champaign, IL: Human Kinetics.

Overby, L., Post, B., & Newman, D. (2005). *Interdisciplinary learning through dance: 101 moventures*. Champaign, IL: Human Kinetics.

Shanahan, J., Morris, M., Bhriain, O., & Saunders, J. (2015). Dance for people with Parkinson disease: What is the evidence telling us? *Arch Physical Medicine Rehabilitation 96*(1), 141-153.

Sterba, J. A. (2006). Adaptive downhill skiing in children with cerebral palsy: Effect on gross motor function. *Pediatric Physical Therapy, 18*(4), 289-296.

Stuart, D. (2001). Creative movement therapy as a therapeutic intervention. *Expanding Horizons in Therapeutic Recreation 19*, 104-111.

Stuart, D. (2006). Inclusive recreation and flow theory. *Expanding Horizons in Therapeutic Recreation 23*, 77-93.

Stuart, D. (2015). Creative movement: Exploring Laban's theories in the classroom. *The Orff Echo, 47*(2), 8-21.

Stuart, D. (2016). Music and creative movement for special needs children. *The Orff Echo, 49*(1), 12-17.

Stuart, D., McDowell, C., & Smith, E. (2006). Therapeutic uses of music, movement, and art. *Expanding Horizons in Therapeutic Recreation 22*, 151-159.

Thacker, E. L., Chen, H., Patel, A. V., McCullough, M. I., Calle, E. E., Thun, M. J., Schwarzschild, M. Q., & Ascherio, A. (2008). Recreational physical activity and risk of Parkinson's disease. *Mov Disord. 23*(10), 69-74.

Ullman, L. (1963). Some hints for the student of movement. in R. Laban. *Modern educational dance*. London: Macdonald & Evans.

Warren, B. (2008). *Using the creative arts in therapy and healthcare: A practical introduction.* New York: Routledge.

Westheimer, O. (2008). Why dance for Parkinson's disease. *Topics Ger Rehabilitation 24*(2),127-140.

17

Writing and Poetry

Writing can meet many needs in therapy settings. Writing techniques range from an introspective and personal process to a way for group members to share their thoughts about a wide range of feelings. Some writing is never to be shared. Other writing activities aim at expressing feelings with a trusted set of people. Between those two extremes we have poetry and journaling. The very process of writing may lead a writer to discoveries about him/herself that lie hidden from conscious thought.

Writing can also be creative, directed, or used for recording events.

Creative writing is a powerful tool for examining and/or exposing personal feelings, attitudes, and beliefs. In creative writing, ideas emerge from our life history, culture, and times, as well as our heart, intellect, and spirit. In writing creatively, an individual makes the statement, "This is me. This is what I believe, see, feel, and think about."

Directed writing also has a place in therapy. In directed writing, clients are asked to look at particular aspects of their situation. Many of the benefits of creative writing, especially self-discovery, are still there. In addition, directed writing asks clients to think about possibilities or ways of looking at a situation that they have never considered. It lets the client explore a whole new way of being.

Journaling keeps a day-by-day record of feelings, actions, treatment successes and failures, and many other aspects of life. It allows clients to see the progress they are making. It also reminds clients of situations that hindered their progress and how they got through those situations in the past.

One huge challenge for a therapist planning to use writing as therapy comes from clients' vastly different attitudes toward the writing process. For some clients, writing is a haven where they can freely express whatever they choose to say and be assured of at least one avid reader … themselves. Others, who struggle to put their thoughts on paper, may perceive writing as an impossible chore. As therapists we need to be sensitive to our clients' attitudes toward writing. We are not trying to teach people how to write well. We are, instead, teaching them how to capture their feelings in a way that preserves them, whether it's on paper, in an electronic file, or with a voice recorder.

Research

Research has demonstrated the efficacy of writing therapy for both physical and mental health.

One of the largest bodies of research that demonstrates efficacy comes from James Pennebaker and his associates, who have been researching what they call Expressive Writing since the late 1970s. In Pennebaker and Evans (2014) book, *Expressive Writing: Words that Heal*, they list 381 studies that demonstrate the effectiveness of Expressive Writing on aspects of health. Here are some samples:

Labs at Ohio State, University of Miami, Auckland Medical School in New Zealand, and elsewhere find that emotional writing is associated with general enhancement in immune function (Koschwanez et al., 2013; Pennebaker, Kiecolt-Glasser, & Glasser, 1988; Lumley et al., 2011).

Asthma patients and rheumatoid arthritis patients showed improvements in lung function and joint mobility (Smyth & Arigo, 2009; Smyth et al., 1999). Higher white blood cell counts were demonstrated among AIDS patients (Petrie et al., 2004). Patients with irritable bowel syndrome achieved a significant improvement in disease severity (Halpert, Rybin, & Doros, 2010).

Depressive symptoms, rumination, and general anxiety tend to drop in the weeks and months after writing about emotional upheavals (Lepore,

1997). Other studies found improvement in overall well-being and improved cognitive functioning (Barclay & Skarlicki, 2009).

At least three studies have found that students make higher grades in the semester following participation in an Expressive Writing study (Lumley & Provenzano, 2003; Cameron & Nicholls, 1998; Pennebaker, Colder, & Sharp, 1990). Expressive writing frees working memory, allowing people to deal with more complicated issues in their lives (Klein & Boals, 2001).

Studies demonstrate that expressive writing helps couples reduce anger, depression, and PTSD symptoms while couples are in psychotherapy after extramarital affairs (Snyder et al., 2004). Soldiers who did expressive writing about being reunited with their spouses and families after deployment improved their marital satisfaction (Baddeley & Pennebaker, 2011).

Positive effects have been found for expressive writing in countries around the globe: United States, Japan, New Zealand, Mexico, Holland, Germany, Spain, England, Hungary, Poland, and Texas. Writing in any language appears to work — either the person's native or learned language. Similarly, people can be in upper, middle, or lower social classes in these countries, and writing continues to bring benefits (Lepore & Smyth, 2002; Pennebaker, Mayne, & Francis, 1997).

Expressive Writing follows a specific protocol that says the writing is never to be shared. This means that these extremely positive Expressive Writing results may not be found in any other kind of writing program. One study that looked at sharing what was written found that trauma patients who write about their traumas and then read their stories to other people in a group were more depressed (Gidron et al., 1996). About this study, Pennebaker (Pennebaker and Evans, 2014, p. 16) says:

> Talking to a real person about a trauma is … complex. If the other person can accept you no matter what you say and you can be completely honest in your disclosure, then talking may actually be better than writing. But therein is the rub. If the person you are confiding in does not react favorably to you and to what you say, then talking may actually be *worse* than not confiding at all.

Writing programs where the writing is shared need to adhere to two rules to get benefits from the writing exercise, as described above:

- No one must be required to show their writing to anyone else, including the therapist.
- The group who reads or hears writing from someone else must accept what is written.

There are situations where required sharing is beneficial in different ways. In a therapy situation it may be necessary to call bullshit on a client's beliefs before the client will see the need to change them. It's is easier to call bullshit on something that is in writing (Pennycook et al., 2015).

Outside of Pennebaker's work, an article in the *American Psychological Associations Monitor on Psychological Studies*, "suggests that writing about emotions and stress can boost immune functioning in patients with such illness as HIV/AIDS, asthma and arthritis" (Murray, 2002).

Researchers at the Dana Farber Cancer Institute and Harvard Medical School found "therapeutic journal writing can improve the mental and physical health in cancer patients" (Laura, 2015).

An article published in *Advances in Psychiatric Treatment* states that journal therapy and therapeutic writing are beneficial for treating severe trauma, body image problems, and grief and loss issues (Baikie and Wilhelm, 2005).

Heimes (2011) reviewed the state of poetry therapy research and found a total of 1129 studies. Two hundred three were used for analysis. A majority of the studies were conducted in the United States in the fields of psychiatry and psychology. Most of the studies corresponded to level 5 on the scale of evidence-based medicine. Findings suggest that connecting with a writing community, having a forum of communication, emotional development, and having an internal drive to write seemed to help the poets to feel balanced in everyday life. Studies in other areas such as oncology point to future ranges of application. The increasing interest in poetry therapy and its scientific establishment has encouraged additional research projects for which appropriate evaluation methods need to be developed.

Swinnen (2016) states that the personhood movement in dementia research has established the theoretical foundation for implementing cultural arts interventions in care practices. An underlying assumption is that people in the expressive arts can see the person behind the condition and focus on possibilities for meaningful relationships through interactions in the here and now. Swinnen draws on participant observations of poetry interventions by Gary Glazner (Alzheimer's Poetry Project, USA) at the New York Memory Center, and identifies the benefits of using the arts for person-centered care. The researchers used a humanities-based approach applying Huizinga's framework: play is the heart of human activity and gives meaning to life. Play is used to explore potential for expression, meaning making, and relationship building in later life. The arts programs (TimeSlips and the Alzheimer's Poetry Project) were conducted at two residential care facilities, Scharwyerveld and DeBeyart, in the Netherlands over 10 weeks. Three benefits or observations were noted: people learned to play again, there is power in playing together, and play often leads to expressions of joy. Overall the researchers concluded the notion of play may be a helpful framework for future research into innovative arts-based approaches to dementia care.

Wexler (2014) describes one kind of poetry program that has therapeutic value. Wexler noticed that the elders were responding. They were becoming more alert and positive in their comments to him and others in the group. Participants were enjoying themselves and connecting to one another. In poetry, participants found validation of their own experiences, and that they are shared. While the contexts changed with each poetry reading session, each session "contained poems that speak to significant and relevant matters — to hope, to courage, to beauty, to love, to trust to spirituality, to loss, to redemption, to belonging, to nature, to family, to time, and what is timeless/the soul" (Wexler, 2014, p. 36).

Reasons for Writing

Clients have many reasons for choosing to write including therapeutic goals of healthcare. Here are some that the therapist should keep in mind when explaining how writing will be beneficial.

- **For venting:** Graffiti — or a private diary/journal — helps the writer to think, reflect, and stay in touch with self. Written from the heart, it may be cathartic. Not meant to be read by others. No editing, just immediate reactions (and possibly fresh insights) regarding daily events or past traumas.

- **For reflection and/or sharing:** May be autobiographical, reminiscing, life history, or oral history. Increases self-esteem — goals may be socialization and improved interactions. Example: group newspaper.
- **For fun:** Humorous narratives, short stories, and descriptive pieces. Perspective leads to more ability to see possibilities.
- **For imagination:** Writing about utopia, a projection of the future, the self in a different setting, and alternate worlds or other people. Opens up possibilities.
- **For self-expression:** Haiku, free verse, sonnets, or simple rhymes — all can carry the feelings and emotions of the writer.

Writing Techniques

Writing techniques vary along three axes: the kind of writing, how directed the writing is, and the amount of sharing among members of the group.

Kinds of writing can vary from just getting words on paper to attempting to write and analyze profound, beautiful poetry and prose. The first tends to provide a written description of feelings or situations so they can be remembered as part of a therapeutic process. Profound, beautiful writing makes writing the purpose of the group rather than the therapy that may come out of the writing. Therapists need to intentionally choose the focus of the group based on the clients' goals. Both extremes of writing have their purpose. It's less likely that a group that aims for sort-of-profound writing that focuses somewhat on the emotional content will be as successful as a group that is focused on one of the extremes.

Writing directions can vary from "Write about this specific topic" to "Write about anything that comes to mind." In the middle is the instruction, "Write about something that is bothering you (or keeps you awake at night)." The last one is directed in the sense that the client is instructed to write about something that is troubling, but the specific topic is left to the client. Any level of direction can be successful, as long as clients are not allowed to ruminate about a problem, over and over, without searching for a solution or a new way to consider the situation.

The *amount of sharing* also depends on the focus of the group. The efficacy found in Expressive Writing research is usually based on unshared writing. However, unshared writing is not really a group exercise. Some research (Pennebaker and Evans, 2014) suggests that sharing can be more effective than unshared writing when the group is accepting. But it is less effective, and can be harmful for working through trauma, when the group is not accepting. On the other hand, shared writing can be helpful when clients are diagnosed as needing attitude and behavior changes. Then calling bullshit, or related confrontational techniques, are based on concrete written statements that can't be changed.

We will now look at some writing techniques that are used in therapeutic groups. We will see that while there are differences between the types of writing, there are also overlaps in how the writing is done.

Expressive Writing

The purpose of Expressive Writing is to heal from a trauma, such as divorce, rape, family abuse, or a suicide attempt. It can also be effective in exploring conflicts or stressors. It is directed writing in the sense that the client is instructed to focus on a particular problem for the writing sessions. It contains the writer's deepest thoughts in totally private writing. The aesthetic quality of the writing is not important. With appropriate adaptations it can be effective for many populations, as described in the research section.

Therapists who want to use Expressive Writing as part of their treatment should read through the detailed explanations of the technique in Pennebaker and Evan's (2014) book, *Expressive Writing: Words that Heal.* The quick description of the technique provided here is not enough to use Expressive Writing effectively, but it does show the time and effort involved. With great care to be accepting, the no sharing rule may be broken. Clients who deeply want to share the experience or clients who are not figuring out how to make the exercise effective may share what they wrote — but with the knowledge that they never have to share their writing again.

Expressive Writing is usually done for twenty minutes a day, four days in a row. Each session can be about the same event or a different, but related, event. Clients must include their deepest thoughts and feelings for the writing to be effective. It is important to write without ever stopping. If clients can't think of anything to say, they need to keep writing anyway, either by repeating what they wrote before or by writing a filler phrase like "still writing… still writing…" until they think of something new to write. There will often be increased sadness immediately after writing. If it continues for more than a few hours, this topic probably is not appropriate for Expressive Writing at this time. When Expressive Writing is effective, each day is slightly different, as the client looks at the event more deeply and from different perspectives.

There is a Flip-Out Rule that must be followed:

If you feel that writing about a particular topic is too much for you to handle, then do not write about it. If you know that you aren't ready to address a particularly painful topic, then write about something else. When you are ready, then tackle the other topic. If you feel that you will flip out by writing, don't write.

When using Expressive Writing, clients may find it useful to measure how they feel before and after sessions. It can be as simple as choosing a number between zero and ten to describe how much the issue they are writing about is bothering them. Zero means not at all and ten means it is driving them out of their minds. It's hard to remember how much something once bothered you after it has been taken care of. Successful writing sessions might see the number move lower from before to after. The best measure of effectiveness is how the numbers change from one day to the next.

Journal Therapy

Journal therapy, also referred to as journal writing therapy, involves the therapeutic use of journaling exercises and prompts to bring awareness and improve mental health conditions resulting from inner and outer conflicts. According to the Center for Journal Therapy it is the "purposeful and intentional use of reflective writing to further mental, physical, emotional, and spiritual health and wellness" (Adams, 1999, p. 1).

Journal therapy originated in the 1960s with psychologist Ira Progoff's Intensive Journal Method (Dialog House Associates, 2019). His work informed the public about the therapeutic potential of journal writing. Prior to this, the primary function of journal writing was to record events and experiences from a narrative point of view.

Today, journal therapy is considered a standalone modality like art or music therapy. Journal therapists can train in programs approved by the National Federation for Biblio/Poetry Therapy or independent programs. Those who are not trained can still use journal writing. One of the major differences between keeping a journal and journal therapy is the way internal experiences, thoughts, and feelings are captured. Journal therapy allows participants to write down dialogue and to analyze their issues and concerns. Therapeutic journal writing uses prompts and exercises to allow clients to be reflective, introspective, and intentional about their writing.

Journal therapy has been used in treatment for conditions including PTSD, anxiety, depression, obsessive-compulsive disorder, grief, and loss. It is used to work on issues related to chronic illness, substance abuse, eating disorders, interpersonal relationships, low self-worth, and communication skill.

Journal therapy is used to increase awareness and insight, promote change and growth, and further develop a sense of self. Through writing prompts and activities, a therapist can guide a person in treatment toward his or her goals. Writing things down can bring clarity to issues. A therapist might request that the group begin each session with a writing exercise to declare their intention for the session or to focus on present concerns and solutions.

Journal therapy and journal writing are not concerned with aesthetics. They both may be personal or shared, but neither is as personal as Expressive Writing. Journal therapy is usually focused. Journal writing may not be focused.

Exercises and Prompts

There are many creative and effective ways to use journal writing in treatment. Some examples of journal exercises and prompts include:

Journaling with Photographs

People chose personal photographs and spend time in session writing responses to questions about the photographs. Questions can include: "What do you feel when you look at these photos?" or "What do you want to say to the people, places, or things in these photos?" For clients with limited verbal and writing skills, see the collage exercise in the Visual and Tactile Arts chapter for how to use photos in reminiscing.

Letter Writing

Participants are encouraged to write a letter to someone about various issues they are experiencing. Participants can choose to write to anyone: people they know, wise people they know about, themselves, or someone they have lost. For example, a client might write a letter to a deceased mother to tell her what the client is going through.

Timed Journal Entries

This is a technique that may be used with people who have difficulty focusing their thoughts. The client and therapist decide on a topic. The participant has five to ten minutes to write about it.

Sentence Stems

The therapist provides open ended sentences for the participant to complete. An example, "My happiest memory is …"

List of 10

The therapist asks the client to list 10 items that relate to a chosen topic or theme. Examples, 10 Reasons to Wake Up in the Morning, 10 Things I Love, 10 Things I Want to Do with My Life.

Writing for Wellness Groups

Writing for Wellness classes create an environment that provides healing for its members with personal or family health issues. It helps those with ongoing illnesses or families recovering from grief. The class is most effective for people with a deep need to express their feelings as a way to address their current struggles.

By providing specific topics for the whole group to write about, and a safe environment in which to write, Writing for Wellness classes help participants improve their physical, mental, and spiritual health as part of a supportive group. Class members are instructed in writing techniques which will help them to relieve grief, forgive hurts, and address frustrations and anger.

Participants in Writing for Wellness classes often say they never liked writing before. However, with the help of the lessons, samples from previous participants, and prompts, they find an ease in writing. They begin to share their stories, thus fostering the sense of community, a vital element in wellness. Writing together creates a unique healing experience.

What Happens in the Classes?

Writing for Wellness classes can be adjusted to fit many different settings and group dynamics. Most of them will follow the general format described here:

First, everyone is welcomed and asked to briefly introduce themselves. The leader of the class then describes the topic for the session and offers readings, sometimes from the *Writing for Wellness* book (Davey, 2007) and other times from previous groups. Each chapter in the book contains "Healing Words," which are examples of writings completed by those in earlier Writing for Wellness classes.

After the readings, the leader reiterates the writing topic for the session and gives some introductory sentences to help even the reluctant writer get started. Members of the class are given some time to write, at least 20 minutes. After most of the writing is finished, members are asked if anyone wants to share what they have written. No one is required to share, but there are usually plenty of volunteers. To close the meeting, an appropriate quote may be offered.

The number of sessions in a group varies greatly with the setting. Some places offer only four or five sessions for a group. Others, such as the City of Hope where Julie Davey has taught, have offered classes continuously. It is important to have the same members for all the sessions because sharing is facilitated by increasing trust in other members of the group. Members who are not able to refrain from critical comments must be removed to allow trust to form.

Step-by-Step Procedures

What follows is a simple step-by-step plan for a class session. It may be adapted to suit your purposes.

1. Greet each person as they enter. Create a relaxed and supportive atmosphere, realizing that coming to class may, in itself, be an achievement for some people.
2. Take care of introductions and check-ins.
    - In session one, describe your own background and why you are teaching the class. Allow everyone else to introduce themselves.
    - In later sessions, offer a chance for people to share a brief summary of what has happened since the last meeting.
3. Prepare for the lesson. In session one, distribute a class syllabus.
4. Set the stage for this session's topic. Read parts of the "Healing Words" examples and any other writings you choose, or share your own experience, if you feel it is appropriate.
5. Distribute writing materials (pens, paper, etc.) to anyone who doesn't have them.
6. Initiate some low-key, impromptu discussion about this session's "It's Your Turn" writing prompt. This is a good time to remind the class that you won't call on anyone unless they volunteer.
7. Allow 20 minutes to write about the prompt. Ask everyone to be quiet, since many people cannot concentrate on writing if others are talking. Write your own response to the prompt.
8. After about 18 minutes, announce that time is almost up. This gives everyone a chance to finish up a thought or make notes about something they may want to write more about later.
9. At the end of the writing time, ask if anyone would like to share what they have written. If there is complete silence, break the ice by reading what you wrote. Tell how writing about it made you feel. When someone volunteers to read, provide a small reward for their courage.

Ask the others what they liked best about the writing that was shared, with the reminder that there will be no criticism. The objective is getting one's feelings out and onto paper, not creating literary masterpieces.

10. Point out that they may continue to write about the topic. No homework is ever assigned. It's enough to simply come to class and write.
11. Close with an appropriate inspirational quote and a smile.

Poetry

Poetry therapy is based on the principle that by writing poetry, reading it, or both, clients will be encouraged to express their thoughts and find greater awareness and self-understanding.

In *Poetry Therapy* edited by Dr. Jack Leedy (1969), the purpose of poetry therapy is twofold:

- By writing verse, the individual is encouraged to voice fears, doubts, and anxieties that s/he might otherwise not share with others. The individual may also be able to use writing as a source of emotional release (e.g., if you can't say it, write it).
- By reading poetry others have written, an individual may find:
    - someone with whom to identify
    - a springboard for discussion
    - the opportunity to share with others

Stylized Forms of Poetry

Other uses of poetry can be effective in the therapy process. This section looks at several stylized forms of poetry. The structure of the poems helps clients who have difficulty with more free-form types of expression. Experimenting with any of them provides a good learning activity and an effective means of expressing thoughts and feelings.

Syntu

Goals: To think creatively. Express emotions and feeling about others in writing.

Directions: Have clients pair up or form groups. Each client then tells the other member(s) of their group something really nice about themselves that s/he has refrained from saying during previous sessions. Ask the group to think about how they feel when they're giving a compliment and/or receiving one. After the compliment-giving is over, explain to clients that they may write a syntu about friendship. A syntu is a five-line poem written in the following form with one or two words to as line:

subject: friends
descriptive word: comforting
emotion felt by writer: loving
descriptive word: necessary
synonym for subject: support system

Materials: Paper, crayons, pencils.

Setting: The leader should explain what a syntu is and read one example to the group.

Haiku

Goals: To be able to express emotions and feelings about others in writing. To think creatively.

Description: A haiku is a tightly structured, three-line, 17 syllable verse form with an emphasis on images from nature and rhythms. Haikus attempt to evoke a feeling and create an image with a minimum of words. They are originally found in Japanese literature as part of the Japanese love of nature and beauty. Haikus evolved during the 14th century. Zen monks adopted the form during the 15th century. One of the monks, Yamazaki Sakon (1465-1553) is known as the father of Haiku because he was the first poet to use the form separately from the larger body of poetry in which it originally appeared. There are five important things to remember when creating a haiku.

- It should provide a clear image.
- It must come from the heart and be sincere.

- It should not preach.
- It must be a simple statement of what is.
- It is usually associated with a season of the year.

The following example shows the structure of a haiku with the syllable count shown.

1 2 3 4 5
Hungrily searching
1 2 3 4 5 6 7
Seagulls swirling overhead
1 2 3 4 5
Rising with the wind

Materials: pens/pencils, paper, examples of haikus, (optional) Japanese music.

Setting: The leader reads some examples of haikus and gives a brief background on its history.

Diamonte

Goals: To think creatively. To be able to express emotions and feelings about other people, places, or things in writing.

Description: A diamonte is a seven-line poem with an ascending and descending number of words. When the lines are centered, the words form the shape of a diamond (*diamonte)* on the page.

- one noun (name of person, place, or thing)
- two adjectives describing the first noun
- three verbs that are actions of the first noun
- four nouns (associated with the nouns at top and bottom)
- three verbs that are actions of the last noun
- two adjectives describing last noun
- one noun which is the opposite of the first noun

Materials: Paper, crayons, pencils.

Setting: The leader should explain what a diamonte is and read one example to the group.

Poetry Themes

Holidays, seasons, families, pets, or life issues are examples of themes that can be very effective as the basis for poetry. Use the senses to engage memory and begin the writing process. If the topic is "summer," bring in seashells, tanning lotion, and/or sand — anything that evokes the essence of summer. Ask the group to suggest other things that symbolize summer. These suggestions could be the basis for individual poems or even a group poem such as a *renga* (everyone writes one line, word or phrase on an agreed upon theme). Contributions to the renga may be public (e.g., stating them out loud to the group) or private (e.g., each person writes a line without seeing the other lines). Often, in the private method, the other lines are masked from each writer until the whole piece is revealed by the leader who reads all the lines together. The lines always seem to come together as a whole.

Poetry Readings

Reading poetry inspires writers of poetry. Having group members recite and listen to poetry will help them learn new language and ways of expressing ideas and sensitize them to the rhythms of poetry. In conducting poetry readings, remember to:

- Choose poems with understandable language.
- Choose poems that represent a variety of emotions and experiences.
- Provide each person with a copy of the poem, if possible or appropriate (and if permissible, given copyright laws).
- Ask how the group responded to the poem: feelings, opinions.
- Bring poetry books and ask participants to find a favorite poem to share.
- Record the poetry reading and then play it back for people to hear.
- Ask for someone whose native language is not English to read a poem in his/her native language and to translate it.

Marvin Wexler (2014) describes another kind of poetry reading program using poems that speak to hope, courage, beauty, love, trust, spirituality, and other timeless issues. It has been especially effective for the elderly in long-term care. Many of the poems are selected by the residents. Some readings become singings as with "Amazing Grace." Power point pictures accompany each poem, a field of daffodils in front of a lake for Wordsworth's "Daffodils," a cardinal for Dickinson's "Hope is the Thing with Feathers," and cherry trees in bloom for AE Housman's "Loveliest of Trees." Wexler encourages people who care for the elderly, whether professionally or on a personal level, to consider including poetry as part of that care. As the Irish poet Seamus Hearney remarked (as cited in Kerrigan & Wylie, 1999), "The aim of the poet and poetry is finally to be of service to ply the effort of individual work into the larger work of the community as a whole" (p. 127). Wexler reminds us, "You do not have to be a poet to do poetic service" (p. 46).

Inter-Being

If the therapist wishes to discuss the interconnectedness of all things, one place to start is Thich Nhat Hanh's "The Heart of Understanding." Clients can start with any object and write about the interconnections (inter-being) they find in the object. The writing can be poetry or creative writing, as described in the next section.

If you are a poet, you will see clearly that there is a cloud floating in this sheet of paper. Without a cloud, there will be no rain; without rain, the trees cannot grow; and without trees we cannot make paper. The cloud is essential for the paper to exist. If the cloud is not here, the sheet of paper cannot be here either. So we can say that the cloud and the paper inter-are. "Inter-being" is a word that is not in the dictionary yet.

If we look into this sheet of paper even more deeply, we can see sunshine in it. If the sunshine is not there, the forest cannot grow. In fact, nothing can grow. Even we cannot grow without sunshine. And so we know that the sunshine is also in this sheet of paper. The paper and the sunshine inter-are. And if we continue to look, we can see the logger who cut the tree and brought it to the mill to be transformed into paper. And we see the wheat. We know the logger cannot exist without his daily bread, and therefore the wheat that became his bread is also in this sheet of paper. Looking even more deeply, we can see we are in it too. This is not difficult to see, because when we look at a sheet of paper, the sheet of paper is part of our perception. Your mind is in here and mine is also. So we can say that everything is in here with this sheet of paper. You cannot point out one thing that is not here — time, space, the earth, the rain, the minerals in the soil, the sunshine, the cloud, the river, the heat. Everything co-exists with this sheet of paper. To be is to inter-be. You cannot just be by yourself alone. You have to inter-be with every other thing. This sheet of paper is, because everything else is.

Creative Writing

Creative writing is like poetry therapy in that it also encourages clients to express their thoughts and find greater awareness and self-understanding. Therapists may choose one or the other, or both, depending on what they think will be best for the people in the current group.

Some of the ways creative writing works include how it encourages:

- sharing with others to establish a sense of community
- using writing when it is easier than speaking
- learning about ourselves
- learning about others
- writing spontaneously to find what is in our unconscious
- sharing our writing to invite others to look through our eyes

Guidelines

The objectives of creative writing include:

- offer comfort or support
- increase insight into self or others
- increase empathy
- foster creative growth
- encourage imagination
- build self-confidence in writing abilities
- increase socialization skills
- amuse

The following ideas give clients permission to write by unblocking some of the blocks:

- Anything they have written is acceptable.
- The focus of the group is on creative expression only.

- No one will care about spelling, grammar, punctuation, or handwriting.
- There will be no red pencils or grades.
- Sharing is optional.
- The group is only interested in your ideas, not in analyzing your creation. Analysis is only important in terms of what the writer does with his/her own work.

People may respond:

- as they really are
- as they would like to be
- with whatever pops into their minds

Group Process

Creative writing groups generally follow this structure:

- **Warmup:** This is optional. As with other creative arts groups, a warmup activity helps focus the group before they do the main activity.
- **Introducing the activity:** Be able to give the group an accurate idea of what to expect and how long the activity will take (familiarize yourself with it beforehand).
- **Doing the activity:** Allow enough time — everyone thinks and writes at a different rate.
- **Closing:** Provide time for sharing a gentle closing, feedback, and validation.

Creative Writing Warmup Exercises

Even experienced writers need to warm up as they prepare to write. These exercises focus the mind and/or produce ideas that can be used in the main activity. These warmups also eliminate the fear of the blank piece of paper — once they're done, the page is no longer empty, and the individual has begun writing.

One excellent exercise is *free writing.* In this technique, the person is instructed to write a stream of consciousness (whatever comes to mind) for a limited time. Some writers start every day with 10 minutes of free writing to clear their mind of all the things which distract them, "to give the barking dog a bone," as one writer put it. Another excellent warmup comes from a book by Gabriele Rico (2000) called *Writing the Natural Way* and it is called *clustering*. In this technique, one word acts as the stimulus for recording all the associations that spring to mind in a brief time.

Ideas for Writing

Ideas for writing can come from almost anywhere. The following is a list of some of the ways to stimulate group writing.

Word Associations

Stereotypes

- women
- men
- mountain folk
- city people
- bigots
- ethnic groups

Themes

- holidays
- life issues

Free Association

- summer
- life
- men
- love
- women
- pain
- happiness
- death
- hope
- I am
- ambition

Writing in Response

Describe feelings related to a story, poem, statement, song, picture, etc.

Autobiography

- life histories
- oral histories
- reminiscing
- life review

Letter Writing

- to others
- to self

Newspaper/Newsletter

- about the facility, its participants or events

Personal Reflection

- sharing of wisdom
- journal
- epitaph

Projection and Association

- statement completion
- clustering

Writing Groups

Groups that are interested in writing can form for non-therapeutic reasons, as well as for therapy. Creative writing groups or poetry groups are organized to develop writing skills related to poetry, short stories, or any kind of narrative writing. Some groups get together to produce a newspaper or newsletter to publicize information about the facility, participants, or upcoming events. Other groups, especially in long-term care settings, get together to compile life histories or life reviews, and for reminiscing. Therapists should support these groups when they are helping clients.

Writing Activities

Writing can be used for particular purposes. The rest of the chapter includes individual activities that are not part of a larger writing program. There are warmups for groups doing writing or other kinds of creative arts. Other activities are designed to introduce a therapeutic concept. Some are intended to increase cohesion of the group. They can be mixed and matched by the therapist to meet therapeutic goals.

Writing Games

Games that help individuals sharpen creative thinking and word skills include: *Shufflebook, Mad Libs,* and *Flabbergast.* These are available in toy and specialty stores. Crossword puzzles and other word games may also help in developing writing and thinking skills. Advanced groups can try creating their own crossword puzzles.

Writing Exercises

The exercises listed below are for the most part short and to the point. There may be a therapeutic aspect to their content, but as a rule they are less psychologically intense than the guided activities which appear in the following section. They are the written equivalent of theater games, meant to foster spontaneity and creative thinking.

- Write a title for the following types of writing:
    - a detective novel

  - a romance novel
  - love poems
  - a great adventure
  - a science fiction story
  - a gothic horror story

- Write your own epitaph.
- Spell names backwards (moorssalc = classroom).
- Create a poem or short story; each person adds a line or a paragraph.
- Write a situation from another person's point of view.
- Write a letter to mother, father, old friend, former teacher, former lover, President, spiritual guide, higher self, someone you resent regarding "unresolved business."
- You are given $500,000 tax free. What would you do?
- The medicine person of a tribe wants to talk to the children about adulthood and growing up. What does s/he want them to know? Parenting? Work? Love? Courage? Fun?
- Make up a dream or fantasy life and write as if you were someone else.
- Design a perfect resort for yourself. Where would it be? What could you do there?
- Recall an embarrassing moment (e.g., getting a traffic ticket). What were you thinking of at the time?

This next set of exercises are formally named but are still basically simple exercises.

Personal Associations/Extensions of Self

Provide a list of ideas or ask participants to come up with their own. What would I be like if I were a:

- book
- period in time
- type of weather
- dance
- piece of clothing
- song

Images of Self

- Are there any images of yourself that get you in trouble sometimes?
- Are there healthy ones you want to retain?
- Is there something from your pocket or purse, or something you are wearing that has meaning for you?

Props — To Evoke Characters

We all have met interesting characters in our lives. The introduction of props can jog memories of people we have known or seen. Ask questions such as these about each piece of clothing: Who wore this? Who would wear this?

- hats
- shoes
- jewelry
- purses
- t-shirt

Three Wishes to Find the One

You are granted three wishes; write down what you wish for. Cross out one, then cross out another. Which wish remains? Which ones did you let go?

Dialogue

Write a dialogue between a person (mother, friend, family, boss, spiritual guide, self) and a drug (your favorite drug or food that is most difficult to refuse or limit).

Three Envelopes

Three envelopes are filled with slips of paper by the leader. Each one deals with a different type of subject and contains:

1. names of things (work, walkie-talkie)
2. names of people/occupations, etc. (story character, a 90-year-old grandfather, female astronaut)
3. names of places or events (marriage, birthday)

Choose one slip of paper from each of the three envelopes and make up a paragraph incorporating the thing, person, and place.

Visualization Journal

Use the script in Chapter 18. Meditation and Creative Visualization called "Advisor." Do the visualization and then write about the gift or advice received from your spiritual guide. Writing about the visualization solidifies the experience, bringing insight and comfort. It can be a good healing exercise.

Writing Activities for Therapy Goals

The following activities are described in the context of particular therapeutic goals that the therapist may have for the group.

Back Drawing and Writing

Goals: A good warmup activity; introductory contact between participants.

Description: The leader divides the group into pairs. One of the partners sits and becomes a "canvas" while the other partner is the "artist." Using one finger, the standing "artist" draws a shape or a figure on the seated person's back. The seated person reproduces that form on a piece of paper. Then together, the partners write what comes to mind about the symbol and the experience.

Materials: pens/pencils, paper

Setting: Chairs (for "canvases" to sit on) generously spaced around a table. The leader demonstrates and explains that the artist should draw slowly so that the "canvas" can understand what is being drawn.

Zen Telegram

Goals: This is a non-threatening activity. Participants work individually as well as together. May be used as an introduction to creative expression.

Description: The group close their eyes and are encouraged to get into a meditative mood. They then make any marking (e.g., symbol, geometric figure, random mark) they care to make on their paper. When they are satisfied that they are finished, participants open their eyes and write any word or phrase on the paper which the marking brings to mind. Discussion follows for those who wish to comment on their reaction to the exercise.

Materials: pens/pencils, paper

Adaptations: A follow-up activity is to mark the paper in the same manner (but not the same configuration), as in the first activity. When eyes are opened, all participants pass their "telegrams" on to the person sitting next to them, who then writes any word or phrase which comes to mind about the marks on the paper. Discussion follows.

You'll Never Believe...

Description: This is an exercise in guided creative writing. The facilitator establishes the parameters of the writing by using a phrase as the format and defining the elements for the clients to include in writing. For example:

1. "You'll never believe who I saw!" — Name one person, one word that describes a person, and one place. The participant could write, "I saw kind Whoopi Goldberg in the kitchen."
2. "You'll never believe what I ate." — Name one food, one word for flavor, and one place. "I ate a sweet strawberry in the back yard." Participants may read their sentences aloud.

Adaptations: In the beginning, the number of elements can be varied (e.g., just name a person) depending on the abilities of the group. Add more elements as the group proceeds through the activity.

Materials: pens/pencils, paper

Group size: Do not make the group too large — a smaller writing group allows the facilitator to give proper attention to each client.

Pictures and Words

Description: Pick a painting that lends itself to storytelling. Put someone in charge of writing down what is said about the painting by the group members. Let your imagination fly. Expand what you see. Example: *Girl, girl crying, girl sitting.*

Now expand the story by asking questions, "Why is she sitting?" *Girl crying, waiting for her mother to come home.*

Finish the project when the time period or story ideas end. Read what was written, as is. For a cohesive finale, hang the picture and story in a common space so all clients can enjoy their project.

Adaptations: Anything that is said about a picture can be written down by the leader; clients can draw, and the leader can write a story about each person's drawing. Sharing the story may be a teaching method to get individuals interested in telling stories about themselves.

Materials: any painting that lends itself to storytelling.

Group Size: Any, but a group numbering over 25 may need to be split up into smaller groups.

Statement Completion

Directions: Write down the following partial statements and complete them:

- It makes me mad when …
- I suppose …
- I have …
- Don't you hate it when …?
- Just when …
- I need …
- When I get mad I …

Adaptations: If the participants are unable to write, the facilitator may write for them. If a participant cannot think of a completion to a statement, move on to another statement. Similarly, if the participant can't think of a response to a word, or any other way to complete the sentence, move on.

Materials: pens/pencils, paper

Group Size: two or more

Word Response

Directions: The leader reads off each word, allowing time for participants to write down the word(s) which each subject brings to mind.

- men
- women
- hope
- summer
- death
- ambition
- pain
- life
- happiness
- love

Adaptations: See *Statement Completion* above.
Materials: pens/pencils, paper
Group Size: two or more

I Am

Directions: Leader instructs participants to write down the phrase "I am…," and complete it as many ways as they would like to. For example:

- I am…lovable.
- I am…blue-eyed.
- I am…lazy.

Adaptations: See *Statement Completion* above.
Materials: pens/pencils, paper
Group Size: two or more

Small Potato Touch

Goals: To facilitate small group cooperation and to foster using senses other than sight, to introduce the senses as a creative medium.

Description: The group is divided into smaller groups which are given a bag apiece. Each bag contains one item — perhaps a piece of rope, a silver dollar, or a dried herb. After closing their eyes, each person in the group feels it, smells it, and passes it on to the others. When all have examined it thoroughly, it is returned to the bag and the group members open their eyes. Each person takes a strip of paper, writes a line about the item, and tapes it onto the full sheet of paper provided. The group may arrange the order of statements to create the group poem. Each completed sheet of paper is hung on the wall, and the collective group discusses its reactions to the activity. The group may wish to guess what was in each bag which did not belong to them by the evidence written on the strips.

Materials: Miscellaneous items of widely varying properties of smell and touch and paper bags for each item. Scotch tape, paper in strips, full sheets of paper.

Setting: Group sits at five separate tables of five chairs each. Facilitator reads the poem, "The Blind Men and the Elephant," which addresses the idea of identifying an object without the sense of sight.

Our Memory Poem

Goals: To facilitate large group participation and cooperation to explore the creation of poetry. To increase awareness through visual stimulation.

Description: Each person writes one line or image that describes a childhood memory. The facilitator collects the lines from each person and randomly places them on a large table or on a bulletin board. Working together, the group decides the order of the lines and arranges them. The group then picks a title for its poem. Another possibility is that the facilitator puts the lines in order and the group creates the title or titles for the work.

Materials: Use whatever helps recall the past. Items could include an old tablecloth, magazines, old toys, clothes, photographs. Old music could be playing. Pieces of paper and pens for individual writing. A place to combine paper — e.g., newsprint, a bulletin board, table.

Setting: Each old item may be discussed by the group or participants may look at items as they wish. The facilitator may read nursery rhymes or poems by Robert Louis Stevenson, Gabriela Mistral, Langston Hughes, and others that evoke childhood.

Resources:

Poems that may be used include:

- "Some Good Things to Be Said for the Iron Age" by Gary Snyder
- "The Language" by Robert Creeley
- "This is Just to Say" by William Carlos Williams
- "Snow" by Lovis NocNeile
- "The Blessing" by James Wright

Thanksgiving Memories

Goals: To share the holiday, recall previous happy holidays, feel connected to the holiday and each other. To stimulate creativity through the senses of taste and smell.

Description: Participants are asked to pick out the most memorable Thanksgiving they can recall and, in half an hour or less, to write about it. Participants are then encouraged to share what they wrote with the group. Writing may be in prose or poetry, and it is stressed that principles of detail are equally applicable to prose or poetry.

Materials: pens/pencils, paper

Setting: If possible, pie (preferably fresh baked) and coffee are waiting in a nearby kitchen to be served during the discussion. The group talks about what Thanksgiving means to them and the pros and cons of holidays in general.

Resources:

- "The First Thanksgiving" by Jennifer Mulondy
- "In Appreciation" by John Silver

Clustering/Wandering with Words

Goals: To teach a brainstorming technique. To involve a participant in a creative experience that can bring insight.

Description: The leader suggests a word for the nucleus of the cluster, or each participant picks a word that holds emotional content for him/her. It could be someone's name, a place, color, food, smell, year, etc. Be sure it's just one word. That word is written down and circled. The participants let their thoughts wander, allowing any connections to the word to come into their heads. Write these down quickly, each in its own circle, with a line connecting it to the nucleus word. As the associations grow, some words that arise may relate directly to the nucleus word; others may relate to an associated word. Connect words with lines to the appropriate association.

Materials: pens, paper, and music

Setting: Facilitator begins by asking participants to share one word. Then questions may be asked to help stimulate "word wandering" such as, "How does your word feel? How does it smell? Is it strong?" Another technique is to simply play music and allow participants to take their time and wander as they wish.

Toy Talk

Goals: To encourage reminiscence. To engage in a fantasy experience.

Description: This is a creative writing exercise based on fantasy. Participants select two toys from those placed in front of the group. Participants become acquainted with their choices, make up names for them, decide where the toys come from, and if the toys have a message for participants. Participants write a paragraph describing a conversation the two toys would have or some experience the toys shared.

Materials: pens/pencils/crayons, paper, a variety of small toys (e.g., dolls, balls, trucks)

Setting: If working with young adults or adults, the leader may need to reconnect the group to childhood and the roles that toys played in their lives. Possibly use creative visualization to take the group back to childhood and "their favorite toys."

I Remember

Goals: To formulate and express appreciation of another person.

Description: This exercise can be done in more than one way. Participants can create their own entire poem or contribute words or lines. The idea is to write a poem honoring someone who has left the group. For this purpose, a poem will be described as: "The simple, clear expression of a fully felt experience."

In writing the poem — I remember [person's name].

1. Describe the person's appearance or demeanor (flowing hair, twinkling eyes, raucous laugh).
2. Describe some quality, value, or attitude of the person (their generosity, willingness to fight, shyness).
3. Describe an experience shared with the person (a conversation, a walk, studying together, riding home, time in class).
4. If possible, summarize with a description of feeling about the person. (This is not always necessary).

Materials: pens/pencils, paper

Setting: The leader may want to start this activity by initiating a brief reminiscence about a person who has left the group, in order to bring this individual into the group's consciousness.

Writing Gifts

Goals: Gain experience in giving and receiving gifts and thoughts; social skills development.

Description: Each person selects a subject on which s/he wishes to receive a thought, a sort of "gift" in writing. For example, if the subject is peace, the thought may be, "have peaceful interactions with family members." Requests are written on pieces of paper, collected, and handed out to other group members randomly. Each group member writes a thought on the paper s/he receives and returns it to the original person. The recipient reads their gift aloud.

Variation: One participant makes a request for thoughts to the entire group and the other group members respond.

Materials: colored pens/pencils, paper

Setting: The leader may give some examples to help clarify the idea.

Making Captions

Goal: To encourage creative thinking.

Description: Tape pictures up on walls around the room. Have participants write a title, remark, or caption for each picture. Allow people to mill about the room — like being at an art exhibit or museum. Set and state a time limit. Give people a few reminders to let them know how much time is left. The leader then has the group sit to talk about the pictures and captions one by one. What similar and different thoughts, ideas, and feelings came up? How do these relate to various issues they are dealing with? How do individuals in the group tend to view things?

Materials: Photos from magazines, pictures of paintings. In order to reuse the photos or pictures, mount them on construction paper or thin foam board. Participants will need paper and pencils/pens for writing captions.

Setting: The leader can start by giving an example of a caption.

Music and Markers

Goals: To encourage expression. To facilitate group interaction. It may be used as an introduction to creative expression.

Description: Each participant has a piece of paper. The music begins and group members close their eyes. They may listen to the music as long as they wish. When each member feels like it, s/he may select a marker and make a mark on the paper with eyes opened or closed. When the music stops, words or other markings may be added. Those who wish to discuss any part of what they wrote or how the music makes them feel may do so. The process may be repeated with different music. After the exercise has been completed, members of the group hold their work in front of them and arrange themselves to form a "rainbow" of colors with the work they've done. The rainbow incorporates all colors and creates splendor that far surpasses the beauty of one color. The facilitator can congratulate the group for the diversity of its artistic expression and how it creates a rainbow of color and creativity.

Materials: CD player or iPod; music without words, perhaps classical or quiet jazz; many markers of as many colors as possible; paper.

Setting: Non-threatening activity; participants work individually as well as together. This is a good activity to use with clients who are functioning at a lower level, or with those who are having difficulty writing down words or thoughts. It will be up to the facilitator to decide how long the music should play. Any kind of music is acceptable as long as there are no words.

Therapist Concerns

Therapists who are thinking about using a writing group need to consider the following issues as they decide what kind of a group to develop:

- What is the goal of this writing group? What is the purpose of writing?
- People are like crystals — with a full range of personalities. Different aspects of people may emerge from their writing.
- Don't be afraid that no one will write.
- If you as the therapist say everything is acceptable/okay, you need to really believe that.
- Writing can give a vision concrete power.
- Honor each person's effort.
- Don't deny anything that is going on, whether it is a new idea or an interpersonal development.
- Be mindful not to set a standard, so that group members are not tempted to compare themselves.
- Try it yourself first. Test a writing activity to see how it works and how long it takes to do it.
- Keep your own journal of thoughts, poetry, and ideas so that you are as involved in the writing process as your clients are.
- Reporting laws about harm or self-harm.

References

Adams, K. (1999). Introduction to journal therapy. In Allison, N. (ed.) *The illustrated encyclopedia of body-mind disciplines*. New York: Taylor & Francis.

Baddeley, J. L. & Pennebaker, J. W. (2011). A postdeployment expressive writing intervention for military couples: A randomized controlled trial. *The Journal of Trauma Stress, 24*(5), 581-585.

Baikie, K. A. & Wilhelm, K. (2005). Emotional and physical health benefits of expressive writing. *Advances in Psychiatric Treatment, 11*(5), 338-346.

Barclay, L. J. & Skarlicki, D. P. (2009). Healing the wounds of organizational injustice: Examining the benefits of expressive writing. *Journal of Applied Psychology, 94*(2), 511.

Cameron, L. D. & Nicholls, G. (1998). Expression of stressful experiences through writing: Effects of a self-regulation manipulation for pessimists and optimists. *Health Psychology, 17*, 84-92.

Center for Journal Therapy. (2019). https://journaltherapy.com/.

Davey, J. (2007). *Writing for wellness: A prescription for healing*. Enumclaw, WA: Idyll Arbor.

Dialog House Associates. (2019). Progoff intensive journal method for self-development. http://intensivejournal.org/index.php. (viewed 20 May 2019).

Expressive Writing Therapy. (2007). In American Holistic Health Association. Retrieved from http://ahha.org/ExpressiveWriting.htm

Gidron, Y., Peri, T., Connolly, J. F., & Shalev, A. Y. (1996). Written disclosure in post-traumatic stress disorder: Is it beneficial for the patient? *Journal of Nervous & Mental Disease, 184,* 505-507.

Halpert, A., Rybin, D., & Doros, G. (2010). Expressive writing is a promising therapeutic modality for the management of IBS: A pilot study. *American Journal of Gastroenterology, 105*(11), 2440-2448.

Heimes, S. (2011). State of poetry therapy research. *The Arts in Psychotherapy, 38*(1), 1-8.

Kerrigan, J. C. & Wylie J. J. (1999). An interview with Seamus Hearney. *Nua: Studies in Contemporary Irish Writing, 2*(2), 125-135.

Klein, K. & Boals, A. (2001). Expressive writing can increase working memory capacity. *Journal of Experimental Psychology: General, 130*, 520-533.

Koschwanez, H. E., Kerse, N., Darragh, M., Jarrett, P., Booth, R. J., & Broadbent, E. (2013). Expressive writing and wound healing in older adults: A randomized controlled trial. *Psychosomatic Medicine, 75*(6), 581-590.

Laura, S. (2015). Expressive writing helps cancer patients. American Holistic Health Association. Retrieved from http://ahha.org/Expressive Writing.htm.

Leedy, J. (1969). *Poetry therapy.* New York: Lippincott.

Lepore, S. J. (1997). Expressive writing moderates the relation between intrusive thoughts and depressive symptoms. *Journal of Personality and Social Psychology, 73*, 1030-1037.

Lepore, S. & Smyth, J. (2002). *The writing cure: How expressive writing promotes health and emotional well-being.* Washington, DC: American Psychological Association.

Lumley, M. A., Leisen, J. C., Partridge, R. T., Meyer, T. M., Radcliffe, A. M., Macklem, D. J., … & Granda, J. L. (2011). Does emotional disclosure about stress improve health in rheumatoid arthritis? Randomized, controlled trials of written and spoken disclosure. *Pain, 152*(4), 866-877.

Lumley, M. A. & Provenzano, K. M. (2003). Stress management through emotional disclosure improves academic performance among college students with physical symptoms. *Journal of Educational Psychology, 95,* 641-649.

Murray, B. (2002). Writing to heal. *Monitor on Psychology, 33*(6), 54. Retrieved from http://www.apa.org/monitor/jun02/writing.aspx.

Pennebaker, J. W., Colder, M., & Sharp, L. K. (1990). Accelerating the coping process. *Journal of Personality and Social Psychology, 58*, 528-537.

Pennebaker, J. W. & Evans, J. F. (2014). *Expressive writing: Words that heal.* Enumclaw, WA: Idyll Arbor.

Pennebaker, J. W., Kiecolt-Glaser, J. K., & Glaser, R. (1988). Disclosure of traumas and immune function: Health implications for psychotherapy. *Journal of Consulting and Clinical Psychology, 56*, 239-245.

Pennebaker, J. W., Mayne, T. J., & Francis, M. E. (1997). Linguistic predictors of adaptive bereavement. *Journal of Personality and Social Psychology, 72*, 863-871.

Pennycook, G., Cheyne, J. A., Barr, N., Koehler, D. J., & Fugelsang, J. A. (2015). On the reception and detection of pseudo-profound bullshit. *Judgment and Decision Making, 10*(6), 549-563.

Petrie, K. J., Fontanilla, I., Thomas, M. G., Booth, R. J., & Pennebaker. J. W. (2004). Effect of written emotional expression on immune function in patients with HIV infection: A randomized trial. *Psychosomatic Medicine, 66*, 272-275.

Porter, H. R. (2016). *Recreational therapy and the international classification of functioning, disability, and health.* Enumclaw, WA: Idyll Arbor, Inc.

Rico, G. (2000). *Writing the natural way: Turn the task of writing into the joy of writing,* 15th anniversary expanded edition. New York: TarcherPerigee.

Smyth, J. M. & Arigo, D. (2009). Recent evidence supports emotion-regulation interventions for improving health in at-risk and clinical populations. *Current Opinion in Psychiatry, 22*(2), 205-210.

Smyth, J. M., Stone, A. A., Hurewitz, A., & Kaell, A. (1999). Effects of writing about stressful experiences on symptom reduction in patients with asthma or rheumatoid arthritis: A randomized trial. *Journal of American Medical Association, 281*, 1304-1309.

Snyder, D. K., Gordon, K. C., & Baucom, D. H. (2004). Treating affair couples: Extending the written disclosure paradigm to relationship trauma. *Clinical Psychology: Science and Practice, 11*(2), 155-159.

Swinnen, A. M. (2016). Healing words: A study of poetry interventions in dementia care. *Dementia 15*(6), 1377-1404.

Wexler, M. (2014). A poetry program for the very elderly: Narrative perspective on one therapeutic model. *The Interdisciplinary Journal of Practice, Theory, Research and Education 27*(1), 35-46.

18

Meditation and Creative Visualization

The creative process seems to take place with greater ease when we are in a state of relaxed awareness. In this state we can be free from our standard responses and beliefs and discover new images and ways of thinking.

There are situations which at first glance seem totally separated from the creative process, but which are actually conducive to creative reflection. Some are relaxing, such as taking a walk or daydreaming, while others demand a person's full attention, such as meditation, writing, house cleaning, or physical labor.

In order to reap the most benefit from the creative process, we should learn to relax and listen to our inner dialogue without judgment or censorship, to be an objective observer. The paradox is that when we're "trying to get an answer," the demand we put on ourselves may defeat our purpose. What is creative may appear as an image, an idea that may seem to be almost wordless, a feeling, intuition, emotional response, an inspiration, or insight. Welcome it, for its true value may not be revealed at once.

Write down with words, drawings, notations, or symbols the thoughts and images that come to mind. Although these messages emerge from deep within us, we can work with them once we allow them to be revealed to us.

Research

A combination of therapy techniques can be more effective than using a single technique when treating clients. Strategies of acceptance and mindfulness meditation with modeling add another dimension to the therapy process. Other techniques include work on healthy coping strategies, such relaxation training.

Yoga and meditation are often recommended for individuals with multiple sclerosis (Morgante, 2005). Hatha yoga has been shown to significantly improve levels of stress and fatigue for individuals with multiple sclerosis (Oken et al., 2010).

Mindfulness-based meditation has been shown to significantly improve health-related quality of life and reduce depression, stress, and fatigue (Grossman et al., 2010)

Endorphins are neurotransmitters that interact with opiate receptors in the brain to reduce perceptions of pain. There are over 20 types of endorphins in the human body (Stoppler, 2007). Activities that help to increase endorphins include exercise, massage, hot baths and showers, laughter, meditation, guided imagery, and music.

Techniques to help cope with chronic back pain include relaxation training to reduce muscle tension, biofeedback to learn how to control body functions, visual imagery, repetition of positive words or phrases, and engaging in activities that distract from painful, negative stimuli (Block, 2007). Pain management is also a common concern for persons with osteoporosis (Mobily & MacNeil, 2002; National Osteoporosis Foundation, 2012). Relaxation techniques of various types, including progressive relaxation, meditation, and biofeedback, contribute to easing the body's response to pain and may result in perceptions of psychological control (Mobily & MacNeil, 2002).

Individuals with post-traumatic stress disorder have reported that prayer, participation in church-related activities, and meditation are helpful in the healing process. These types of experiences are related to self-nurturing, which is a concept addressed by Najavits (2002) and Griffin (2005).

Thorpe (2017) identifies a set of health benefits of meditation. They include reducing stress, controlling anxiety, promoting emotional health, enhancing self-awareness, and lengthening attention span. Meditation may also reduce age-related memory loss, generate kindness, help fight addictions, improve sleep, help control pain, and decrease blood pressure.

In the study "When Science Meets Mindfulness," researchers Shapero and Desbordes (2018) studied how meditation seems to change the brain in depressed clients. Functional magnetic resonance imaging scans detected changes in the subject's brain activation patterns in the part of the brain called the amygdala after an eight-week course in mindfulness-based cognitive therapy.

Meditation

Meditation is any activity that keeps the attention anchored in the present moment. Think of an activity that you really enjoy. I (Ann Nathan) am sitting here at the typewriter on a hot summer day. I'm sweating profusely and I fantasize for a moment. I approach a beautiful lake. I notice the trees, flowers, and grass. The wind is warm as it blows over me. Now I wade into the lake and then dive in. I pause and enjoy my own sense of the cooling water. Ahh. For a moment the world stops. I am no longer concerned with books, bills, shopping, relationships, or any other thoughts. I surrender to the immediate pleasure of the water. That's what enjoyment is. Surrender. Letting go of all the things pulling you out of the moment.

For this time, the mind is not reading its list of things that must happen before we can be happy. It's not reciting the list of awful things that could happen to steal our happiness. It has taken a back seat to just being. This is the meditative state that elicits the relaxation response. It is peace.

Meditation: A Curated Guide (Donna L. Talaga)

There are many different styles or types of meditation available today. Some people use active forms such as yoga, tai chi, or other types of movement meditation. Others prefer simply sitting and breathing with or without a repeating mantra. And others want a concentrated body approach which involves tensing and releasing muscles while sitting or lying down. Whatever the approach, a common theme is being "present."

Meditation offers awareness and the opportunity to just "be," it's a way to enter our basic natural state of human "being" rather than human "doing." One might consider meditation as the art or practice of "non-doing."

Meditation is a journey, not a destination. The benefits of meditation are the byproduct of the practice rather than the goal. These benefits, however, have been increasingly documented. In a scientific review, Goyal et al. (2014) said, "…evidence suggests that mindfulness meditation programs could help reduce anxiety, depression and pain in some clinical populations. Thus, clinicians should be prepared to talk with their patients about the role that a meditation program could have in addressing psychological stress."

Meditation is for everyone. It is universal. There are vast references crossing many different cultures and religions. For example, both Buddhist and Benedictine monks teach meditation techniques. Distinguished brothers His Holiness the Dalai Lama (Buddhist), Fr. Laurence Freeman (OSB) Director of the World Community for Christian Meditation (originated by Benedictine monk and priest John Douglas Main OSB) incorporate meditation as a spiritual practice going beyond one's self. Some of the oldest written records reference meditation originating from Hindu traditions of Vedanta in India from around 1500 BCE.

Although meditation has its earliest roots in ancient religions, secular programs and body-mind studies were made popular in the west by Dr. Herbert Benson with the 1975 bestselling book, *The Relaxation Response*. Transcendental Meditation (TM) was popularized by celebrities like the Beatles under the instruction of Maharishi Mahesh Yogi in the late 1960s. John Kabat Zinn created the research-backed stress-reduction program Mindful-Based Stress Reduction (MBSR) which he describes as an awareness that arises through paying attention on purpose in the present moment non-judgmentally. Jack Kornfield, one of the leading Buddhist teachers in America, introduced mindfulness and meditation to America with an emphasis on compassion and loving kindness.

Today there are meditation programs at your local library, community center, or your church or school. The David Lynch Foundation provides secular TM-based programs for at risk groups, including veterans with PTSD, and uses The Quiet Time Program in schools to reduce stress and violence and help improve performance. Deepak Chopra and Oprah Winfrey regularly offer free meditation programs online along with meditation instruction from The Chopra Center.

If you want to spend more time with animals, you can even find instruction or places to meditate or do yoga with your cat or other animals. While studies have shown a beneficial effect on humans' relaxation response to purring and petting cats and other animal companions, it turns out the cats may also benefit from a shared meditation experience. A year-long study on the effects of yoga meditation music on cats in a veterinary clinic showed that music had an effect of lowering the respirating rates of the cats themselves. Perhaps not surprising to spiritual teacher Elkhart Tolle, the author referred to his cats as Zen masters in his bestselling book, *The Power of Now*.

It's important to note that the abundance of choices can lead to confusion for meditation groups. Group leaders may discover one type that works for everyone. Or they may find a combination of styles works best. Most likely, different members of the group will prefer different methods. It is their practice after all.

Most experts agree that consistency is more important than the style of meditation. Twenty minutes twice a day may be more beneficial, but if your clients can regularly practice just five minutes a day or even introduce a simple breathing technique into their daily lives, they will still benefit. Don't be afraid to explore and try different forms of meditation.

You may want to start with the simple conscious relaxing breath technique illustrated by Dr. Andrew Weil:
https://www.drweil.com/videos-features/videos/breathing-exercises-4-7-8-breath/1/?amp=1

The following exercises will help clients begin their meditation journey: The first is a simple exercise. The second provides details on how to incorporate many of the techniques used to induce a meditative state.

Simple Meditation Exercise

Find a quiet space where you can be undisturbed.

Sit comfortably with your back straight.

Close your eyes and take a few relaxing breaths.

Next you can introduce a mantra or phrase or simply just be aware of your breath.

Don't try to control anything, just observe or be present gently as "the observer."

If your mind starts to wander naturally just observe and simply return to the quiet breath or mantra or phrase.

Begin by practicing for a few minutes preferably twice a day. As you become accustomed you can gradually increase the time of your sessions.

Meditation Exercise

Choose a quiet spot where you will not be disturbed by other people or by the phone.

Sit in a comfortable position, with back straight and arms and legs uncrossed, unless you choose to sit cross-legged on a floor cushion.

Close your eyes. This makes it easier to concentrate.

Relax your muscles sequentially from head to feet. This step helps to break the connection between stressful thoughts and a tense body. As you do this, breath slowly in and out. For now, just become aware of each part of your body in succession, letting go as much as you can with the out breath. Take a second now just to take a deep breath in. Let it go. Notice how your body relaxes as you let go. This is the good old sigh of relief. The pull of gravity is always present, encouraging us to let go, but if there is no awareness of being tense, there can't be any letting go.

Notice your shoulders right now. Is there any room to let them down more, cooperating with gravity and your own out breath? Every out breath is an opportunity to let go. Starting with your forehead, become aware of tension as you breathe in. Let go of any obvious tension as you breathe out. Go through the rest of your body in this way, proceeding down through your eyes, jaws, neck, shoulders, arms, hands, chest, upper back, middle back and midriff, lower back, belly, pelvis, buttocks, thighs, calves, and feet. This need only take a minute or two.

Become aware of your breathing, noticing how the breath goes in and out, without trying to control it in any way. You may notice that your breathing gets slower as the meditation progresses. This is due to the physiological effects of the relaxation response, the fact that your body requires less oxygen because your metabolism has slowed down.

Choose a focus word or phrase that evokes a sense of meaning that is important to you. This could be anything at all. If you cannot think of one, you might want to try a very old Sanskrit mantra, Ham Sah. (Ham means "I am" and Sah means "That.") Repeat your focus word silently in time to your breathing. In the case of Ham Sah, just listen to your breath, imagining that it sounds like "Ham" on the in breath and "Sah" on the out breath.

Don't worry about how you are doing. As soon as you start to worry about whether you are doing it right, you have shifted from meditation to anxiety. If you notice that tendency, try labeling it, saying to yourself "judging, judging." Then let go, coming back to the breath and the focus, which are your anchors in the shifting tides of the mind. Your mind will not stop for more than seconds at a time, if at all, so don't expect it to. What happens is that the part of yourself that can watch or witness the shenanigans of the mind is learning to flex its muscles.

Each time you notice that you've drifted into thought, try labeling where you were. For instance, "thinking, thinking" or "anger, anger" or "judging, judging" and then let it go, getting back to the anchor. In this way, you begin to train yourself in awareness — the antidote to denial and mental unconsciousness. The awareness you develop in meditation will begin to carry over into life, affording you much more choice in how you respond and restoring your ability to enjoy life. The most common experience and complaint about meditation is "I can't stop my mind from wandering." That's fine. Don't try. Just practice bringing it back to concentration on the breath and focus whenever you notice it wandering.

Practice at least once a day for ten to twenty minutes. Remember that practice is required to improve in anything you do. In meditation your goals are twofold. The session itself is the goal. In the true sense, the process is the product. Your main goal is to sit and do the meditation. Even if it seems that the only thing you're doing is chasing after your mind to tie it down again, remarkably, the relaxation response is still most likely occurring. Long before clients think they know "how to do it," they begin to notice that they are generally feeling more peaceful and their symptoms are beginning to improve. That, of course, *is* the second goal. Meditation does become easier and more deeply peaceful after repeated practice. If you can sit twice a day for ten to twenty minutes, so much the better. The preferred times are early morning, after a shower and exercise (if that is part of your regime) but before breakfast, or before dinner. The only times to avoid are when you're tired — simply because meditation is a concentration exercise and, if you're tired, you'll fall asleep — and just after a heavy meal, since the process of digestion makes people sluggish.

Creative Visualization

Creative visualization uses the imagination to help create what you want in your life. When you are visualizing, you use your imagination — your capacity to create images, emotions, and thoughts in your mind — to create a vivid image of something you wish to make real in your life. You create and visit with this image regularly and continue until it becomes objective reality. This is not prayer, and you need not believe in a higher being. What is necessary is to want to expand your experience and understanding of life and be willing to try something new without being cynical or negative. Therapists have said that this technique deals with an image in a conscious way in order to challenge any possible unconscious reluctance to interact directly with the image.

What you want to make real could be cognitive, spiritual, physical, or emotional, or a combination of these elements. Examples include a new home, a home that is easier to keep clean, a new job, recognition for the job you're doing, a promotion, satisfaction at work, feeling calm and focused, being more calm and focused with specific people in your life, a complete and fulfilling relationship, grace under pressure — in general or in a specific situation, acceptance of a difficult reality, or finally getting started on a creative endeavor. Other helpful areas on which to focus creative visualizations include:

Relationships

- conflict resolution
- showing and receiving affection
- loss and letting go

- commitment

Self-Improvement

- being more patient
- better test-taking
- accepting appearance
- stopping smoking

Health

- stress reduction
- eating and weight concerns
- peaceful, refreshing sleep
- recovery from illness or injury
- preparing for surgery or other treatment
- regaining strength after surgery or treatment
- medication — feeling it work
- talking to your body
- going to the dentist

Job and Career

- motivation to seek work
- feeling confident to call
- going on an interview
- asking for a raise
- giving birth or assisting in a birth
- changing careers
- handling conflict with co-workers

Affirmations

Affirmations are one of the most important, productive, and life-changing ways to use creative visualization. An affirmation is a very strong, positive statement that something *is* the way we wish it to be, that it has happened. This adds another dimension to what you are imagining.

Many of us have an almost non-stop monologue (and sometimes conversation) going on in our minds. The mind talks to (some would say "at") itself in an endless commentary about all facets of our physical and emotional life. When we listen to ourselves, we become aware of how our mind works and, often, how negative and self-critical it can be. For example, a person might catch his/her mind saying repeatedly, "This will never work," a thought that could affect the outcome of a situation. In other words, our inner monologue may follow set negative patterns. Just becoming aware of these patterns can be very useful.

Affirmations, which are new and productive patterns, can be expressed in many ways. Some people prefer to say them aloud, while others prefer to say them silently, write them down, sing, or chant them.

The following guidelines have proven helpful:

- Always word your affirmation as if it has already happened, now, in the present.
- Make it positive — what you want. Don't talk about what you do not want.
- Use your own words or take great care that what you say is exactly what you want, that it's just right for you.

Some examples of positive affirmations:

- I do well in class.
- I control my temper.
- I am able to be happy, or I am happy.
- I am a nice person.
- I am passing this test.

If we are able to forgive ourselves and others, if we can let go of disappointment, heartache, resentments, and guilt, the tremendous blessing of emotional healing awaits us. It *is* within our grasp.

Often, we feel that someone has taken something away from us: our faith in ourselves, a job, opportunity, love, money, or optimism. We think we have lost our best selves to someone who has cheated us out of them, who has robbed us of our peace of mind.

The guidelines listed here can be very helpful in creating an effective visualization-affirmation process.

Ho'oponopono

Ho'oponopono makes thing right between two people or groups of people (Blaschko, 2017). It is often done as a visualization.

The practice involves saying four basic phrases:

I'm sorry. What do we have to be sorry for? Here are some thoughts: If you know you hurt someone in any way, mentally, physically, emotionally, or spiritually, you can say you're sorry for doing that. This only works if you really are sorry, though. Thinking that it's all right to hurt others means you have some other work to do before ho'oponopono. Sometimes we are sure that it's the other person's fault — all of it. There is still something we can apologize for. We can say I got to this place where there is a misunderstanding or conflict. I did not see a way to keep this from happening. I was unaware. The Huna practitioners say I did not do this consciously, but my unconscious knew what was going on. My unconscious knew this problematic pattern and did not fix it. When something isn't working, I take my share of the responsibility for the problem. From the Huna perspective it's never all one person's fault.

Please forgive me. What can we ask to be forgiven for? Some possibilities: I was unaware of what I did to hurt or trouble you. I didn't realize what I was doing. I could have done better. I could have cleaned up this pattern before we ever met.

I love you. The Huna point of view is that the essence of God is love. When we say I love you, we move toward God. They speak of the new pattern of this age as Aloha. Aloha translates as many things, including love. Along with all the other possibilities for love, we recognize each other as part of the divine. Then we love that in each of us.

Thank you. Saying thank you is how each part of the healing is sealed. For me it's like this: I recognize the change, I welcome the change, and I acknowledge accepting the new way I am. I do this with gratitude.

The basic technique is actually quite simple. You repeat four phrases: *I'm sorry. Please forgive me. I love you. Thank you.* Specify why you are sorry and what you want to be forgiven for. There is no particular order to the phrases. You just pick the phrase that works for what you are feeling in the now of the healing. Whatever shows up for you, including your own resistance, is what you say these phrases about. You can expect it to take several minutes to clear up the misunderstanding.

Don't do this exercise to help an abusive relationship. If you are being abused, find someone to help you. If they guide you in using ho'oponopono, they will let you know that you must not take the blame for the abuse and you do not forgive the abuser when you say you are sorry. You can say (to yourself) that you are sorry for being in a place where another person chooses to abuse you. Then you make sure to get completely away.

You can say these phrases aloud to the person you are asking to forgive you, or you can say them to yourself as a visualization. Saying them to the other person feels good to the person who receives the apology, especially when the other person is working in your best interest. But there will be times when you do not want to say the phrases to the other person. This is especially true when the other person will use what you say against you in the future. One young woman apologized to her mother for everything she had ever done that the mother didn't like. But she didn't say a word to her mother. It was all done privately. And it really helped the young woman free herself from the mother-daughter conflict.

Note that the young woman did not ask her mother to apologize for what the mother had done. That puts the mother in control. This practice works because we do everything we can to clean up our side of the relationship, even when it means totally leaving the relationship. We don't give the other person control by expecting anything from them. If they ask for forgiveness, too, it's a sign that the relationship is better. If they don't ask and continue to do the same things that hurt you, it's time to dissolve the relationship.

There is also a question about who receives these phrases. They are usually directed at the relationship. Specifically, they should be phrased for the person you have the conflict with, even if you are saying them to yourself. The following exercise is one way to do ho'oponopono.

Visualization of Forgiveness

This exercise helps you find forgiveness for what you have done to harm another person. Relax your body and mind. Follow relaxation techniques found in this book or elsewhere. Breathe deeply through your center which is just below your navel. Close your eyes.

Imagine a beautiful, peaceful setting which is calm and without distractions. You can imagine yourself walking, or swimming, as well as in a reclining position.

Visualize the person you have a conflict with. S/he is walking toward you. You see this person as a human being, like you, moving through life and trying to learn, as you are. If the usual negative thoughts begin to emerge, reset the scene to the peaceful moment just before the person shows up. Then have the person walk toward you again until s/he can approach you without causing negative feelings in you. Remember that your feelings are within your control.

Think of a thing you have done or not done that has hurt the other person. Say "I'm sorry I [acted this way]. Please forgive me." Repeat this process for everything you can think of. There will probably be a lot. Add an "I love you" and "Thank you" when it feels right.

If the process begins to feel insincere or if you're making apologies through clenched teeth, then this is something you are not ready to apologize for. Perhaps it's something you do not need to apologize for. You might need to forgive yourself for something before you ask someone else to forgive you. You can do ho'oponopono and ask yourself for forgiveness, too.

It's normal to have unresolved feelings come up later. Continue to ask for forgiveness for anything that comes up. Each session will help, so do the exercise again when you feel the need. A better life awaits you. It's already yours, you need only claim it.

Sample Scripts

These sample scripts using creative visualization can be used and modified as required for individual situations.

Meeting an Adviser

The goal of this exercise is to find or imagine someone outside of the physical world who can advise you about a problem or situation.

Allow yourself to totally relax your mind and body. When you feel yourself deeply relaxed, imagine a place that is beautiful and peaceful. It might be a quiet isolated beach, a lovely meadow on a spring afternoon, or a spectacular view from a mountain top. It might be a place where you have vacationed and where you remember being very happy and relaxed.

When you feel very comfortable in this beautiful place, look for the person whom you have come here to see. If you don't see that person at first, keep looking. When a figure appears, ask first is s/he is the advisor you are looking for who will act in your best interest. If the answer is no, continue to look for someone else.

When you find someone who answers yes, tell the person that you have come looking for him/her to ask for advice. Allow yourself to be with this person as comfortably as you would be with a friend in your own home.

When you feel comfortable and accepting of your adviser, ask him/her the question or questions that you have been wanting to ask. Then wait patiently for the answer. If an answer doesn't come immediately, ask your adviser how you can find the answer to your question.

Keep asking questions until you have the answers you sought. When your answers come, and you feel satisfied that they are what you sought, thank your adviser and tell him/her that you will return. Know that this place is always within your reach.

Allow yourself to return to the physical world and feel good — to feel that you have found out what you wanted to know and have the ability to use the information you have received.

Remember the beautiful place and use the adviser within you.

Relaxing the Body

Close your eyes. Get comfortable and concentrate on your breathing.

Pay careful attention to your breathing. Recognize how slow and deep breathing will help to induce relaxation. Exhale. Then take a deep breath in through your nose and blow it out through your mouth. Breathe from your abdomen; deeply and slowly.

As you concentrate on your breathing, focus your attention on an imaginary spot in the center of your forehead. Look at the spot as if you were trying to see it from inside your head.

You will begin to realize that your eyelids have become tense. Get a sense of how tense the eyelids can become as you stare at the spot so that you can compare this feeling with relaxation.

When your eyelids become strained and uncomfortable, let them drop.

Notice the feeling of relaxation that radiates all through and around your eyes. Allow that feeling of warmth and relaxation to move out to the temples and across the forehead.

Let the relaxation then radiate to your scalp, to the back of your head, to your ears, temples, cheeks, nose, to your mouth and chin.

As you feel the tension leave your face, relax your jaw muscles. Let your jaw open slightly, so all the tension can smoothly flow away.

Relax the muscles in your neck. As you do, let your head tip forward gently so your chin just about touches your chest.

Let this feeling of relaxation flow down into your shoulders and from there into the muscles of your arms and hands, then down your back, over to the front of the chest, on down to the abdomen, and then allow it to reach all the way down to the base of the spine.

Let the buttocks go completely loose and limp. Allow the warmth and relaxation to spread to the thighs, on down the legs, down to the ankles, and down through the feet to the tips of the toes.

Now you feel completely relaxed. Take a moment, starting from the top of your head and working down, to check if any part of you is not yet fully relaxed.

If you find any part of your body not fully relaxed, simply inhale a deep breath and send it into the area, bringing soothing, healing, relaxing, nourishing oxygen to comfort that area. As you exhale, imagine blowing out through your skin any tension, tightness, or discomfort. By inhaling a breath into that area and exhaling right through the skin, you replace tension in any part of your body with gentle relaxation.

When you find yourself quiet and fully relaxed, take a few moments to enjoy it.

Meditation and Creative Visualization Resources

Books

Dinuri, M. (2016). *Meditation for beginners: The ultimate and easy guide to learn how to be peaceful and relieve stress, anxiety and depression*. Dallas, TX: CreateSpace Publishing.

Meditation-Mindful.org
books, websites, audio, and video.
https://www.mindful.org/downloads/your-guide-to-meditation.pdf

Mindfulness Meditation for Beginners
meditation e-book for beginners (how to incorporate mindfulness into your daily life)
https://mindfulnessexercises.com/ebook-mindfulness-meditation-beginners/

CDs, Videos, and Downloads

Halpern, S. Steve Halpern Inner Peace Music. Belmont, CA.
The "Mozart of the New Age." Selection of relaxing music with and without subliminal messages from reducing pain to increasing memory.
https://www.stevenhalpern.com/

Helland, P. Relaxing Harp Music for Meditation
https://www.youtube.com/watch?v=-BvhR1M2K9Q

Helland, P. Relaxing Music "Our Future" piano, guitar, and cello
https://wwwyoutube.com/watch?v=D4BZshNWJMc

Miller, E. MD. Menlo Park, CA
High quality tapes from pain relief to surgery preparation and healing etc.
https://www.drmiller.com/

Additional Resources

Benson-Henry Institute. History of the Institute.
https://www.bensonhenryinstitute.org/mission-history/

Cats in Meditation
https://www.dailyinfographic.com/the-healing-power-of-cat-purrs-infographic
https://paulocoelhoblog.com/2016/09/26/cat-in-meditation-3/
https://www.telegraph.co.uk/news/newstopics/howaboutthat/7898325/Yoga-meditation-music-helps-cats-relax.html

Chopra, Deepak. How to Meditate.
https://Chopra.com/free-programs/how-to-meditate

Chopra, Deepak. Oprah & Deepak 21-Day Meditation Experience.
https://chopracentermeditation.com/
also available on Google Play or iOS App Store.

Dalai Lama
https://www.dalailama.com/news/2013/dialogue-between-his-holiness-the-dalai-lama-and-fr-laurence-freeman-about-the-teacher-and-disciple-in-sarnath-varanasi

David Lynch Foundation. Healing Traumatic Stress and Raising Performance in At-risk Populations
https://www.davidlynchfoundation.org/

Franciscan Meditation
https://www.franciscanmedia.org/why-should-we-meditate/
Junger, Alejandro. 5-Minute Meditation.
https://soundcloud.com/cleanprogram/dr-jungers-5-minute-meditation
Kabat-Zinn, Jon. Defining Mindfulness
https://www.mindful.org/jon-kabat-zinn-defining-mindfulness/
Kornfeld, Jack. Loving Kindness Meditation
https://jackkornfield.com/loving-kindness-meditation/
Mead, Elaine. The History and Origin of Meditation
https://positivepsychology.com/history-of-meditation/
National Institutes of Health. Meditation.
https://nccih.nih.gov/health/meditation/overview.htm
Weil, Andrew. Breathing Exercises.
https://www.drweil.com/videos-features/videos/breathing-exercises-4-7-8-breath/1/?amp=1
World Community for Christian Meditation
https://www.wccm.org/ and https://wccm-usa.org/

References

Blaschko, T. (2017). *We all have souls and I think we can prove it.* Enumclaw, WA: Pine Winds Press.

Block, A. R. (2007). Chronic pain coping techniques: Pain management. Retrieved from http://www.spinehealth.com/conditions/chronic-pain/chronic pain-coping-techniques-pain management.

Goyal, M., Singh, S., Sibinga, E. M., et al. (2014). Meditation programs for psychological stress and well-being: a systematic review and meta-analysis. *JAMA InternMed. 174*(3), 357-368. Doi:10.1001/jamainternmed.2013.13018

Grossman, P., Kagen, L., Gensicker, H., D'Sousa, M., Mohr, D. C., Penner, I. K., & Steiner, C. (2010). MS quality of life, depression & fatigue improve after mindfulness training: A randomized trial. *Neurology, 75*(13), 1141-1149. doi-10.1212//WNL.obo13e3181f4d80d.

Griffin, J. (2005). Recreation therapy for adult survivors of childhood abuse: Challenge to professional perspectives & the evolution of a leisure education group. *Therapeutic Recreation Journal 39*, 207-228.

Mobily, K. E. & MacNeil, R. D. (2002). *Therapeutic recreation and the nature of disabilities*. State College, PA: Venture.

Morgante, L. (2005). Healthy living with multiple sclerosis. *MS in Focus 5*, 4-5.

Najavits, L. M. (2002). *Seeking safety: A treatment manual for PTSD and substance abuse.* New York: Guilford Press.

National Osteoporosis Foundation. (2012). Bone health basics. Retrieved from: http://www.nof.org/aboutosteoporosis/bonebasics/whybonehealth.www.nof.org.

Oken, B. S., Kishiyma, S., Zajdel, D., Bourdette, D., Carlsen, J., Haas, M., & Mass, M. (2004). Randomized controlled trial of yoga & exercise in multiple sclerosis. *Neurology, 62*(11), 2058-2064.

Porter, H. R. (2015). *Recreational therapy for specific diagnoses and conditions*. Idyll Arbor Inc. Enumclaw, WA.

Shapero, B. & Desbordes, G. (2018). When science meets mindfulness. *The Harvard Gazette.* https://news.harvard.edu/gazette/story/2018/04/harvard-researchers-study-how-mindfulness-may-change-the-brain-in-depressed-patients/.

Stoppler, M. C. (2007). Endorphins: Natural pain and stress fighters. Retrieved from: http://www.medicinenet.com/script/main/art.asp?articlekey=55001.

Thorpe, M. (2017). 12 science-based benefits of meditation. *Healthline.* https://www.healthline.com/nutrition/12-benefits-of-meditation.

Tolle E. (1997). *The power of now: A guide to spiritual enlightenment.* Vancouver, BC: Namaste Publishing. Republished (1999) New World Library.

19

Puppetry

Storytellers have used puppets to illustrate and entertain for centuries, animating and conveying society's thoughts and wants. While the ancient history of puppetry is not completely known, it is thought to have its origins in either China or India.

Western society has seen puppetry through plays, movies, and television with characters like Punch and Judy, Lamb Chop, Howdy Doody, Sesame Street, and the Muppets. Puppetry is a powerful tool for communicating with all ages, cultures, and levels of language (Peck, 2005). The advantages of puppetry are numerous: they stimulate imagination, invite you into a world of fantasy, allow you to pretend to be someone or something else, and stimulate various learning styles. But most of all, puppets are fun (Northern California Association of Kodaly Educators, 2000).

Psychiatrists Adolf Woltmann and Lauretta Bender began experimenting with puppetry for therapy at Bellevue Hospital during the 1930s. Their work involved children whose behavioral problems stemmed from unfavorable home or school conditions, unhappy emotional experiences, or inconsistencies in emotional growth. "The chief need of these children is a psychotherapeutic one, an opportunity to work out their problems, the chance to give some free expression to their aggressive tendencies, to verbalize and clarify the difficulties in their relationship to their life with their mother, father, and siblings, and to be relieved from feelings of guilt and anxiety" (Bender & Woltmann, 1936, p. 341). Puppet plays and puppet classes were a great help as an active psychotherapeutic method.

Puppets can amuse, educate, wonder out loud, and express feelings (Dalton, 2007). Puppets fascinate and engage people in ways that few other art forms can, maybe because they allow us to see ourselves, or parts of ourselves in them. "Puppets protect: What is expressed can be denied and blamed on the puppet, so that inner emotional worlds are revealed in nonthreatening ways" (Aronoff, 2005, p. 118). Because puppets often reveal the inner world of the person, a great deal can be accomplished in therapy by using puppetry.

Jane Geiser (2015) has a wonderful vision concerning puppetry. She states:

> Puppets are real. They are nothing but themselves. They ground us in their relationship to the material world, yet they move freely between life and nonlife. Their breath comes from elsewhere, but they can leave us breathless.... They say what we won't say and do what we can't do. They tell truth to power, they make us laugh, they help us grieve, they embody our stories. They tell us things about ourselves that we forget to understand until we see it through them. We need them to do this.... How will puppets survive into the future? Simply by being themselves (p. 18).

Therapy Settings

Therapeutic puppetry may be adapted to a variety of people of all ages (individuals, couples, groups, and families) in order to meet various treatment goals. Bernier (2005) further describes how puppetry can work as a therapeutic tool in various settings and modalities:

Hospitals: Assist a patient to better understand a medical procedure, hospital environment, or personnel. Puppets also help families cope with emotional stressors of illness and hospitalization.

Psychotherapy (includes play, art, and drama therapies): Puppets are used to express feelings and thoughts, which might otherwise be hidden or repressed, in situations such as divorce, accidents, domestic violence, and child abuse.

Drama and play therapies: Clients engage in their own puppet play, where they are encouraged to work through emotional conflict or share confusing thoughts or experiences. Clients choose from a selection of puppets, while the therapist notes which puppet was chosen, the role the puppet plays, the plot or narration of the stories told, and the themes that evolve.

Group puppetry: Clients produce an original puppet play around a common theme, which will hopefully provide an emotional outlet to a situation (such as divorce). The Family Puppet Interview is an example of group puppetry where families create an original story together and act it out for the therapist by speaking through the puppets (Sori, 2018).

Art therapy: Clients design their own puppet for use in a puppet play.

Music therapy: Clients can extend vocal range, match pitch, overcome stuttering, or develop the ability to sing (when they are unable to speak) after suffering a stroke.

Speech therapy: Puppetry assists clients in language development and speech modification by reinforcing letter sounds, blends, word recognition, and listening skills. A puppet with a mouth and a tongue is ideally suited to demonstrate articulation exercises.

Physical therapy: Puppets challenge and coax clients in order to assist with exercises, pain management, and stress relief.

Research

Hospitals

In a study by Reid-Searl, Dwyer, Nancarrow, and Walker (2017), thirteen nurses described using puppets in a pediatric unit when caring for children who were sick. Puppet use was found to be an effective way to distract children from unpleasant procedures, reduce fears, and help to describe how a particular procedure would be performed.

Sposito et al. (2016) used finger puppets with ten children (five boys, five girls) between the ages of seven and 12 years old who had been diagnosed with cancer. Data collection occurred between April 2010 and May 2011 in the pediatric oncology ward at a Brazilian public teaching hospital. The treatment and was structured in two steps: children making their own puppets and children being interviewed using their puppets. The researcher used a puppet representing herself and the children used the puppets they made. The puppets allowed the children to express their feelings and experiences in the hospital. Some children used their puppets to talk about anything except their treatment or illness. It was also interesting that the children designed their puppets to look like they had looked before their illness, or with features totally different from themselves. The use of puppets as a playful resource enriches communication with children who have cancer. This communication enhances clinical practice by assisting health professionals with assessments and interventions and also reaffirms the value of health professionals using creative techniques (Sposito et al., 2016).

Psychotherapy

Talnova (2018) designed a puppet therapy treatment with 27 juvenile offenders between the ages of 15 and 17 with delayed mental development. Fourteen teenagers were part of the experimental (treatment) group and 13 comprised the control group. Participants began by producing a puppet from craft paper, then sculpting a puppet from plasticine, manipulating the puppets, writing a script, and filming it as a cartoon. The puppet was a device for self-examination and correction of the teenagers' self-image. The Piers-Harris Children's Self-Concept Scale, the Who Am I? test, and the World Assumptions Scale were used for evaluating the puppet therapy's effectiveness. A comparative analysis revealed that the juveniles became more honest and more realistic, the perception of school became more positive, and they increased their ability to control their life events and be successful.

Another resource, developed by puppeteer Raven Kaliana (2018), was the Love vs. Trauma: Puppet-Based Resilience Project for people facing trauma. *Love vs. Trauma* is a 45-minute live shadow-puppet play for adults and teens about child abuse. This is followed by a 30-minute post-show discussion. *Rehearsing Resilience* is a two-hour puppet-based workshop, mostly for young people, where they learn about effects of trauma and its recovery stages, and then act out a scene in which a puppet must seek assistance to handle the situation. This project can help young people recognize and manage posttraumatic responses. Kaliana's work has received support from numerous agencies in the United Kingdom.

Group Puppetry

Benefits of shadow puppetry are demonstrated in the Stichting Droomtheatre, which organizes presentations and workshops for special target groups. The theater's director, Joanne Ousseren, describes a theater show with residents of a dementia care unit. Participants may draw, color, and cut out characters and tell stories. This allows interaction between the residents. Caregivers and nursing staff may hear memories from their patients that they never knew before. Learning about the patient's past experiences unlocks the doors to new conversations for all.

Each person's story becomes part of the puppet show, and the topic may be anything — politics, traveling, gardening, a walk in the park, etc. The resident's response will sometimes activate an emotional experience, which helps to develop a new rapport between residents, their caregivers, and their surroundings (Ousseren, 2018).

Music Therapy

Musical skill is a vital component for a puppeteer working with the Doctor-Puppet approach, which provides psychological aid for seriously ill children. The Doctor-Puppet is approximately 36 inches tall and looks like a doctor with a clown face. The puppet interacts with children individually, twice a week for 20 to 40 minutes throughout their entire treatment.

The puppeteer must be able to improvise this interaction based on the child's reaction to the Doctor-Puppet. This includes playing musical instruments, reciting nursery rhymes, singing, making a toy or musical instrument out of any object, etc. Props that mimic medical instruments are also part of the visit, with the puppet performing a procedure on the child, or vice-versa. The puppet prepares the children for the challenges that they face during a prolonged, difficult, and painful treatment in the hospital (Gref, Sokolova, & Slonimskaya, 2018). Gref and Sokolova (2003) provide case notes for two areas where the Doctor-Puppet program helped during treatment. In the first area doctors used puppets as surrogates to give children truthful information about their medical procedures and their illness. The second area was to continue school during the hospital stay. Children who continued the normal routine of going to school exhibited greater mental functioning, strengthening the child's motivation for treatment.

Speech Therapy

Remer and Tzuriel (2015) conducted a study using puppets for interviews with 145 kindergarteners (age five to seven), 68 from special education kindergartens and 77 from regular kindergarten classes. The special education children had major speech deficiencies in addition to other learning disabilities, and most also had emotional difficulties. These regular and special education students were divided into two groups: an experimental group that included mediation using a puppet and a control group that received mediation without a puppet. Mediation using puppets increased the children's cooperation, interest, and attention span, and developed a dialogue that encouraged their learning. The use of "childish" language with the puppet allowed for more participation from children who are introverted and quiet and from children with special needs who found it difficult to respond to regular instruction. The researchers also recommended using puppets to promote language and to encourage verbal expression and conversation among children with language difficulties.

Puppets in Therapy

Before using puppetry in a session, a therapist should consider the goals s/he wants to accomplish by using the puppets. King (2017) suggests that puppets be used as a tool for:

- **Communication:** Puppets can be whoever or whatever you want them to be.
- **Problem-solving:** Puppets are empathetic listeners.
- **Conflict resolution:** Puppets are good problem-solvers.
- **Storytelling:** Puppets are wonderful conversationalists.
- **Education:** Puppets are a great teaching tool.
- **Building relationships:** Puppets can interact with people or with other puppets.

- **Advocating for social change**
- **Enhancing creativity:** Puppets add a sense of safety.
- **Having fun and playing:** Puppets create an atmosphere of playfulness.

Puppet Play Therapy Fundamental Approaches

Puppet play therapy "involves the use of puppets by mental health professionals for diagnostic and therapeutic purposes" (Schaefer & Drewes, 2018, p. 3). Puppet play has also provided benefits in medical, educational, and home settings for all ages—infancy to old age. Schaefer and Drewes (2018) describe ten fundamental approaches where puppet play promotes or reaches a therapeutic goal with clients:

- **Self-expression:** talking through puppets
- **Access the unconscious:** projection (project one's feelings or desires onto a puppet), symbolization (one item stands for another), and displacement (direct negative feelings toward the puppet instead of a person)
- **Catharsis:** acting out feelings of violence or frustration though the puppet
- **Direct teaching:** maintain attention span and interest in academic and social behaviors
- **Abreaction:** reenactment of stressful or traumatic events
- **Awareness of feelings:** confide in or do something to please the puppet that they would not normally do for another person
- **Rapport:** build trust and motivation
- **Problem-solving:** therapist uses a helper puppet to converse with the child's puppet
- **Behavioral rehearsal:** model coping strategies
- **Assess family dynamics:** observe patterns of communication and roles in family interactions.

Puppetry in a Therapeutic Setting

The use of puppetry in therapy combines a verbal and nonverbal means of expression. Determining which type of interaction the client will have with the puppet depends on the goal and/or approach a therapist wishes to use. Therapists may choose from the following puppet interactions (Passmore-Godfrey, 2005):

- client puppet making (either for themselves or another)
- client puppet using (in puppet play, conversations, scripted plays, speeches)
- client interacting (client talks to a puppet used by the facilitator)
- client assessment

There are several puppet assessment techniques that may prove beneficial when working with children. The Berkeley Puppet Interview (BPI) allows the therapist to ask questions using two puppets. Clients respond to the questions by indicating which puppet is most like them. For example (Measelle & Ablow, 2018, p. 31):

- *Puppet One: I have lots of friends.*
- *Puppet Two: I don't have lots of friends.*
- *Question to client: How about you?*

A connection usually occurs more quickly if the therapist knows the client's interests (e.g., music, movies, gardening) and the puppet can begin an interaction from the same mood or temperament as the client. Once this connection is made, the therapist can try to shift the general mood to positive and playful exchanges with statements like, "Wow! That is really interesting. Tell me more." Puppets may nod, tip their heads in funny ways, act surprised, and ask questions to keep the conversation going. The therapist may also elect to have a three-way conversation between himself, the puppet, and the client.

Puppet Creation

If a therapist decides to have the client make a puppet, The Kohler Puppetry Method (TKPM), created by Marc Kohler in 1966, suggests that the process of making the puppet take no more than 20 to 30 minutes. After the puppet is finished, Kohler asks the puppet creator six questions:

- What is the puppet's name?
- What is the puppet's age?

- Where is the puppet from?
- What is the puppet's job?
- What does the puppet like to eat?
- What is the puppet feeling?

Other questions may be added to this list, "helping puppet-makers create puppet biographies, life histories, family trees, and personalities that will lead to play and story-writing with actual writing or taping!" (Kohler, 2017, p. 22).

There are six general types of puppets (Schaefer & Drewes, 2018):

- **Hand puppets:** worn on the hand and have a moveable mouth
- **Marionettes:** a small figure of a person or animal with jointed parts and operated from above by pulling strings and rods
- **Shadow puppets:** a flat rod puppet that casts a silhouette when manipulated between a light and a screen
- **Muppets:** mouth is operated like a hand puppet, but limbs are operated by strings and rods like a marionette
- **Dummies:** operator's hand fits inside the dummy and manipulates its jaw, arms, and legs with strings and rods
- **Finger puppets:** fit over a finger

Making puppets together is a way to build a connection between therapist and client. Cornett (2007) describes some simple puppets that can be made from readily available materials:

- **Finger puppets:** Cut off fingers of inexpensive work gloves to make individual puppets, using fabric paint for faces.
- **Glove puppets:** Each finger becomes one character or object in the story.
- **Stick puppets:** Popsicle sticks, tongue depressors, wooden rulers, spoons, or dowel rods can serve as a base for a character made from paper, papier mâché, or cloth.
- **Paper-lunch-bag puppets:** The puppet's mouth is placed at the fold to look like it is talking. Yarn or paper shreds can serve as hair, and the head can be stuffed with newspaper.
- **Sock puppets:** Sock may be cut at the toe to create a mouth or held at the toe so that a mouth is created by the fold.

- **Paper-plate puppets:** Plate may serve as a face. It needs a stick attached to the back for a base.
- **Clothespin puppets:** These can be clipped to a ruler or stick to add height.
- **Paper-cup puppets:** These need a stick attached to the back for a base.
- **Index-card puppets:** These need a stick attached to the back for a base. Index cards may be placed in a pocket chart as a story is told.

Manufactured puppets are available for purchase at toy stores, thrift shops, consignment stores, or garage sales. You can search on-line by type of puppet, character name, or manufacturer. Websites for these puppets include (Schaefer & Drewes, 2018):

- The Puppet Store: www.thepuppetstore.com
- Folkmanis: www.folkmanis.com
- PuppetU: www.puppetu.com

Puppet Selection

Carter and Mason (1998) recommend that therapists have fifteen to twenty puppets in their everyday collections. More puppets than this may overwhelm the client with too many choices, and fewer may not offer enough variety. Types of puppets in a collection should include family figures, wild and tame animals, human characters (doctor, police officer), and fantasy figures (witch, fairy, superhero).

A survey of play therapists revealed that certain puppets were most useful with their clients (Schaefer, 2017). Following is the top ten list of puppets and their representations:

- dragon: scary experiences
- turtle: shyness
- family: interactions between family members
- shark: hostility
- bird: can fly away and escape
- dog: a friend and comfort
- dinosaur: power
- alligator: anger

- snake: power
- wizard: magical powers

Puppets should have different skin colors and moveable mouths, and should be washable or cleanable, soft, visually appealing, and easy for children to manipulate (Schaefer & Drewes, 2018, p. 8).

Puppet Manipulation

The way the puppet is held, moves, looks, and speaks is important to the part it will play in a session. The arm has four puppet duties — movement of the fingers, wrist, elbow, and shoulder (Schaefer & Drewes, 2018; Puppet Manipulation, 2017).

Fingers control the puppet's jaw. If the fingers are pulled back, the puppet scrunches its face. Opening and closing the fingers is how the puppet talks. Try to move the puppet's lower jaw more than the upper jaw. By combining finger movement with wrist movement, the puppet can shake its head "yes" or "no" or perform neck exercises. Practice different facial expressions. Add elbow and shoulder movements and the puppet can do almost anything.

Fingers control the puppet's speech, so the puppet's mouth and the therapist's mouth movements must match. Lip and hand coordination is not easy. Practice by having the puppet (and therapist) say the ABCs, recite a nursery rhyme, or sing a favorite song in front of a mirror. Practice using different voices with the puppet as well. Would the client be convinced that the puppet is talking? The puppet should establish eye contact with the client when it is speaking.

Find a natural position for the puppet so that it is looking straight ahead. With most mouth puppets, the therapist's wrist needs to be bent slightly forward. Practice having the puppet look at the floor, the ceiling, around a corner, out a window, or at a book. Practice walking movements (up and down, not a sliding motion). Make sure that your puppet is "awake" at all times. If your arm goes limp, it appears that your puppet has fallen asleep.

Puppet appearance should resemble its character. Give each puppet a name. Facial expression, hair type, glasses, clothing type, accessories, mouth, nose shape, eyelashes, and eyebrows can be determined by the puppet maker.

Puppet Storage

Puppets should be displayed in a bookcase, on a shoe rack that hangs on the back of a door, in a pocket chart, or on a puppet rack. Simply throwing them into a box does not portray the puppets as "real" (Schaefer & Drewes, 2018).

Planning a Puppet Session

Therapists can create a simple puppet stage by placing a blanket over the back of a chair or table or turning a table on its side, crouching down behind, and placing the puppet-manipulating hand above the stage. Therapists may use these guidelines when planning a puppet session with their clients.

1. Select a story — a familiar fairytale with a different twist, a takeoff on a familiar film or television show, or make up your own.
2. Limit the story to four characters with three scenes. Each character should have a name.
3. Write the dialogue (who, what, where, when).
4. Have each group member choose a character from the story.
5. Create the puppet head and costume.
6. Rehearse the story with the group. Music and sound effects may be added.
7. Perform for the group (Jenkins, 1980).

Planning a session for children may be more difficult for the therapist due to their shorter attention spans and lack of expressive skills.

O'Hare summarizes the process: "A puppet play requires understanding of the topic to be portrayed, sequencing of events, dialogue, props, movement, articulation, volume, expression, sharing, thinking quickly, and using bodies and voice simultaneously. It also requires listening, responding, reacting, sharing, and supporting one another. It requires constructing puppets and learning new ways to use familiar materials to make an inanimate object, which can move and talk. It requires fully understanding the topic which is being presented and internalizing the events and characters so that they can be recreated with conviction with puppets" (O'Hare, 2005, p. 65).

Helpful Hints

Jenkins (1980) also offers the following suggestions for practicing and creating a session with puppets.

Things a puppet can do:

- act frightened
- gallop
- put head on
- take head off
- bow
- hammer
- read
- think
- brush hair
- touch something hot
- remove hat
- throw kiss
- brush itself off
- kneel
- rise
- wake up
- carry
- laugh
- scold
- walk
- clap
- lead songs
- scratch
- wash hands
- climb
- lie down
- scrub
- wave

- come to life
- limp
- search
- write
- cry
- look behind
- shake or nod head
- yawn
- dance
- march
- sit down
- die
- pick up things
- skip
- eat
- play music
- sleep
- exercise
- point
- sneeze
- fall down
- pray
- sweep
- fly
- push
- swim

Things puppets can do in pairs:

- carry something together
- chase one another
- dance together
- embrace or kiss
- hand objects back and forth
- have a tug-of-war
- play catch

- shake hands
- talk together

When creating a session, keep the following in mind:

- The play needs a plot, which consists of a conflict or apparently insoluble problem with an ingenious solution.
- Like any play, it should have an introduction, body, and conclusion. The problem is introduced, there are attempts to solve it, and a satisfying ending is reached. The play should end as soon as possible after the problem is solved.
- The story should have plenty of action. Puppets are not good for long, talky material.
- The script lines should not be memorized but improvised in keeping with the structure.
- The puppets should keep in character (funny, worried, bossy) throughout the entire play.
- Take advantage of the unique ability of puppets to do things that are impossible for people, like fly, disappear, etc.
- It is best to get the audience involved whenever possible. Having them help the characters adds to their enjoyment of the play. This is one of the strengths of puppetry — it gets everyone involved, not just the performers.
- Avoid lengthy plays. A good puppet story can be told in five or ten minutes.

Puppet Adaptations

Puppets may need to be modified due to a person's developmental skill level or other limitations. Salmon and Sainato (2005) suggest attaching the puppet to a mitten using Velcro or hook-and-loop tape. Mittens are easier to put on and easier to manipulate with the wave of a hand. Attaching bells, beads, or other noisemakers to a sock, glove, or finger puppet can also provide some auditory feedback. For persons in wheelchairs, a glove marionette on a flexible dowel rod may be attached to the wheelchair tray using a C-clamp, allowing the puppet to move when the person kicks or swings his feet, bumps, or throws his head back.

Puppetry Resources

Center for Puppetry Arts — www.puppet.org
Jim Henson Foundation — www.hensonfoundation.org
Puppeteers of America — www.puppeteers.org
Puppetry Home Page — www.sagecraft.com/puppetry/questions.html
UNIMA — www.unima-usa.org/
Puppetry International Magazine

References

Aronoff, M. (2005). Puppetry as a therapeutic medium: An introduction. In Bernier, M. & O'Hare, J. (eds.). *Puppetry in education and therapy: Unlocking doors to the mind and heart*. pp. 117-124. Bloomington, IN: Authorhouse.

Bender, L. & Woltmann, A. G. (1936). The use of puppet shows as a psychotherapeutic method for behavior problems in children. *American Journal of Orthopsychiatry, 6*(3), 341-354. https://doi.org/10/1111/j.1939-0025.1936.tb05242.x.

Bernier, M. (2005). Introduction to puppetry in therapy. In Bernier, M. & O'Hare, J. (eds.). *Puppetry in education and therapy: Unlocking doors to the mind and heart*. Bloomington, IN: Authorhouse.

Carter, R. & Mason, P. (1998). The selection and use of puppets in counseling. *Professional School Counseling, 1*(5), 50-53.

Cornett, C. E. (2007). *Creating meaning through literature and the arts: An integration resource for classroom teachers* (3rd ed.). New York: Pearson.

Dalton, J. (2007). The art of puppetry. *School Arts, 106* (8), 64.

Geiser, J. (2015). The future of the puppet is inevitable. *Puppetry International, 37*, 18.

Gref, A. & Sokolova, L. (2003). *Doctor-Puppet: The program of psychological help to children with oncological diseases in hospital and in hospice*. Moscow: Author.

Gref, A., Sokolova, L., & Slonimskaya, E. (2018). Doctor-Puppet: An approach to psychological aid for sick children. *Puppetry International, 43*, 30-33.

Jenkins, P. (1980). *The magic of puppetry: A guide for those working with young children*. New York: Prentice Hall.

Kaliana, R. (2018). Rehearsing resilience. *Puppetry International, 43*, 8-11.

King, S. (2017). The power of using puppets with people living in long term care homes — part one. Retrieved on January 18, 2018, from: http://puppeteria.ca./blog/?p=2792.

Kohler, M. (2017). Puppets for education and therapy. *Puppetry International, 42*, 22-23.

Measelle, J. & Ablow, J. C. (2018). The Berkeley puppet interview for child assessment. In Drewes, A. A. & Schaeer, C. E. (eds.), *Puppet play therapy: A practical guidebook*. pp. 29-47. New York: Routledge.

Northern California Association of Kodaly Educators. (2000). *Puppet power! Songs and games using puppets in the classroom*. Oakland, CA: Northern California Association of Kodaly Educators.

O'Hare, J. (2005). Puppets in education: Process or product? In Bernier, M., and O'Hare, J. (eds.). *Puppetry in education and therapy: Unlocking doors to the mind and heart*. pp. 63-67. Bloomington, IN: Authorhouse.

Ousseren, J. (2018). Shadow theatre: A suitable means of developing the talents of the impaired elderly. *Puppetry International, 43*, 24-25, 28.

Passmore-Godfrey, W. (2005). Accessing the power of puppets in therapeutic and educational settings. In Bernier, M. & O'Hare, J. (eds.). *Puppetry in education and therapy: Unlocking doors to the mind and heart*. pp. 167-176. Bloomington, IN: Authorhouse.

Peck, S. (2005). Puppet power: A discussion of how puppetry supports and enhances reading instruction. In Bernier, M. & O'Hare, J. (eds.). *Puppetry in education and therapy: Unlocking doors to the mind and heart*. pp. 73-81. Bloomington, IN: Authorhouse.

Puppet manipulation. (2017). Retrieved January 14, 2018, from: http://legendsandlore.com/puppetmanipulation.html.

Reid-Searl, K., Dwyer, T., Nancarrow, L., & Walker, B. (2017). Puppets in an acute paediatric unit: Nurse's experiences. *Collegian, 24*(5), 441-447. http://dx.doi.org/10.1016/j.colegn.2016.09.005.

Remer, R. & Tzuriel, D. (2015). "I teacher better with the puppet" — Use of puppet as a mediating tool in kindergarten education — An evaluation. *American Journal of Educational Research, 3*(3), 356-365. Available at: http://pubs.sciepub.com/education/3/3/15; doi:10.12691/education-3-3-15.

Salmon, M. D. & Sainato, D. M. (2005). Beyond Pinocchio: Puppets as teaching tools in the inclusive early childhood classrooms. *Young Exceptional Children, 8*(3), 12-19. https://doi.org/10.1177/109625060500800303.

Schaefer, C. E. (2017). Play therapists report their most useful puppets. *Play Therapy Magazine, 12*(3), 25-27.

Schaefer, C. E. & Drewes, A. A. (2018). Fundamental concepts and practices of puppet play therapy. In Drewes, A. A. & Schaefer, C. E. (eds.), *Puppet play therapy: A practical guidebook*, pp. 3-16. New York: Routledge.

Sori, C. F. (2018). The family puppet interview. In Drewes, A. A. & Schaefer, C. E. (eds.). *Puppet play therapy: A practical guidebook*. pp. 48-58. New York: Routledge.

Sposito, A. M. P., Sparapani, V. de. C., Lima R. A. G. de., Silva-Rodrigues, F. M., Nascimento, L. C., Pfeifer, L I., & deMontigyn, F. (2016). Puppets as a strategy for communication with Brazilian children with cancer. *Nursing and Health Sciences, 18*(1), 30-37. doi:10.1111/nhs.12222.

Talnova, L. (2018). Effectiveness of puppet therapy in changing the self-image of adolescents in conflict with the law. *Puppetry International, 43*, 12-13, 19.

20

Integration

The arts have been a part of every known society. Since people first sang, danced, painted on the walls of caves, and acted out stories for their children, people have considered the arts worthy of study and practice. The arts begin early in a child's life in the form of play, for a child's work is play. "Playing consists of pretending (drama), drawing (art), moving (dance), and singing (music). The arts form a base from which the child explores the world and his/her relationships to it" (Coates, 1983, p. 32).

Therapists using creative arts, educators, artists, and arts organizations have a growing interest in the relationship between the arts and the healing processes. Medical professionals and arts leaders have been researching and documenting how using the creative process in a therapy situation impacts illness prevention, disease treatment, and recovery (National Arts Policy Roundtable, 2013).

History

Expressive arts therapy has a relatively short history, beginning in the 1970s with faculty members at Lesley College in Cambridge, Massachusetts (Estrella, 2007). The faculty began to document their use of this integrated arts approach as therapy. In 1981, McNiff's book, *The Arts and Psychotherapy,* was published, establishing a foundation for the field.

This book explored the "historical, aesthetic, and philosophical applications of the arts to psychotherapy," and is still used in expressive arts training programs today (Estrella, 2007, p. 184).

While this integrated approach was developing, others were questioning who should use it. Must the expressive arts therapists have mastery skills in one or more of the established arts therapies, such as art, drama, dance, or music therapy? Rather than require expressive therapists to obtain additional education or certification, the profession chose to focus on common factors within each arts area — the creative process, sensory-based expression, and aesthetics (Estrella, 2007). This focus recognizes the value of specialized as well as integrated use of the arts as a therapeutic device.

Research

Expressive arts therapies are tools that can bring about change in our life experiences and relationships. Therapies offered most often include art, dance/movement, and music. Poetry and writing therapy are also possibilities. Stuckey and Nobel (2010) conducted a review of literature (1995-2007) to determine what is known about the arts and health. In all four categories of music, visual arts, movement, and writing, there were definite indications that artistic engagement has significantly positive effects on health.

Megranahan and Lynskey (2017) conducted a literature review to see if expressive arts therapies reduced substance misuse. This review was unable to reach conclusive results about beneficial outcomes of this treatment but did indicate strong positive effects of music therapy in treatment of substance misuse.

Another literature review was conducted by Dieterich-Hartwell and Koch (2017). They investigated the role that arts therapies can play for refugees. Hearing, playing, and singing music, as well as drawing or sculpting, may assist these persons in maintaining their cultural identity while in their temporary home, serve as a bridge, and providing strength for integration into a new country.

An integrated arts therapy program (music, art, movement, and drama) was developed, applied, and tested with young female delinquents (ages

14-17) at a correctional institution. Twelve females were part of the experimental group who received this intervention twice a week during a five-week period while seventeen females in the control group received no intervention. Sessions consisted of three activities — an opening activity to establish the main topic for the day (fear, anger, self-esteem, communication barriers); a core activity to engage participants in art, music, and drama experiences that targeted the main topic; and a final activity to share a sense of achievement and support from others. A self-report version of Strengths and Difficulties Questionnaire and a modified Behavior Checklist was given before and after the treatment. The results indicated that the integrated arts therapy sessions decreased frequencies of aggressive behavior and emotional and conduct problems (Kõive & Kaudne, 2015). A session outline utilized in this study is given below.

Sample session

Aim of the session: Increase effective interaction in relationships promoting positive emotions.

- Opening activity: Circle time — express current thoughts and emotions through drawing, movement, rhythm, and voice.
    - Preparing for the arts activity (brainstorming a topic or theme)
    - Discussing benefits of helping behavior and agreeing on prosocial rules
- Main activity: Art making — express positive emotions through movement, mimicry, rhythm instruments, body sculptures.
    - Drawing and free-writing positive emotions
    - Making mood cards (drawing and collage), labeling emotions to the pictures, expressing two chosen emotions
    - Writing a letter to someone close
    - Preparing an improvised drama with the theme of "helper"
- Ending activity: Discuss content of the mood cards.
    - Relaxation and imaginary journey
    - Closing activity to affirm trust among members of the group (Kõive & Kaudne, 2015)

Integrated arts therapy can generate memories and stir emotions that catch a client's attention and distract him/her from negative thoughts. "The more we understand the relationship between creative expression and healing, the more we will discover the healing power of the arts" (Stuckey & Nobel, 2010, p. 261).

Common Factors within the Arts

There are three common factors that are seen in all the arts: similar modes in the creativity process, the sensory basis of the experience, and the dominance of aesthetic feelings over cognitive responses.

Groen-Bar's Creativity Axis

The first common factor is that the creative process is similar for each of the arts. Groen-Bar (1997) describes how each of the categories of arts relates to each stage of the creativity process. The stages in his six-stage creation axis are outlined below.

Contact

Definition: First contact with art materials
Art: Touch and examine materials
Movement: Choose a place to move
Drama: Try on costumes or tell a story
Music: Select instruments or voices
Emotions: Hesitation, enthusiasm, curiosity

Organization

Definition: Define scope
Art: Separate materials
Movement: Flex and relax limbs
Drama: Set the stage
Music: Tune instruments, attempt a scale, chord, or rhythm
Emotions: Irritation, carelessness, recklessness

Improvisation

Definition: Approach by trial and error
Art: Push fingers into clay
Movement: Explore limbs in space
Drama: Change voice or text into a "role"

Music: Test the range and dynamics of the instruments

Emotions: Embarrassment, criticism, laughter

Central Theme

Definition: "Figure" emerges from the background

Art: Attention to color, shape, or scribble

Movement: Focus on repeated movement or expression

Drama: Improvised activity can become part of the story

Music: Emphasis on rhythm, melody, or form

Emotions: Obligation, effort, destruction

Elaboration (Variation)

Definition: Develop, modify, improve, decorate — the client has control of the medium

Art: Bring into shape or form

Movement: Movement turns into a dance

Drama: Scene expands into a story

Music: Musical theme develops into a piece

Emotions: satisfaction, productivity

Preservation

Definition: Separate from the work, put it away, and preserve it; praise, criticize, and present work

Art: Find a place to display the work

Movement: Rest

Drama: Share, draw conclusions with audience help

Music: Perform and record the musical work

Emotions: Criticism, fear, pride, satisfaction

(Groen-Bar, 1977, p. 413-416)

Noting the client's emotional responses, mood changes, delays, regressions, or amount of time spent in each level helps the therapist determine the client's limitations and strengths.

Observations by Groen-Bar (1997) found that certain clients experience difficulties at particular stages. These observations are based solely on his clinical experience with the creation axis.

- Persons with learning disabilities experience difficulties with stages one through three due to organizational breakdown.

- Persons with behavioral and personality disorders tend to stay at the improvisational level or stop work during the central theme stage as an effect of weak ego.
- Narcissistic clients demonstrate strong self-criticism or suspicion concerning the medium during the initial stages. Approval and mirroring from the therapist in the contact and organizational stages are crucial.

Knowing the tendencies of these populations as they progress along the creation axis provides the therapist reference points during a creative therapy session. More detailed scientific analysis on a wider range of populations still needs to be done.

Sensory-Based Expression

The second common factor within each arts area, sensory-based expression, allows therapists to connect with a client's thoughts, feelings, and experiences in a nonverbal way. This can be especially helpful for clients "with whom verbal language is inaccessible" such as persons with Alzheimer's and those who have suffered a stroke (Estrella, 2007, p. 187). It is also useful for clients who have fears related to a traumatic experience or a mental health problem.

Aesthetics

The third common factor is aesthetics. It is often referred to as the "world of feeling," and defined as a reaction to what is seen or heard. Aesthetics deals with experiences and feelings that often have more effect on people than rational, cognitive thinking (Hoffer, 1993). Aesthetic experiences differ from ordinary experiences in that they (Hoffer, 1993):

- Are an end in itself — they are valued for their enjoyment, not for any practical benefits.
- Involve intellect, emotion, and a focus of attention.
- Must be experiences — a second-hand description many provide insight, but it doesn't provide a similar aesthetic experience.
- Result in a richer, more meaningful life.

An example of how an aesthetic experience is different from a second-hand description might be explaining a scene in a movie to someone, a scene which gave the viewer goosebumps, but the other person simply does not understand. Your response is, "You just had to be there," a reaction the movie producer would be thrilled to hear.

When we look at a painting aesthetically, we are consciously aware of the lines, shapes, and colors involved. The same holds true for listening to a piece of music (what instruments are playing, the volume of the music), and watching a dance performance (the number of dancers on stage, the shape of their movements). This is the intellectual portion of the aesthetic, but at the same time, one is also reacting with feelings to what is seen or heard.

Common Elements among the Arts

The lines, shapes, and colors are part of the intellectual aesthetic, but they are also common elements among the visual arts, movement, and music. Each art has their own set of symbols and technical demands, but they also share these same features. Expressive arts therapists may consider an integrated approach that combines two arts areas simultaneously, sequentially, or transitioning from one area to the other (Malchiodi, 2007). Berke (2000) defines integration as "the combining of two equal groups into a unified whole" (p. 9). Integration represents a shift away from emphasizing the differences between the arts and other subjects toward making connections between them. This ability to transfer and connect knowledge from one subject to another is essential for meaningful learning to occur (Barry, 1996).

For meaningful integration to occur, therapists should understand the different integration methods. Gerber (1999) describes three integration approaches:

- Elemental — common components
- Historical — events in history
- Thematic — ideas, events, or relationships

Common Elements among Movement, Music, and Art

Some of the qualities each of the arts share are shown below. The common elements help us explore connections between the arts.

Music

Rhythm: Patterns of tones
Contour: Shape of the melody
Color: Sounds of voices or instruments — tone color
Harmony: Blending of sounds
Form: Different sections of music
Balance: Interplay of loud and soft
Texture: Thickness and thinness of sounds

Movement

Rhythm: Organization of patterns in time
Contour: Shape of the body
Color: Mood and emotion evoked by movement
Harmony: Blending of motions
Form: Arrangement of movements or dance steps
Balance: Interplay of visible and hidden
Texture: Number of dancers

Visual Art

Rhythm: Similar visual patterns
Contour: Visual shapes
Color: Hue or pigment
Harmony: Blending of colors
Form: Volume, mass, or three-dimensional aspects of objects
Balance: Interplay of shapes and colors
Texture: Surface quality of artwork

Additional correlated elements may include continuity, emphasis, variety, tension, division, tempo, dynamics, duration, and technique (Barret, McCoy, & Veblen, 1997; Crystal Productions, 1995; Gerber 1999).

Integration Sessions

Two examples of an integrated arts activity are shown below. The arts areas may be presented in a different order from what is listed here. The therapist may choose to begin the session with the arts area s/he feels most comfortable with.

Discipline-Based Art Education

One type of integration approach is the Discipline-Based Art Education (DBAE) model, a model advanced by the Getty Center for Education in the Arts in 1985. This model expanded teaching and learning in the arts beyond production and performance. It was designed to provide exposure to, experience with, and knowledge about the arts from four disciplines — production, criticism, history, and aesthetics.

Production involves improvising and composing as well as performing. Criticism asks the question why — why did the composer, artist, performer, or conductor choose or interpret the artform a certain way? History examines the lives of composers and performers, countries and cities in which they lived, what events were taking place during their lifetimes, and when the relevant works were created. Aesthetics helps people reflect on their responses to an artform through writing, discussing, and producing similar art. Each discipline provides a different perspective from which to view, understand, and value works of art (Patchen, Lindsey, Wheetley, & Duling, 1995).

The following example uses the historic approach to allow clients to examine an artwork (painting, music composition, or dance) as it relates to other people, places, events, and cultures. The historic discipline, combined with the aesthetic aspects, would work like the following in a therapy setting.

Route 66

This is an example of a historical approach combined with aesthetic aspects as an integrated arts lesson. Possible therapy-session questions are shown in italics (modeled on Patchen, 1996a):

- Listen to Nat King Cole's 1946 version of the song "Route 66." All the cities listed in the song are places that one passes while travelling on the historic Route 66 from Chicago to Los Angeles. Highlight these cities on a road map.
- Listen to Nat King Cole's daughter, Natalie Cole, singing "Route 66" in 1991. *Was there a difference between the two recordings? (Yes:*

more instruments, louder, drums were added.) The recording technology advancements result in a clearer sound.

- Consider the following historical questions, paired with possible session questions:
    - Music and history: What events were happening in the world during the 1940s? 1990s? *What events do you remember when you travelled away from home?*
    - Historical thought: What events caused changes in the music recording or the song's lyrics? (Recording techniques, interstate construction, air travel). *Have you always listened to the same style of music? If so, what style? If not, why did you change?*
    - Historical imagination: Pick a main street in your community and list all the places that were there in years past and that are present today. *What memories do you have of visiting these places?*
    - Diversity: "Route 66" is jazz style of music, an American art form with a European musical background influenced by African rhythms and syncopation. How would this song sound if it were written in a gospel or classical style? *Could you perform a song in a style different from the way it was recorded or is normally performed? How would you change the music?*
    - Historical higher-order thinking: Compare and contrast events that occurred in the 1940s and 1990s and/or the two versions of this song. *Compare and contrast an original recording of a song and a more recent remake. For example: Layla* by Derrik and the Dominos (1971) and Eric Clapton (1992), *Drift Away* by Dobie Gray (1973) and Uncle Kracker (2002), *To Make You Feel My Love* by Bob Dylan (1997) and Garth Brooks (1999).
    - Roles of women and minorities: Discuss how Nat King Cole and his band were restricted during the days of segregation. For example, African American bands could not perform in the same venues or travel in the same way that Caucasian bands could. *Imagine how these performers felt. What would you ask them if you had the opportunity to interview these performers?*
- Additional questions:

- What does this musical piece reflect about the everyday life of the culture?
- Identify one of the cities mentioned in the song. How might the music of this region be different from yours? Take a musical tour of the state where that city is located.
- Movement activity: What dances were performed during the 1940s? 1990s? Try to perform one of the dances from that time period.
- Artwork: Who were artists living during the 1940s? What were characteristics of the Modernism era (1920-1945) and the twentieth-century trends in art history?

Thematic Approach

Themes can deal with human characteristics and behaviors, relationships with others and the world, rituals and traditions, philosophy, ethics, moral issues, and the cycle of life (Patchen, 1996b). The arts fit well with a thematic approach because the arts are a means of human expression and communication that reflect our culture.

Therapists do not need expert knowledge in the arts areas. Rather, they can ask simple but powerful questions to help their clients reflect upon experiences. How does a piece of music, artwork, or dance connect to a particular theme? Therapists need to understand that a thematic approach requires extensive research and preparation in order to lead a session. Using the "Route 66" example again, a possible theme could be oppression and the treatment of African American musicians during the 1940s.

Some other examples of themes include:

Adulthood, old age, death
Beauty
Birth, childhood, adolescence
Chance
Change
Chaos
Community
Destiny
Emotions
Ethics

Evil
Failure
Faith
Fame
Family
Freedom
Friendship
Good
Hardship
Honor
Humility
Ignorance
Law and Justice
Man/Woman
Man/Woman Relationships
Nature
Order
Patience
Peace
Poverty
Prejudice
Reality
Respect
Rites of Passage
Stability
Success
Technology
Time
Tradition
Trust
Truth
War
Wealth and Prosperity

An integrated approach to a therapy session has the therapist presenting information about the arts and using the arts as teaching and learning tools. The arts engage, motivate people, and support healing by providing creative outlets for expression.

Other Interventions

Darewych and Bowers (2017) describe a set of art interventions that therapists can integrate into their sessions. The interventions include:

- *Scribble Drawings* to arouse imagination
- *My Strengths Collage* to illustrate one's strength and become aware of strengths of others
- *The Tree of Life* to view life as a tree, with the roots representing roots in the past, the trunk as skills/strengths, the branches as hopes, the leaves as special people, and the fruits as gifts such as acts of kindness
- *Bridge Drawing with Path* to link the past to present and future goals
- *A Favorite Kind of Day* to illustrate what makes a person happy
- *My Sources of Meaning* with photos of what makes life meaningful
- *Spiritual Pathway* to represent the journey from life towards death

References

Barrett, J. R., McCoy, C. W., & Veblen, K. K. (1997). *Sound ways of knowing: Music in the interdisciplinary curriculum.* New York: Schirmer Books.

Barry, N. H. (1996). Integrating the arts into the curriculum. *General Music Today, 9*(2), 9-13.

Berke, M. K. (2000). Curriculum integration: A two-way street. *General Music Today, 14*(1), 9-12.

Coates, P. (1983). Alternatives to the aesthetic rationale for music education. *Music Educators Journal, 69*(7), 31-32.

Crystal Productions. (1995). *Principles of design poster set.* Glenview, IL: Crystal Productions Co.

Darewych, O. H. & Bowers, N. R. (2017). Positive arts interventions: Creative clinical tools promoting psychological well-being. *International Journal of Art Therapy, 23*(2), 62-69, doi: 10.1080/17454832.2017.1378241.

Dieterich-Hartwell, R. & Koch, S. C. (2017). Creative arts therapies as temporary home for refugees: Insights from literature and practice. *Behavioral Sciences, 7*(4), E69. doi: 10.3390/bs7040069.

Estrella, K. (2007). Expressive arts therapy: An integrated approach. In Malchiodi, C. A. (ed.). *Expressive therapies.* New York: Guilford Press.

Gerber, T. (1999). Art and music together in the curriculum. Workshop presented at the St. Louis Art Museum, February 19, 1999.

Groen-Bar, A. (1997). The "creation axis" in expressive therapies. *The Arts in Psychotherapy, 24*(5), 411-418.

Hoffer, C. R. (1993). *Introduction to music education* (2nd ed.). Belmont, CA: Wadsworth Publishing.

Kõive, K. & Kaudne, L. (2015). Impact of integrated arts therapy: An intervention program for young female offenders in correctional institution. *Psychology, 6*, 1-9. doi: 10.4236/psych.2015.61001.

Malchiodi, C. A. (ed.). (2007). *Expressive therapies*. New York: Guilford Press.

McNiff, S. (1981). *Arts and psychotherapy*. Springfield, IL: Charles C. Thomas Publishers.

Megranahan, K. & Lynskey, M. T. (2017). Do creative arts therapies reduce substance misuses? A systematic review. *The Arts in Psychotherapy, 57*, 50-58. doi: 10.1016/j.aip.2017.10.005.

National Arts Policy Roundtable. (2013). Arts and healing: Body, mind, and community, the 2013 report and recommendations. Retrieved January 15, 2018 from: www.americansforthearts.org.

Patchen, J. H. (1996a). History and culture context in a discipline-based approach to music education. In Patchen, J. H. & Harris, L. D. *A discipline-based education handbook*. Chattanooga, TN: The Southeast Institute for Education in Music.

Patchen, J. H. (1996b). Thematic teaching and discipline-based music education. In Patchen, J. H. & Harris, L. D. *A discipline-based education handbook*. Chattanooga, TN: The Southeast Institute for Education in Music.

Patchen, J., Lindsey, A., Wheetley, K., & Duling, E. (1995). *Discipline-based arts education: A conceptual framework for learning and teaching the arts*. Chattanooga, TN: The Southeast Institute for Education in Music.

Stuckey, H. L. & Nobel, J. (2010). The connection between art, healing, and public health: A review of current literature. *American Journal of Public Health, 100*(2), 254-263. doi:10.2105/AJPH.2008.156497.

Index

About the Authors

Ann Argé Nathan was a vibrant woman who lived her life fully for 47 years. In her short life she accomplished much, experiencing life to the fullest and leaving a mark on the lives of everyone she touched. A recreational therapist, educator, consultant, and author, Ann received degrees from, and taught at both San José and San Francisco State Universities. She practiced at Langley Porter Neuropsychiatric Institute at the University of California, San Francisco, and other clinical settings.

While teaching at San Francisco State University, Ann was the coordinator for therapeutic recreation along with clinical supervisor for internships. Ann served as a trainer/consultant on more than a score of projects throughout Northern California, including recovery services for the developmentally disabled and "at risk" youth and families. She was a co-therapist in an eating disorders group

Ann died of breast cancer on January 8, 1995. Her work and her love of students will be remembered for many years to come. The Ann Argé Nathan Spirit Scholarship Award continues to honor her love of teaching by presenting three or four students whose studies have a special emphasis in therapeutic recreation with a scholarship award yearly during the California Parks and Recreation Convention.

Suzanne Mirviss has a master's degree in recreation with emphasis in therapeutic recreation from San Francisco State University. She has taught courses in the Recreation and Leisure Studies Department at both San José State and San Francisco State Universities. For over twenty years she worked with many groups including the San Francisco VA Medical Center as an art consultant in the Psychiatric Day Treatment Center.

Ms. Mirviss received her training in drawing and painting from the San Francisco Academy of Art. She is currently a glass artist, but also engages in painting and jewelry making. She is the author and illustrator of two books for elementary-aged children: *Hello from Sammi* and *Aloha from Sammi*. These books focus on the importance of friendship, cooperation and cultural education/appreciation. Ms. Mirviss lives in Marin County, California, with her husband and family pets.

Deborah Ann Stuart

Deborah Ann Stuart, M.S., CTRS. RSW, completed a bachelor of science and master of science in therapeutic recreation at Michigan State University with Dr. Carol Ann Peterson and Dr. Marsha Carter as mentors. She is presently a research analyst specialist at Michigan State University. Deborah has a thirty-five-year career as a nationally certified therapeutic recreation specialist and registered social worker using movement for therapeutic goals. Deborah was the Director of Therapeutic Recreation Leisure Services for Michigan School for the Blind and Director of Therapeutic Programs for Miami Jewish Home and Hospital for the Aged and Stein Gerontological Research Institute. While Assistant Professor at Southeast Missouri State University, she coordinated the establishment of nationally accredited programs in Therapeutic Recreation. She studied summers at Harvard University in Dance performance and Movement Therapy while teaching at Perkins School for the Blind. Deborah is a United States Figure Skating Test Gold medalist in figures, free style. and ice dancing. She assisted the publication of the USFSA Therapeutic Ice-Skating manual.

Thanks to my father Roger Stuart for encouraging us to add our therapeutic arts materials to this book and to my mother Barbara Stuart for proofreading the therapeutic textbook at 91 years young.

Carol J. McDowell

Carol J. McDowell, Ph.D., is a veteran music teacher of over thirty years for students ranging in age from preschool through graduate school. She has presented workshops for national and state music conventions and served on the editorial boards for *The Missouri Journal of Research in Music Education, The Orff Echo, General Music Today.* Her research articles have been published in various music-education journals. Carol has also completed training in several early-childhood music courses and holds degrees from Southeast Missouri State University and Florida State University.